Myocardial Perfusion Scintigraphy— Clinical Aspects

INTRODUCTION

During its initial 20 yr, exercise myocardial perfusion scintigraphy (MPS) became established as an effective clinical tool for the detection of coronary artery disease (CAD). The method provided diagnostic information and accuracy beyond that of clinical and exercise data, particularly in patients with an intermediate likelihood of CAD (1–6). For more than 15 yr, the technique has been widely applied to the assessment of patient prognosis in CAD. It has now been demonstrated thoroughly that MPS, performed in association with either exercise or pharmacologic stress, yields clinically important and influential prognostic information beyond that of all other methods. The ability to risk stratify CAD patients is at the basis of its clinical success (7–14). Today, in an era of unprecedented cost containment in health care, the clinical applications of nuclear testing are being further redefined and applied throughout its spectrum to resolve the puzzle that is CAD (15–21) (Fig. 1). The need for efficient, cost-effective patient evaluation and management requires physicians to assess carefully the medical applications of testing methods, both in light of current data and from their objective experience with the methods. The value of nuclear cardiology within this clinical and economic framework lies in its ability to provide the most accurate and relevant clinical information and in more safely and favorably influencing overall diagnostic and management costs compared with other methods.

More than 3.3 million MPSs were performed in 1997 and more than 4 million in 1998, with the number increasing each year. This is occurring despite growing competition and claimed disadvantages of the method, severe regulation of radioactive substances and their users by federal and state agencies and close scrutiny and intermittent restrictions applied by some third-party payers. The scientific and clinical advantages of the method are clear and are the reasons for its continued and growing popularity. The exercise perfusion imaging protocol is shown in Figure 2.

DIAGNOSIS OF CORONARY ARTERY DISEASE

The Exercise (Treadmill/Bicycle) Test

Exercise testing is a time-honored method for diagnosing CAD and risk stratifying coronary patients and is based on the presumed identification of the

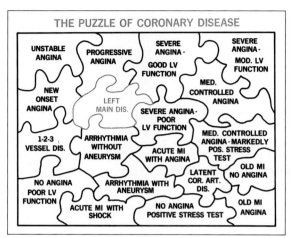

Figure 1   The puzzle of coronary artery disease (CAD). CAD is not a single entity but a spectrum of clinical problems and presentations. The diagnostic puzzle of CAD and the management problems that it presents are graphically illustrated. ART = artery; COR = coronary; DIS = disease; LV = left ventricular; MED = medically; MOD = moderate; MI = myocardial infarction; POS = positive. (Reproduced, with permission, from M. Cheitlin.)

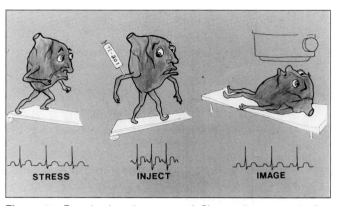

Figure 2   Exercise imaging protocol. Shown diagrammatically is the generic exercise perfusion imaging protocol. This cartoon was made when thallium-201 was the only option.

presence and extent of myocardium at ischemic risk (MIR) (Table 1). Exercise test parameters that suggest the presence of extensive, high-risk CAD and a related poor prognosis include: deep (2-mm) ST segment depression, especially when seen early, within the first 6 min of the Bruce Protocol and at a low achieved heart rate and blood pressure; widespread and persistent ST depression; and a low achieved workload (4 metabolic equivalents [METs]). Researchers also have demonstrated that the functional capacity (*22*), the achieved double product (heart rate × systolic blood pressure) (*23*) and the extent of the perfusion defect (*9–11*) are strong and independent predictors of cardiac mortality (Table 2).

Exercise stress permits the correlation of induced symptoms with hemodynamics, electrocardiographic (ECG) ST changes and image findings and provides the best opportunity to understand and objectify presenting patient symptoms manifested in their own environment. Also, exercise is necessary to generate an exercise prescription after infarction and is helpful in the assessment of the effects of therapy. Yet, both the diagnostic and prognostic values of exercise testing are limited. In those able to exercise to a level needed to answer the clinical question, dynamic exercise testing, rather than pharmacologic stress, is the method of choice, providing valuable symptomatic, hemodynamic and ECG data (see *Self-Study Program III. Cardiology. Topic 2: Pharmacologic Stress*).

The sensitivity and specificity of exercise treadmill testing in 24,074 patients reported in 147 studies are 68% and 77%, respectively (*24*). Perfusion image findings are used to clarify stress test findings. When reversible thallium-201 (²⁰¹Tl) defects were applied as the standard of ischemia to determine the importance of horizontal versus upsloping ST segment depression in 199 patients, the criterion of horizontal depression was more specific but less sensitive to induced ischemia than was upsloping ST depression (*25*).

Nuclear Medicine
Self-Study Program III:
NUCLEAR MEDICINE CARDIOLOGY

Topic 6: Myocardial Perfusion Scintigraphy—Clinical Aspects

Series Editor

Elias H. Botvinick, MD
University of California at San Francisco, California

Contributors

Elias H. Botvinick, MD
Jamshid Maddahi, MD
University of California at Los Angeles, California
Ernest Garcia, MD, PhD
Emory Medical Center, Atlanta, Georgia
Erwin A. Rodrigues, MB
Cedars Sinai Medical Center, Los Angeles, California
Kenneth Van Train, BS
Cedars-Sinai Medical Center, Los Angeles, California
Daniel S. Berman, MD
Cedars-Sinai Medical Center, Los Angeles, California
Rory Hachamovitch, MD

Society of Nuclear Medicine
1850 Samuel Morse Drive, Reston, Virginia 20190-5316

Made in the United States of America.

Library of Congress Cataloging-in-Publication Data

Myocardial perfusion scintigraphy : clinical aspects / contributors, Elias H. Botvinick ... [et al.].
   p. cm. -- (Nuclear medicine self-study program III. Nuclear medicine cardiology ; unit 6)
   Includes bibliographical references and index.
   ISBN 0-932004-58-X
   1. Coronary heart disease--Radionuclide imaging. 2. Myocardium--Radionuclide imaging.
I. Botvinick, Elias H. II. Society of Nuclear Medicine (1953-   ) III. Series.
  [DNLM: 1. Coronary Disease--radionuclide imaging--Bibliography. 2. Coronary Disease
--radionuclide imaging--Examination Questions. 3. Coronary Circulation--physiology
--Bibliography. 4. Coronary Circulation--physiology--Examination Questions.   1998 E-255
Unit 6/WG 18.2 N964 1997 Unit 6]
RC683.5.R33 N855 unit 6
[RC685.C6]
616.1'20757 s--dc21
[616.1'23075]

                                       2001049114

Contents

A prospective analysis was conducted among 420 patients with left ventricular ejection fraction (LVEF) >50% at rest and 1- or 2-vessel CAD (*26*). The study demonstrated an inability to risk stratify between those with (n = 56) or without (n = 208) evidence of exercise-induced ischemia based on 1-mm horizontal ST segment depression, the exercise workload achieved (600 kg-m/min) or a decrease in LVEF on exercise blood-pool imaging. These parameters of increased ischemic risk also failed to correlate with event-free survival and overall outcome. Perfusion scintigraphy provides a more discriminating option.

In a study by Bogarty et al. (*27*), stress ECG indices of high-risk CAD were prospectively compared with the findings on ^{201}Tl perfusion imaging in 66 consecutive patients with stable angina and 70% stenosis of 1 or more coronary arteries. Exercise indices of disease failed to correlate with either the extent of coronary involvement or the extent of perfusion defect. The extent of ST depression could not distinguish between patients based on the number of vessels involved, but the correlation of image findings with angiography was well maintained. ECG and image parameters appeared to measure different aspects of ischemia. Although many researchers take the extent of induced ST segment depression as an indication of the extent of MIR, in this study there was no correlation between the extent of ST depression and the extent of induced perfusion defect, a more direct index of MIR. Similar results regarding prognosis were independently suggested by Brown and Taylor (*7,28*). Among 100 patients without prior infarction studied by planar exercise ^{201}Tl imaging, multivariate analysis revealed that death correlated best with the number of reversible segmental defects. Next most prognostic was the total perfusion image defect size, followed by the number of diseased vessels. However, after these were extracted, the positive stress ECG and other stress testing variables were not contributory. Fixed defects and LVEF were not prognostic, but the study excluded those with prior infarction, and most patients had normal left ventricular function. Similarly, Taylor et al. (*28*) saw no difference between the size of induced perfusion defects or their total extent in those with exercise-induced ST depression of any magnitude. Here, abnormalities on the SPECT perfusion scintigram that suggested extensive MIR included: stress-related perfusion defects >15%–20% of the left ventricle, multivessel defect patterns, multiple reversible defects, transient ischemic left ventricular dilatation and increased lung uptake.

The Duke Treadmill Score, developed and validated by Mark et al. (*29*) and Shaw et al. (*30*) is an index derived from stress test parameters. It combines elements of exercise test performance, including the exercise time or METs (multiple of the baseline metabolic equivalent), the amount of induced ST depression and the severity of induced angina, to derive a single index related to the likelihood and risk of CAD. It has been found to be a reliable method for risk stratification in CAD and was applied for this purpose in the Unstable Angina Guidelines (*31*). Even those who are risk stratified by the Duke Treadmill

---

Table 1
PARAMETERS TO EVALUATE IN STRESS TESTING

Exercise performance—protocol, stage

Parameters of ischemia—chest pain or "equivalent," electrocardiogram, blood pressure, heart rate, rhythm

---

Table 2
EXERCISE TEST PARAMETERS ASSOCIATED WITH HIGH-RISK CORONARY ARTERY DISEASE

Deep (≥2 mm), early horizontal or downsloping ST depression

Poor exercise capacity

Low exercise time

Low workload

Ischemic ST changes at low double product (heart rate × systolic blood pressure)

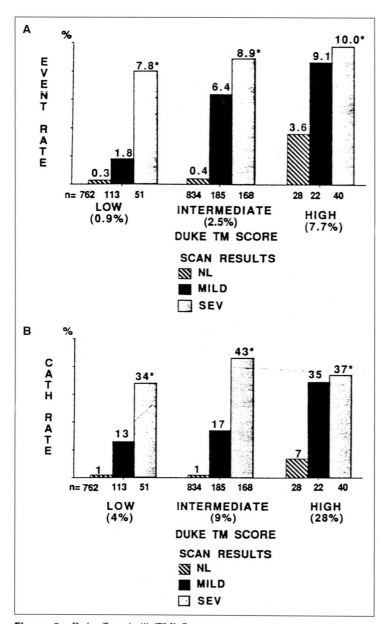

Figure 3 Duke Treadmill (TM) Score category and scan result. (A) Rates of hard events (myocardial infarction and cardiac death) over the follow-up period in patients in low, intermediate and high Duke score categories with normal (NL), mildly abnormal (MILD) and severely abnormal (SEV) scans. (B) Duke Treadmill Score category and scan result versus the rate of catheterization. Rates of referral to early catheterization, within 60 days after scintigraphy, in patients in low, intermediate and high Duke Treadmill Score categories with NL, MILD and SEV scans. Numbers in parentheses indicate hard event rates in these groups. *P = 0.05 across scan results. (Reproduced, with permission, from Hachamovitch R, Berman DS, Kiat H, et al. Exercise myocardial perfusion SPECT in patients without known coronary artery disease: incremental prognostic value and impact on subsequent patient management. *Circulation* 1996;93:905–914.)

Score may be further substratified by MPS. Hachamovitch et al. (*21,32*) were able to substratify patients well in all categories (low, intermediate and high risk) of the Duke Treadmill Test Classification (Fig. 3). Many patients are classified by Duke criteria as intermediate, with ambiguous risk and associated management decisions. Among 1187 patients classified by the Duke Treadmill Score to an intermediate coronary risk group (34%–70%) by Shaw et al. (*33*), 84% could be reclassified to low- or high-risk subgroups (70.3% to low- and 14.2% to high-risk groups) with MPS.

Exercise Testing in Women

ECG specificity for CAD often has been found to be lower in women (64%) than men (74%) (*34–36*), with women having a higher false-positive rate (38%–67%) than men (7%–44%) (*37*) (Table 3). In an extensive study, the Duke Treadmill Score was applied to the diagnosis and prognosis of CAD in 976 women and 2249 men who had symptoms of known or suspected CAD and who had undergone angiography (*38*). Although the scores differed between men and women, as did CAD prevalence and mortality, they were equally predictive of the diagnosis and risk related to CAD, beyond clinical indicators, in both sexes. The method excluded disease better in women. However, extensive studies already have shown the strong ability of MPS to risk stratify within Duke Score subgroups of both sexes (*32,33*) (Fig. 4). The specific cause of a false-positive treadmill test in women may include: a lower achieved workload and double product more likely bringing these subjects to "gold standard" coronary angiography; a higher incidence of baseline ECG abnormalities; or the low CAD incidence in subgroups tested, bringing a low predictive value of a positive stress test by Bayes's theorem (*5*). A postulated estrogen effect on the ECG would not necessarily explain induced ST abnormalities (*39*). Rarely, stress test sensitivity was also reduced (*40*).

However, the key to appropriate application of this and any testing method in CAD is the assessment of pretest CAD likelihood (Tables 4, 5). It is a mistake to perform stress imaging of any kind in men or women who can exercise and have low likelihoods of CAD and a normal or modestly abnormal ECG (*41*). Here, as with modest baseline ST depression <1 mm, even in the presence of mild left ventricular hypertrophy (LVH) or digoxin effect, a negative stress test response at a high achieved double product provides a high negative predictive value and strong assurance that the patient has no CAD and a good prognosis. If imaging is performed routinely, it will be normal in the overwhelming majority of such cases but, when abnormal, could be associated with an unacceptably high false-positive rate (*41*). It is induced horizontal ST depression, the ST response generally taken as positive for ischemia, that is nonspecific in these settings with baseline ST abnormalities and that is best supported in these selected cases by repeat study with MPS. Conversely, a positive stress test

Table 3
CAUSES OF FALSE-POSITIVE STRESS TESTS*

Digoxin

Electrolyte abnormalities (hypokalemia)

Left ventricular hypertrophy

Conduction abnormalities (left bundle branch block, "pre-excitation")

Nonspecific ST abnormalities

Position

Patient motion

Prior infarction (aneurysm)

Cardiomyopathy (hypertrophic, congestive)

Aortic stenosis

Electrical or technical artifacts

Being female?

Mitral valve prolapse?

Small-vessel coronary artery disease?

*Other explanations should be sought before invoking these "causes."

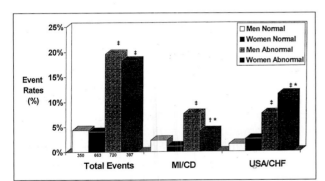

Figure 4 Relationship of events to SPECT findings. Shown are cardiac events in relation to SPECT image results among 2130 patients. Abnormal images relate to a higher rate of all forms of coronary-related events. In this and other studies, the event rate increased linearly with defect size. The catheterization rate increased in relation to defect size (see Fig. 86), and this was mirrored in the revascularization rate (see Fig. 87). Numbers below columns are numbers of patients in each group. *$P < 0.05$, compared with men; †$P < 0.01$, compared with normal images for the same sex; ‡$P < .001$, compared with normal images for the same sex. CD = cardiac death; CHF = congestive heart failure; MI = myocardial infarction; USA = unstable angina. (Reprinted, with permission, from Travin MI, Duca MD, Kline GM, et al. Relation of gender to physician use of test results and to the prognostic value of stress technetium-99m sestamibi myocardial single photon emission tomography scintigraphy. *Am Heart J* 1997;134:73–82.)

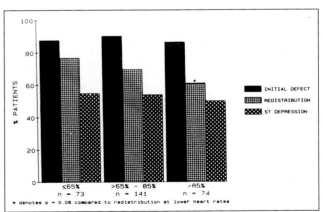

Figure 5 The persistent sensitivity of myocardial perfusion scintigraphy at low stress-related heart rate. Shown is the overall prevalence of initial, postexercise defects, the extent of redistribution and exercise-induced ischemic ST-segment depression based on the maximal heart rate achieved by patients undergoing exercise testing for evaluation of chest pain syndrome. The prevalence of ST-segment depression is reduced compared with thallium-201 scintigraphic abnormalities at each level of heart rate response. (Reprinted, with permission, from Esquivel L, Pollock SG, Beller GA, et al. Effect of the degree of effort on the sensitivity of the exercise thallium-201 stress test in symptomatic coronary artery disease. *Am J Cardiol* 1989;63:160–165.)

Table 4
INDICATIONS FOR EXERCISE TESTING (IMAGING)

Diagnosis of coronary artery disease (consider imaging with intermediate likelihood)*

Evaluate chest pain or equivalent (in ambiguous and low-likelihood emergency department patients)*

Evaluate patients with stabilized unstable angina

Risk stratification of coronary artery disease (imaging with intermediate likelihood)* (Post-myocardial infarction [uncomplicated]/submaximal exercise after 4–6 days; symptom-limited exercise after 10 days; dilator pharmacologic stress after 2–3 days)

Identify cause of chest pain or anginal equivalents (shortness of breath)*

Identify arrhythmia in patients with high risk

Evaluate the function of pacemakers

Detect labile hypertension

"Screening" asymptomatic high-risk patients*

Assess functional limitations (exercise prescription)

Differentiate cardiac from pulmonary disease

Assess effects of therapy (revascularization)*

Exercise imaging when baseline electrocardiography is abnormal (uninterpretable)

Pharmacologic stress imaging when patient cannot exercise adequately

Imaging in all groups to improve risk stratification, add localization and improve magnitude of regional infarction, myocardium at ischemic risk or salvaged after revascularization

*Deal most directly with coronary artery disease. Not recommended by American Hospital Association/American College of Cardiology guidelines.

in the setting of right bundle branch block (RBBB), especially involving lateral leads, generally maintains its specificity for CAD. Yet, occasionally RBBB may obscure ischemic ST changes, which may be seen in recovery after resolution of a rate-related RBBB (*41*).

Advantages of Perfusion Imaging

Among the earliest and most widely accepted abilities of MPS was its documented diagnostic accuracy, superior to that of stress testing, whether performed in association with exercise or pharmacologic stress (*1–6,42*) (Table 6A–E) (Figs. 5–7) (see *Self-Study Program III. Cardiology. Topic 2: Pharmacologic Stress*). This was again documented by Iskandrian et al. (*43,44*) who found that, among 834 patients studied with exercise MPS and coronary angiography, there was a poor relationship among exercise-related variables, ST changes and the coronary anatomy, whereas MPS correlated well with anatomic findings in both sexes.

MPS is most advantageous for CAD diagnosis in the presence of an uninterpretable stress ECG (Table 7). This includes any stress ECG with significant induced ST depression in the setting of rest ST depression or any condition (such as digoxin use) that may itself cause exercise-induced changes and false-positive test results (Table 3). Some studies demonstrated also the ability of MPS to diagnose CAD at a suboptimal achieved double product (*1,43*). As noted above, excluding left bundle branch block (LBBB) and severe LVH, a high-level stress test without further induced ST depression is a reliable method to exclude ischemia. Because a positive response in these settings is nonspecific, it may be cost effective to gain diagnostic security by first performing stress with MPS in some cases. However, the negative test remains generally reliable, and judgment must be applied to the need to perform MPS with the initial stress test. Generally, the more abnormal the ST segments at outset, the greater will be the difficulty in their diagnostic interpretation at stress and the more likely that MPS will be needed. Similarly, those with intermediate pretest CAD likelihood present the greatest need for the diagnostic security provided by MPS. Alternatively, such patients can be exercise tested with the radionuclide at the ready, to be used if the double product is less than optimal or the ST response is uninterpretable. Because most treadmills have a 300-lb limit, pharmacologic stress perfusion imaging with a technetium-99m (^{99m}Tc)-based radiopharmaceutical is recommended for the heavy patient who cannot exercise satisfactorily. If the double product is severely blunted, perhaps the dose should be held and applied with pharmacologic stress. Such flexibility is a desirable feature of a stress imaging laboratory. Although MPS should be considered in the setting of RBBB, this is usually not indicated except in those situations recommended to benefit from accompanying MPS, as with a negative test with a high pretest likelihood of CAD (Table 8). Stress-induced ST depression has no reliable localizing value and a weak ability to risk stratify in CAD. If these are the indications for stress testing, MPS with its strong localizing abilities and prognostic value should be performed in all cases, except those with lowest likelihood.

Analysis of the Diagnostic Accuracy of Stress Perfusion Scintigraphy

Pathophysiologic Considerations. Stress MPS is applied during a hyperemic response seeking to identify stress-induced alterations in the regional coronary flow reserve (CFR). A variety of methods have been designed to induce a hyperemic response using different mechanisms. A heterogeneous flow response will produce a heterogeneous distribution of the perfusion radiotracer. If great enough, a defect developed at stress and "reversible" at rest or with redistribution will identify a region of induced ischemia or ischemic potential. Defects persisting at rest usually indicate the presence of an element of scar but, in some cases, may be seen with viable "hibernating" myocardium. Such image abnormalities are correlated with the findings on coronary angiography to derive the diagnostic accuracy of the method. With such an approach, MPS correlates well with the anatomic evaluation of lesion severity in patients with known CAD (*21,32,43,44*). Abnormalities of CFR and indicators of myocardial ischemia, especially as assessed by MPS, must be treated as continuous variables and not simply as positive or negative, normal or abnormal, findings (see *Self-Study Program III. Cardiology. Topic 2: Pharmacologic Stress* and *Self-Study Program III. Cardiology. Topic 5: Myocardial Perfusion Scintigraphy. Technical Aspects*).

Statistical Considerations. After widespread clinical acceptance of a test, an important factor influencing apparent test sensitivity and specificity is the preferential selection of patients for coronary angiography in the presence of a positive test. The performance of coronary angiography often is based on a positive scintigraphic result. This, with the general lack of angiography in patients with a negative test result, produces a post-test referral bias. The results of the test to be assessed, in this case MPS, are used as the basis for performance of selective coronary angiography, the "gold standard" examination, which serves to define true-positive and true-negative results. Such behavior will increase the incidence of true positives, favorably affecting sensitivity, which is the percentage of positive tests among those with disease (the ability to identify disease):

$$\text{Sensitivity} = \frac{\text{True positives}}{\text{True positives} + \text{false negatives}},$$

Table 5

INFLUENCE OF CORONARY DISEASE PREVALENCE ON TEST ACCURACY IN 1000 PATIENTS*

	Prevalence of coronary disease							
	90%		50%		10%		2%	
Test result	CAD	No CAD	CAD	No CAD	CAD	No CAD	CAD	No CAD
Positive (no. of patients)	810	10	450	50	90	90	18	98
Negative (no. of patients)	90	90	50	450	10	810	2	882
Predictive value		.99		.90		.5		.18
Risk ratio		2		9		40		82

*Varying predictive value of a positive test and risk ratio of an abnormal test with varying prevalence, the basis of the pretest likelihood of coronary artery disease (CAD), with constant sensitivity of 90% and specificity of 90%.

Table 6A
SENSITIVITIES AND SPECIFICITIES OF EXERCISE MYOCARDIAL PERFUSION IMAGING

Radionuclide planar/SPECT (reference nos.)	Method	Years of study	Sensitivity	Specificity
201 Tl planar (57,60,253)	Qualitative	1976–1981	1002/1196 (84%)	435/562 (77%)
(51,85,883)	Qualitative*	1981–1985	255/333 (80%)	69/80 (87%)
(51,85)	Quantitative*		308/333 (93%)	74/80 (93%)
SPECT (120)	Qualitative planar* Qualitative SPECT*†	1989	ROC analysis	ROC analysis
(119,121,123)	Qualitative	1984–1990	442/482 (92%)	98/128 (77%)
(119,121,128)	Quantitative		442/482 (92%)	108/128 (84%)
99mTc sestamibi (planar) (66,112,113,884,885)		1989–1992	154/171 (90%)	14/20 (70%)
201Tl (planar) (66,112,113,884,885)			157/171 (92%)	13/20 (65%)
99mTc sestamibi (886,887)	Qualitative*	1994–1995	74/82 (90%)	51/68 (75%)
99mTc sestamibi (886,887)	Quantitative*		74/82 (90%)	55/68 (81%)
99mTc sestamibi (SPECT) (139,140,170, 888)	Qualitative	1989–1992	225/250 (90%)	35/58 (60.3%)
201Tl (SPECT) (139,140,170, 888)	Qualitative*		221/250 (88%)	29/58 (50%)
99mTc sestamibi (889,890)	Qualitative*	1995–1996	122/143 (85%)	11/14 (79%)
99mTc sestamibi (889,890)	Quantitative*		121/143 (85%)	11/14 (78%)
99mTc sestamibi (890)	Not attenuation corrected*	1996	50/60 (83%)	—
99mTc sestamibi (890)	Attenuation corrected*†		53/60 (88%)	—

*Direct comparison in the same patients.
†Superior by receiver operating characteristic (ROC) analysis.
Adapted, with permission, from Gerson MC. *Cardiac Nuclear Medicine.* 3rd ed. New York, NY: McGraw-Hill; 1997.

and its correlate:

$$\text{Likelihood or risk ratio of an abnormal test} = \frac{\text{Percentage of patients with abnormal test who have disease}}{\text{Percentage of patients with abnormal test without disease}}.$$

Such behavior also will increase the incidence of false positives, causing an adverse effect on specificity, which is the percentage of negative tests among those

Table 6B
DETECTION OF STENOSES IN INDIVIDUAL CORONARY ARTERIES BY VARIOUS
THALLIUM IMAGING METHODS

Method	Author (reference no.)	LAD	CIRC	RCA
		Sensitivity (%)		
Planar (subjective)	Lenaers et al. (60)	84	49	79
	Maddahi et al. (51)	56	34	65
	Rigo et al. (89)	83	35	62
	Massie et al. (68)	78	45	73
	Starling et al. (892)	61	32	64
	Fintel et al. (120)	58	37	64
Planar (quantitative)	Maddahi et al. (51)	80	63	94
Tomographic (subjective)	Tamaki et al. (123)	83	63	88
	Mahmarian et al. (121)	68	60	82
	Fintel et al. (120)	70	55	66
	DePasquale et al. (119)	70	50	88
Tomographic (quantitative)	Tamaki et al. (123)	87	78	92
	Mamahmarian et al. (121)	81	77	75
	DePasquale et al. (119)	78	65	89
	Kahn et al. (140)	62	53	64
	Van Train et al. (113)	78	71	83
		Specificity (%)		
Planar (subjective)	Lanaers et al. (60)	95	89	88
	Maddahi et al. (51)	92	97	91
	Starling et al. (892)	88	91	97
	Fintel et al. (120)	~90	~90	~90
Planar (quantitative)	Maddahi et al. (51)	85	9	82
Tomographic (subjective)	Tamaki et al. (123)	95	96	89
	Mahmarian et al. (121)	89	90	90
	Fintel et al. (120)	~90	~90	~90
	DePasquale et al. (119)	82	98	81
Tomographic (quantitative)	Tamaki et al. (123)	98	96	93
	Mahmarian et al. (121)	92	91	99
	DePasquale et al. (119)	83	95	87
	Kahn et al. (140)	83	63	71
	Van Train et al. (113)	67	66	65

LAD = left anterior descending artery; CIRC = left circumflex artery; RCA = right coronary artery.
Adapted, with permission, from Gerson MC. *Cardiac Nuclear Medicine*. 3rd ed. New York, NY: McGraw-Hill; 1997.

without disease (the ability to exclude disease):

$$\text{Specificity} = \frac{\text{True negatives}}{\text{True negatives} + \text{false positives}},$$

and its correlate:

$$\text{Likelihood or risk ratio of a normal test} = \frac{\text{Percentage of patients with a normal test who have no disease}}{\text{Percentage of patients with a normal test with disease}}.$$

Table 6C
NORMALCY RATES OF MYOCARDIAL PERFUSION IMAGING

Method	Combined normalcy rate (%)	Reference nos.
^{201}Tl qualitative planar	11/11 (100%)	131
^{201}Tl quantitative planar	11/11 (100%)	131
^{201}Tl qualitative SPECT	214/242 (88%)	51,133,893,112
^{201}Tl quantitative SPECT	94/115 (82%)	894
^{99m}Tc sestamibi planar (qualitative)	21/22 (95%)	894,139
^{99m}Tc sestamibi SPECT (qualitative)	87/103 (84%)	893,112
^{99m}Tc sestamibi SPECT (quantitative)	30/37 (81%)	895
^{99m}Tc sestamibi stress/^{201}Tl rest	119/124 (96%)	896,897
^{99m}Tc sestamibi SPECT (attenuation corrected)		151

Adapted, with permission, from Gerson MC. *Cardiac Nuclear Medicine*. 3rd ed. New York, NY: McGraw-Hill; 1997.

This effect is further exaggerated by the low incidence of true negatives coming to coronary angiography, as has been clearly documented by Rozanski et al. (*45*). Working with another nuclear cardiology method, they noted the influence of a post-test referral bias on the apparent decrease in the specificity of exercise radionuclide ventriculography over several years. When fully operational, this bias can dramatically affect apparent test specificity, which, by definition, would fall to 0 if only patients with a positive test went to angiography. In their literature review, Detrano et al. (*46*) found a significant negative relationship between referral bias and test specificity. They showed that studies that attempted to reduce referral bias by not allowing the results of exercise MPS to influence the decision to perform a coronary angiogram had significantly higher specificities than studies that did not (85% versus 78%). Therefore, the actual specificity of exercise ^{201}Tl planar scintigraphy may be higher than that reported by many investigators. Post-test referral bias also will influence apparent diagnostic sensitivity (*46,47*). This effect has become even more pronounced recently, as studies have shown the ability of MPS to stratify risk in patients beyond the ability of stress testing or other factors, increasing even more the tendency to base the performance of angiography on the scintigraphic findings (*47,48*). Although correction of data for referral bias has been suggested (*49*), all must be aware of the fact that true sensitivity is likely lower and true specificity much higher than calculated in clinical data sets in which angiography is the "gold standard" and referral to angiography is influenced by MPS results. Although similar considerations apply to other stress imaging methods, their accuracy will be affected only in proportion to the confidence the public places in the method, demonstrated by the frequency with which positive tests lead to angiography (*50*). No method is more heavily relied upon or the more frequent basis for management decisions than MPS. Nonetheless, even in this setting, stress MPS specificity has increased to relatively high levels, with better training and the application of technetium-based perfusion tracers.

In an attempt to determine a more representative specificity of MPS, the "normalcy rate" has been applied (Table 6C). This value is calculated like specificity but is determined in patients with a low likelihood of significant CAD based on their age, sex, coronary risk factors, symptoms and the results of the exercise ECG, rather than in patients found to have normal coronary angiograms (*51,52*). Rather than studying normal healthy volunteers, if this method is to have its full validity, the population selected for normalcy evaluation should demographically resemble the population to be tested. Normalcy is generally in the range of 90%–95% and may be viewed as a substitute for specificity when the process of selection bias is active.

The initial mean literature sensitivity and specificity for planar dipyridamole ^{201}Tl MPS (*53–56*) were 82% and 83%, respectively (Tables 6A–E). These results

Table 6D

SENSITIVITIES AND SPECIFICITIES OF EXERCISE TETROFOSMIN MYOCARDIAL PERFUSION IMAGING

Radionuclide-planar/SPECT (reference no.)	Method	Year	Sensitivity	Specificity	Per-vessel sensitivity
^{201}Tl versus ^{99m}Tc tetrofosmin (planar) (*898*)	Qualitative	1993	Both 46/50 (92%) 32 of 50 patients with prior MI	—	—
^{201}Tl versus ^{99m}Tc tetrofosmin (SPECT*) (*899*)	Qualitative	1994	20/23 versus 20/23 $P = $ NS	11%	20/32 (63%) versus 21/32 (63%) $P = $ NS
^{201}Tl versus ^{99m}Tc tetrofosmin (SPECT*) (*900*)	Qualitative	1994	24/26 (92%) versus 25/26 (96%) with prior MI	—	Both 16/28 (57%) No prior MI $P = $ NS
^{99m}Tc tetrofosmin (SPECT*) (*901*)	Qualitative	1994	19/22 (86%)	—	80% LAD, 93% RCA, 75% LCX
^{201}Tl versus ^{99m}Tc tetrofosmin (SPECT†) (*902*)	Qualitative	1994	22/23 (96%) versus 23/23 (100%) $P = $ NS	88% versus 100% $P = $ NS	63% versus 69% $P = $ NS
^{201}Tl versus ^{99m}Tc tetrofosmin (planar*) (*899*)	Qualitative	1994	18/23 versus 19/23 $P = $ NS	100%	18/32 (56%) versus 19/32 (59%) $P = $ NS
^{201}Tl versus ^{99m}Tc tetrofosmin (planar*) (*903*)	Qualitative	1995	83% versus 77% (224 patients)	48% versus 58%	80% LAD, 93% RCA, 75% LCX
^{99m}Tc tetrofosmin (SPECT) (*904*)	Qualitative	1995	—	—	85% LAD, 78% RCA, 69% LCX
^{99m}Tc tetrofosmin (SPECT) (*905*)	Qualitative	1996	17/18 (96%)	—	77% LAD, 94% RCA, 80% LCX
^{99m}Tc tetrofosmin (planar versus SPECT) (*906*)	Qualitative	1996	68% versus 87% (72 patients)	78% versus 89%	51% versus 59%
^{99m}Tc tetrofosmin (SPECT) (*907*)	Quantitative	1996	60/61 (98%)	12/13 (83%)	77%
^{99m}Tc tetrofosmin (SPECT) (*908*)	Qualitative	1996	93% (142 patients)	38%	64% LAD, 86% RCA, 49% LCX
^{99m}Tc tetrofosmin (SPECT) (*909*)	Qualitative	1997	85% (59 patients)	55%	53%
^{99m}Tc tetrofosmin (SPECT) (*910*)	Qualitative	1997	22/25 (88%)	—	79% LAD, 88% RCA, 83% LCX

Table 6D
(CONTINUED)

Radionuclide-planar/SPECT (reference no.)	Method	Year	Sensitivity	Specificity	Per-vessel sensitivity
^{99m}Tc tetrofosmin (SPECT) (*911*)	Qualitative	1997	— (80 patients)	—	80% LAD, 100% RCA, 58% LCX
^{201}Tl versus ^{99m}Tc tetrofosmin (SPECT) (*260*)	Quantitative	1998	Both 25/26 (96%)	—	—
^{99m}Tc tetrofosmin (SPECT) (*912*)	Quantitative	1998	89% (65 patients)	86%	89%
^{99m}Tc tetrofosmin (SPECT) (*913*)	Qualitative	1998	34/36 (94%)	19/24 (66%)	78% LAD, 91% RCA, 50% LCX
^{99m}Tc sestamibi versus tetrofosmin (SPECT) (*914*)	Qualitative	1998	17/25 (68%) versus 19/25 (76%) P = NS	P = NS	—
^{201}Tl versus ^{99m}Tc tetrofosmin (SPECT) (*915*)	Quantitative	1998	Both 96%	Both 93%	—
^{99m}Tc tetrofosmin (SPECT) (*916*)	Quantitative	1999	95% (235 patients)	76%	71% LAD, 73% RCA, 61% LCX
^{99m}Tc tetrofosmin (SPECT) (*917*)	Qualitative	1999	— (38 patients)	—	85% LAD, 78% RCA, 87% LCX

*Direct comparison in the same patients.
†With first pass analysis of left ventricular function.
LAD = left anterior descending coronary artery; LCX = left circumflex coronary artery; MI = myocardial infarction; RCA = right coronary artery.
Adapted, with permission, from Azzarelli S, et al. (*141*).

are similar to those noted with planar exercise ^{201}Tl scintigraphy (*5,7,8,46,51, 57– 97*). This observation has been confirmed by analysis of the results of several reports in which exercise and dipyridamole ^{201}Tl MPS were compared in the same patient population (*56,98–101*).

The Interaction of Statistics and Population Sampling. Bayes's theorem expresses the post-test likelihood of disease as a function of test sensitivity and specificity and the prevalence of disease in the population being studied. Stated differently, if the sensitivity and specificity of a test and the prevalence of disease in the population under study are known, one can calculate the likelihood of CAD in a given patient on the basis of a normal or abnormal test result (Table 5). Using Bayes's theorem, the positive and negative predictive accuracy of ^{201}Tl scintigraphy for the presence of CAD depends on the prevalence of disease in the patient population or the pretest likelihood of angiographically significant CAD in the

Table 6E
PROGNOSTIC VALUE OF A NORMAL MYOCARDIAL PERFUSION SCAN

Author (reference no.)	Type of stress	Imaging (S/P)*	Patients (no.)	Mean follow-up (mo)	Cardiac death/ myocardial infarction rate (%/yr)
Brown et al. (7)	Ex	P	100	46	0.8
Iskandrian et al. (917)	Ex	P	402	13	1.1
Pamelia et al. (336)	Ex	P	345	34	1.1
Wackers et al. (918)	Ex	P	344	22	1.0
Wahl et al. (919)	Ex	P	455	14	0.8
Staniloff et al. (9)	Ex	P	374	12	0.5
Gill et al. (312)	Ex	P	192	91	0.8
Heo et al. (920)	Ex	P	519	27	0.5
Koss et al. (921)	Ex	P	309	36	0.5
Kaul et al. (313)	Ex	P	39	64	0.5
Bairey et al. (922)	Ex	P	144	12	2.1
Stratmann et al. (923)	Ap	P	85	19	2.2
Younis et al. (12)	Dp	P	36	24	1.5
Fleg et al. (618)	Ex	P	352	55	0.9
Hendel et al. (13)	Dp	P	271	21	1.7
Brown and Rowen (343)	Ex	P	281	24	0.9
Brown et al. (924)	Ex/Dp	P	234	10	0.5
Burns et al. (925)	Ex	S	137	37	0.2
Herman et al. (926)	Dp	S	80	6	0.5
Steinberg et al. (927)	Ex	P	288	120	0.6

*P = planar; S = SPECT; Ex = exercise; Ap = atrial pacing; Dp = dipyridamole. Normal S studies would be expected to be superior to P methods in their ability to exclude disease.

Adapted, with permission, from Heller GV. Radionuclide imaging in the risk assessment of patients with stable CAD. In: *Myocardial Perfusion Imaging. Part III: Use of Imaging in Risk Assessment.* American Journal of Cardiology Continuing Education Series. Washington, DC: American Journal of Cardiology; 3–10.

patients being studied. From an extensive literature search of almost 29,000 patients, Diamond and Forrester (102) have reported and presented in a tabular form the prevalence of CAD based on age, sex and chest pain symptom classification from large populations at risk. Familiarity with this concept helps define the appropriateness of a test for a given individual (2,102–105). The likelihood of disease resulting from the application of a test with 90% sensitivity and 90% specificity to populations with varying disease incidence is simply calculated in Table 5. This principle is well applied to stress testing as shown in Figures 8 and 9.

Application of Bayes's theorem assumes that the sensitivity and specificity of a test are not affected by the prevalence of disease in the patient population being studied. Although this may not always apply (106), Uhl et al. (81) presented data supportive of this hypothesis when they demonstrated that the sensitivity and specificity of ^{201}Tl MPS is as high in a low-prevalence (21%) population as in the high-prevalence populations that have been more widely reported.

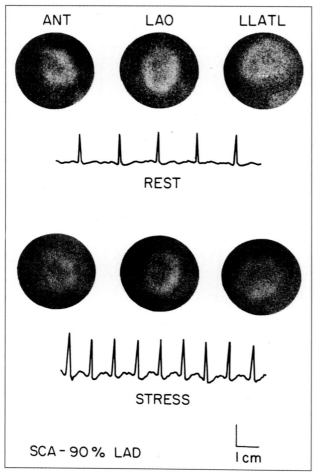

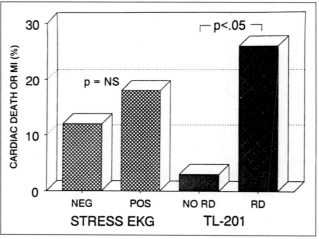

Figure 7 Prognostic value of exercise electrocardiography. Shown is the lack of predictive value of the stress electrocardiogram (EKG) compared with the excellent risk stratification of thallium-201 redistribution (RD) for cardiac death or myocardial infarction (MI). NEG = negative ST-segment depression; POS = positive for ST-segment depression. (Reproduced, with permission, from Brown KA. Prognostic value of thallium-201 myocardial perfusion imaging in patients with unstable angina who respond to medical treatment. *J Am Coll Cardiol* 1991;17:1053–1057.)

Figure 6 False-negative stress electrocardiogram. Shown is scintigraphic evidence of stress-induced septal ischemia in a patient with a 90% left anterior descending (LAD) stenosis. The stress electrocardiogram was normal. ANT = anterior; LAD = left anterior oblique; LLATL = left lateral; SCA = percentage of coronary artery sclerosis. (Reprinted, with permission, from Botvinick EH, Taradash MR, Shames DM, et al. Thallium-201 myocardial perfusion scintigraphy for the clinical clarification of normal, abnormal and equivocal electrocardiographic stress tests. *Am J Cardiol* 1978;41:43–49.)

When Bayes's theorem is applied to subjects at the extremes of pretest CAD likelihood, with the sensitivity and specificity values established with early planar studies of ^{201}Tl imaging, an abnormal or a normal test result changes the post-test likelihood much less than when the pretest likelihood is in the midrange (Table 5). For example, using a simple mathematical model, if stress MPS is 90% sensitive and 90% specific, than in a patient with a low, 10% pretest likelihood of CAD (for example, in a 50-yr-old asymptomatic man with a negative stress ECG), a positive stress MPS increases the likelihood to only 50% and a negative test decreases the likelihood to ~1%! At the other extreme, in a patient with a high, 90%, pretest likelihood of CAD (for example, a 65-yr-old man with typical angina and a positive stress ECG), a positive MPS increases the likelihood to ~99%, but a negative test decreases the likelihood to only 50%. In a patient with an intermediate (50%) likelihood of CAD (for example, a 50-yr-old man with atypical chest pain), a positive MPS increases the likelihood to 90% and a negative test decreases the likelihood to ~10%. These values are further augmented in real populations by concordant stress test results and are also influenced heavily by the severity of the induced abnormality, as shown in Figures 8 and 9. A positive MPS in a patient with a low likelihood of CAD does not always establish the presence of CAD. Similarly, although associated with an excellent prognosis (14), a negative image may not eliminate CAD from consideration in a high-likelihood patient. As in the mathematical models, maximum diagnostic efficacy of the test is noted in patients with an intermediate likelihood of CAD and in whom a positive or a negative perfusion image strongly increases or decreases the post-test likelihood of disease. These patients are considered to be the most appropriate group to benefit diagnostically from stress-perfusion MPS (Table 7).

In practice, the considerations above must be set in terms of the interpretive criteria applied by the reader. These criteria influence the sensitivity and specificity and can be defined by a receiver operating characteristic (ROC) and related ROC analysis (10,11,107). Here, the reader interprets a group of normal and abnormal images by a spectrum of thresholds for abnormality. This yields a ROC curve that establishes the relationship between test sensitivity and test specificity. Optimally, the reading should utilize criteria to maximize these parameters and can be altered to maximize either sensitivity or specificity. By Bayes's theorem, the positive and negative predictive values generated by any sensitivity value on the ROC curve will vary with the prevalence of CAD in the population.

Not considered here, but to be factored into the equation translating pretest to post-test CAD likelihood, are the findings on exercise testing, not available with pharmacologic intervention. Although the pretest (pre-MPS) probability discussed previously was determined after stress test results were known, this is often not the case, and the stress test performed with MPS may be the initial stress test for patient evaluation. In that case, when in parallel with scintigraphic results, the presence or absence of induced chest pain or ST changes polarizes further the post-test likelihood. In the patient described previously with an intermediate pretest disease likelihood, a negative stress test and the absence of induced chest pain or equivalent

---

Table 7
SOME MAJOR CLINICAL ADVANTAGES
OF THE STRESS PERFUSION METHOD

1. Suitability for use with indirect- (dynamic stress/dobutamine) as well as with direct- (dipyridamole) acting coronary dilators to test the coronary flow reserve

2. Excellent diagnostic sensitivity and specificity in both sexes

3. Excellent localizing information. The method provides a "roadmap" of ischemic pathophysiology, of great value to the angiographer.

4. Reproducibility and objectivity of the method

5. The high predictive value of a negative test and the best reassurance of a good outcome when normal

6. Ability to risk stratify and substratify within categories of the quantitative Duke Treadmill Score and within coronary anatomic subgroups

7. The direct relationship between coronary risk and defect size in patients of both sexes

8. The added importance and prognostic impact of scintigraphic and stress testing parameters

9. The importance of defect size to risk stratification of patients before noncardiac surgery, the postinfarct patient and the patient with unstable angina

10. The obvious reliance on the scintigraphic method, with the incidence of coronary angiography paralleling scintigraphic risk

11. The recent relationship drawn between defect size and cardiac death and nonfatal myocardial infarction and its impact on clinical management (21)

12. The clinical and cost advantages of management of well-treated patients with unstable angina and uncomplicated patients with non-Q infarction (and others), based on the results of stress myocardial perfusion scintigraphy as a "gatekeeper" (683,685,825)

Table 8
CLINICAL APPLICATIONS OF STRESS PERFUSION
(OR BLOOD POOL) SCINTIGRAPHY

Diagnosis of coronary artery disease

   Evaluate abnormal electrocardiography (ECG)
   With an equivocal or uninterpretable stress test with baseline ECG abnormalities
   When the diagnosis is ambiguous and disease likelihood is intermediate
   Where the stress ECG is abnormal in a patient with a low likelihood of disease, or the converse
   When the stress ECG is negative for ischemia at a low achieved double product
   Unsatisfactory exercise performance
   To establish the pathophysiologic significance of coronary lesions of questionable significance
   Determine the "culprit" coronary lesion
   Screen relatively low-likelihood patients presenting with chest pain
   Application of vasodilator pharmacologic stress

Risk stratification

   Aids identification of left main and multivessel coronary artery disease
   Provides an estimate of myocardium at ischemic risk
   Assists in the evaluation and management of patients after uncomplicated infarction
   Assists in the selection of patients for catheterization and angiography
   Assists in the selection of patients for revascularization
   Aids identification of patients at risk for ischemic perioperative complications of extensive, high-risk noncardiac surgery

Evaluation of therapy

   Localizes ischemia to specific vessels
   Aids evaluation of symptoms after revascularization procedures
   Aids assessment of bypass graft patency
   Determines the effectiveness of collaterals
   Determines regional viability, differentiating ischemia from infarction
   Evaluates new anti-ischemic therapies in clinical trials

---

symptoms added to the negative image would drive down the post-test likelihood even further. It would make CAD unlikely and put it at the likelihood level of that in an asymptomatic patient, presenting a basis for management. When contrary to the clinical findings or when the stress ECG is frankly uninterpretable or nonspecific, MPS is even more valuable as a diagnostic tool and is then, again, a necessary adjunct of stress testing. The scintigraphic method is of even more general value when applied for prognostic assessment and risk stratification in patients with high likelihood of CAD or known disease (Table 7).

Planar Imaging. Many observations made in the analysis of the accuracy of planar MPS have more widespread applications to single-photon emission-computed tomography (SPECT) MPS and to the evaluation of testing methods in general (Fig. 10) (Tables 6A–E). The diagnostic accuracy of stress MPS is modified by several technical and imaging factors, such as: the perfusion agent, whether acquired by planar or SPECT methods, analyzed visually and qualitatively or quantitatively, gated or not (108–123), or related to exercise or pharmacologic stress. In addition and as noted above, characteristics of the patient population, the coronary anatomy test parameters and interpretation criteria may affect the apparent sensitivity and specificity reported in different studies at different centers. Some of these factors include: the presence of prior myocardial infarction (MI), the severity and extent of CAD, the presence of coronary collaterals, the level of achieved myocardial flow demand related directly to the double product and indirectly to the workload achieved and the definition of significant CAD. Interestingly, among both planar and SPECT studies, there appears to be no significant difference in data acquired by cameras made by different manufacturers from similar generations and with similar specifications.

A large and early literature, which can only be summarized here, relates to exercise and redistribution ^{201}Tl MPS by planar acquisition and qualitative analysis (2,5,7,8,48,52,53–97,102–105,115). The overall sensitivity and specificity of this technique in a total of 4678 reported patients were 82% and 88%, respectively. In an analysis of the factors affecting sensitivity and specificity of exercise ^{201}Tl testing, Detrano et al. (46) demonstrated that, among 56 published reports, the mean sensitivity of ^{201}Tl MPS was 86% and the mean specificity was 85%. In the subgroup of patients without MI, the sensitivity was 79%. This was significantly lower than the 96% among patients with prior MI.

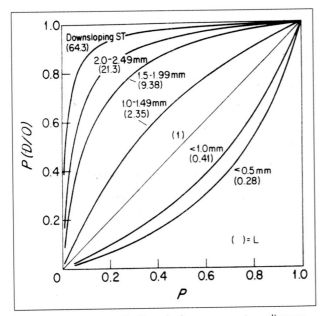

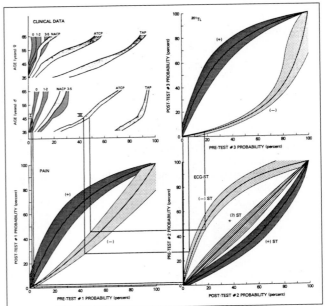

Figure 8 Post-test likelihood of coronary artery disease (CAD). Shown is the post-test likelihood of CAD [P(D/O)] after exercise electrocardiographic (ECG) testing as a function of the pretest CAD likelihood (P). Curves are plotted for varying levels of ECG ST-segment depression in which greater degrees of ST-segment depression produce an increasing likelihood ratio (L) for the presence of CAD. For any given level of exercise-induced ST-segment change, the post-test likelihood will be altered most in relation to the pretest likelihood for patients with an intermediate pretest disease likelihood. (Reproduced, with permission, from Rifkin RD, Hood WB Jr. Bayesian analysis of electrocardiographic exercise stress testing. *N Engl J Med* 1977;297:681–686.)

Figure 9 Diagnosis of coronary artery disease. Illustrated is the interaction of clinical data (upper left) and noninvasive stress-induced pain (lower left), ischemic electrocardiographic changes (lower right), and perfusion defects (upper right) in formulating the likelihood of coronary disease. The type of presenting pain, nonanginal (NACP), atypical (ATCP) or typical angina (TAP), in addition to patient age and sex, present an initial estimate of disease likelihood according to the data of Diamond et al. (*103*). Thereafter, the results of noninvasive stress testing influence likelihood assessment. Shown are examples of patients presenting clinical findings related to low and intermediate coronary likelihood. The effects of negative noninvasive results are traced and have little impact on the patient with an initial low likelihood of disease. However, a patient presenting with initial intermediate (40%–50%) likelihood relates to a 2% (lower with more recent scintigraphic studies) likelihood of coronary disease after negative noninvasive tests. This incidence is not significantly different from a similar asymptomatic population. (Reproduced, with permission, from Patterson RE, Eng C, Horowitz SF, et al. Practical diagnosis of coronary artery disease: a Bayes' theorem nomogram to correlate clinical data with noninvasive exercise tests. *Am J Cardiol* 1984;53:252–261.)

In the published reports of 11 studies of planar stress ^{201}Tl imaging that specified the effect of the extent of disease on test sensitivity (*1,58,60,61,68–70,74,80,81,90*), the mean test sensitivity increased from 79% for single-vessel disease to 88% for double- and 92% for triple-vessel disease. Similar findings relate to SPECT imaging but with increased accuracy and additional advantages (Tables 6A–E).

With the advent of SPECT, planar imaging is performed less frequently. However, planar images remain the basis for SPECT acquisition, and familiarity with the planar method and its interpretation remains important. Planar imaging remains of great value for the acquisition of bedside portable studies in patients who cannot safely be moved, in uncooperative patients who cannot lie still for the complete SPECT acquisition and especially in large patients who exceed

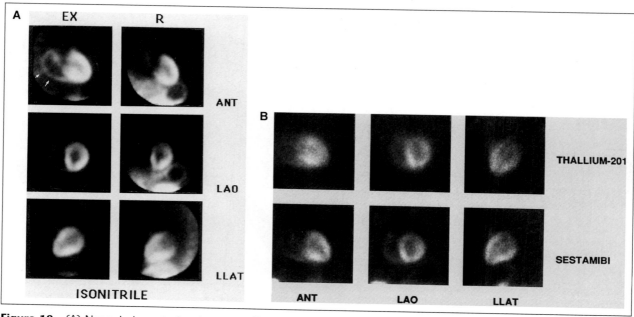

Figure 10 (A) Normal planar technetium-99m (^{99m}Tc) sestamibi images after exercise and at rest. Compared with thallium-201, these images show greater anatomic detail. The right ventricle and right atrium are visualized (anterior [ANT] view, arrows). Because of less low-energy scatter, these images have a crisper quality. Apical thinning can be noted on the left anterior oblique (LAO) view. (B) Normal planar thallium images (top) are compared with those of ^{99m}Tc sestamibi (bottom). Note the thinner, better-resolved walls on ^{99m}Tc imaging and the apparently larger cavity size. In addition, the normal apical slit is seen only in the better-resolved ^{99m}Tc image. Similar findings are seen with imaging ^{99m}Tc tetrofosmin. LLAT = left lateral. (Reproduced, with permission, from Wackers FJTh. Artifacts in planar and SPECT myocardial perfusion imaging. *Am J Cardiol Imaging* 1992;6:42–58.)

SPECT imaging-table limits. Planar ^{99m}Tc sestamibi imaging has been reported to be less sensitive than planar ^{201}Tl imaging, possibly because of the higher ^{99m}Tc emission energy, with which well-perfused walls behind and defects closer to the camera may "shine through" such defects and make them less evident. Such defects may be visible with the more highly attenuated ^{201}Tl. However, most researchers apply planar ^{99m}Tc sestamibi with good results and even gate these studies (*108,124,125*).

SPECT Imaging. Today, these diagnostic relationships have been refined and extended with SPECT data (*48,114,126–138*). Reports suggest a well-maintained diagnostic sensitivity, better than that of planar imaging, in the presence or absence of prior infarction using the SPECT method (*112,114,129*) (Fig. 11). Diagnostic and prognostic ability have held up well in the "post-thrombolytic" era (*133*).

The normal SPECT myocardial perfusion scintigram is illustrated in *Self-Study Program III. Cardiology. Topic 5: Myocardial Perfusion Scintigraphy. Technical Aspects* and elsewhere in this volume. As a measure of the qualitative, visual analysis of SPECT ^{201}Tl imaging, in a total of 2818 patients reported (*119–126*) the sensitivity and specificity were 90% and 77%, respectively. Based on the results of objective, quantitative analysis involving 1627 patients, the average diagnostic sensitivities and specificities of treadmill exercise SPECT ^{201}Tl myocardial perfusion imaging were 90% and 70%, respectively, with a normalcy rate of 89% (*121,131–134*). These findings are further supported by others generated in hundreds of individuals (*119–121,134,135*).

It is noteworthy that the specificity of the test appeared to be lower in some SPECT than planar studies and lower in the study by DePasquale et al. (*119*) in

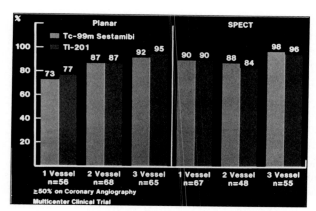

Figure 11   Accuracy of sestamibi. Shown in this multi-center trial is the comparative diagnostic sensitivity of stress planar and SPECT technetium-99m sestamibi and thallium-201, for the diagnosis of 1-, 2- and 3-vessel disease. Although SPECT sensitivity was no more accurate than planar imaging for overall diagnosis, it was equally sensitive for 1-, 2- and 3-vessel disease, an example of the strength of the SPECT method. In general, the application of SPECT technique does add to diagnostic accuracy. (Reproduced, with permission, from Taillefer R, Lambert R, Dupras G, et al. Clinical comparison between thallium-201 and technetium-99m methoxyisobutyl isonitrile (hexamibi) myocardial perfusion imaging for the detection of coronary artery disease—multicenter trial. *Eur J Nucl Med* 1989;15:280–288.)

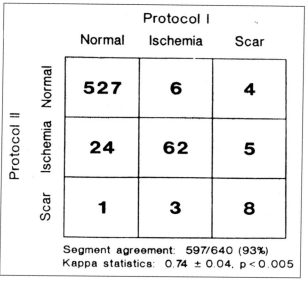

Figure 12   Rest/stress and stress/rest protocols. A comparison of the same-day technetium-99m sestamibi rest-exercise sequence (protocol 1) and the exercise–rest sequence (protocol 2) performed in the same patients. Although there was concordance of results in 93% of the segments, there was a higher incidence of discordant negative results among the rest-first studies, probably as a result of an inability to recognize stress-induced defects with background activity related to the previous exam. (Reproduced, with permission, from Heo J, Kegel J, Iskandrian AS, et al. Comparison of same-day protocols using technetium-99m sestamibi myocardial imaging. *J Nucl Med* 1992;33:186–191.)

1988 than in the study by Tamaki et al. (*123*) in 1984. A similar trend also is noted for the quantitative SPECT method, with a decrease in specificity from 1984 to 1989, despite an insignificant change in sensitivity of 98% compared with 94% during the same period. This apparent decline of specificity with time is again probably the result of increased referral bias in the more recent studies related to a justifiable increase in clinical dependence on the method for patient management and its use as gatekeeper for angiography. Although the true, unbiased specificity of the SPECT technique has not been determined, it may be implied from the "normalcy rate." In some studies performed at the same time, the specificity of the SPECT technique was slightly lower than that for the planar imaging method. This may be a result of the fact that the SPECT method is technically more demanding and leaves more room for artifacts during acquisition and processing. It has improved with new technology and experience, and its current ability far surpasses the planar method.

Fintel et al. (*120*) compared the visual diagnostic performance of planar and SPECT methods in 136 patients. In subgroup analysis, they found that ^{201}Tl tomography was superior in males and in patients with milder disease, such as those with no prior MI or with single-vessel disease or in patients with 50%–69% coronary stenosis. The increased contrast resolution of SPECT provided a greater ability to identify more abnormal regions and related coronary beds. Its dissemination into the community with increased experience and the advent of new methods to correct for attenuation artifact promise a further increase in specificity (*136,137*) (Tables 6A–E).

Comparative Diagnostic Accuracy: Thallium-201 and Technetium-99m–Based Perfusion Radiotracers. Thallium-201 and (even more so) ^{99m}Tc sestamibi underestimated the magnitude of the flow disparity between stenotic and normal beds induced with adenosine-related hyperemia in a canine model (*138*). This may be a result of the reduced linearity of sestamibi (and tetrofosmin) distribution to flow compared with that of thallium. However, the greater scatter and redistribution of ^{201}Tl may reduce any clinical advantage.

As shown above, diagnostic sensitivity generally falls with decreased vascular involvement. Yet, several studies evaluating SPECT perfusion imaging, including a multicenter trial comparing both ^{99m}Tc sestamibi and ^{201}Tl planar and SPECT imaging (Fig. 11), show similarly maintained high SPECT sensitivity and specificity, in the range of 90%, regardless of the number of vessels involved (*118,139*). This multicenter trial, evaluating imaging methods among 294 patients at several centers in the United States and Canada, demonstrated sensitivity, specificity and normalcy rates for SPECT ^{99m}Tc sestamibi to be 85%, 95% and 100%, respectively, and, for ^{201}Tl, to be 87%, 55% and 100%, respectively. Reduced specificity probably related to technical factors and referral bias (*45,50–52*) and appeared to be improved with the ^{99m}Tc-based agent. For the detection of a perfusion abnormality in the presence of 1-, 2- and 3-vessel disease, planar sensitivities averaged 75%, 87% and 93%, without interagent differences. In this study, planar imaging of both ^{99m}Tc sestamibi and ^{201}Tl demonstrated an incremental sensitivity for CAD diagnosis in the presence of 3-vessel disease (92% and 95%, respectively) compared with that in single-vessel disease (73% and 77%, respectively). However, SPECT image analysis demonstrated similar high sensitivities for ^{99m}Tc sestamibi and ^{201}Tl in the presence of single- (90% and 90%), double- (88% and 84%) and triple-vessel disease, (98% and 96%, respectively). Additional multicenter studies and many clinical evaluations have demonstrated the diagnostic accuracy of SPECT ^{99m}Tc sestamibi images to be equal to or greater than that of ^{201}Tl, with greater contrast and spatial resolution than planar imaging. SPECT advantages derive from physical factors and from the tomographic display, which separates myocardial regions that overlap in planar images, presenting a "fingerprint" of regional perfusion. Most prominent is the ability of SPECT with either agent to better recognize defects in the left circumflex region, deep in the chest.

Several individual studies compared the relative accuracies of SPECT ^{201}Tl and ^{99m}Tc sestamibi protocols for detection of disease in individual vessels (Table 5) and for the diagnosis of CAD overall (*112–114,118,131,139–140*) (Table 6A–E). For CAD detection, ^{201}Tl evaluation presented an average sensitivity of 83% versus 90% for ^{99m}Tc sestamibi and an average specificity of 80% versus 93% for sestamibi, with respective normalcies of 77% and 100% (*112,114,118,131,139, 140*). For detection of CAD in individual vessels, average ^{201}Tl sensitivities and specificities were 70% and 75%, respectively, whereas those for ^{99m}Tc sestamibi were 83% and 77%, respectively (*112,114,118,131,139,140–171*). When the rest/stress and stress/rest sestamibi protocols were performed in random order in the same patients, there was concordance of results in 93% of the segments. There was a higher incidence of discordant negative results among the rest-first studies, probably because of an inability to recognize stress-induced defects with background activity related to the previous study (Figs. 12–14).

Tetrofosmin. Technetium-99m tetrofosmin (Table 6D) has been approved by the United States Food and Drug Administration (FDA) as a perfusion radiotracer for clinical use. According to the literature, the diagnostic abilities of the method are fully preserved, regardless of whether ^{201}Tl, ^{99m}Tc sestamibi or tetrofosmin is used as the imaging agent. However, the 3 current agents do differ

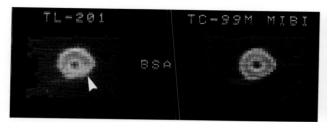

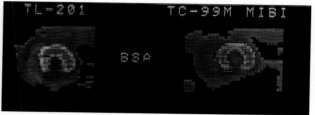

Figure 13 Inferior attenuation. Shown are tomograms of postexercise basal short-axis (BSA) sections for thallium-201 (^{201}Tl) and technetium-99m sestamibi (MIBI) from a normal volunteer. The ^{201}Tl study shows reduced activity (arrowhead) in the inferoposterior segments, probably as a result of diaphragmatic attenuation and only evident in the lower-energy ^{201}Tl image. (Reproduced, with permission, from Khan JK, McGhie I, Akers MS, et al. Quantitative rotational tomography with Tl-201 and Tc-99m methoxy-isobutyl-isonitrile: a direct comparison in normal individuals and patients with coronary artery disease. *Circulation* 1989;79:1282–1293.)

Figure 14 Inferior defect. Basal short-axis (BSA) thallium-201 (^{201}Tl) and technetium-99m (^{99m}Tc) sestamibi (MIBI) slices from the postexercise tomograms of a patient with an occluded right coronary artery and a 75% stenosed left anterior descending coronary artery. Both studies show an inferoposterior defect, but an anterior defect is evident only on the sestamibi study. (Reproduced, with permission, from Kahn JK, McGhie I, Akers MS, et al. Quantitative rotaional tomography with Tl-201 and Tc-99m methoxy-isobutyl-isonitrile: a direct comparison in normal individuals and patients with coronary artery disease. *Circulation* 1989;79:1282–1293.)

widely in their methods of production, availability, emission energies, half-lives, permitted administered doses, attenuation and scatter, extraction fractions, intracellular localization, linearity with flow, excretion patterns and other factors (see *Self-Study Program III. Cardiology. Topic 5: Myocardial Perfusion Scintigraphy. Technical Aspects*). This should lead to an active choice of the agent and protocol to apply in any given clinical setting. The diagnostic accuracy of ^{99m}Tc tetrofosmin was demonstrated in 235 consecutive patients (*141*). Yet the extraction fraction of these agents at high flow rates and resultant linearity with flow are greatest for ^{201}Tl and least for ^{99m}Tc tetrofosmin. This may make a diagnostic difference when assessing limited stenoses at high flow rates, as usually seen with coronary dilator pharmacologic stress. With dipyridamole, myocardial uptake is 20% less with tetrofosmin than sestamibi.

Kapur et al. (*142*) evaluated image characteristics among more than 2500 patients randomized for study by ^{201}Tl, ^{99m}Tc tetrofosmin or sestamibi stress MPS. Although there were expected differences resulting from the agents' physical characteristics, diagnostic sensitivities were similar (*142*). Perfusion and viability information were the same when evaluated by exercise MPS performed with ^{99m}Tc tetrofosmin and ^{201}Tl in 33 patients with left ventricular dysfunction (*143*).

To test agent sensitivity at the limits of stenosis significance, Taillefer et al. (*144*) prospectively compared dipyridamole stress ^{99m}Tc sestamibi and tetrofosmin in 81 patients without previous MI and with mild-to-moderate (50%–90%) coronary stenoses. The patients were studied serially and randomly at 2 centers within 1 wk using same-day or 2-day stress/rest protocols and waiting 60 min after injection before imaging. Image concordance was evident in 66 of 88 (76%) patients. Although the overall sensitivities for MPS with both agents were not significantly different, sestamibi identified 363 ischemic segments compared with 285 for tetrofosmin, with higher ischemic-to-normal wall activity ratios and larger defect size. Sestamibi images more often identified multivessel CAD. A multicenter study performed with 81 patients supported the superiority of dipyridamole ^{99m}Tc sestamibi compared with ^{99m}Tc tetrofosmin for identification of mild but significant coronary lesions (*145*). These differences could have important clinical consequences. Nonetheless, evidence in animal studies supports the application of tetrofosmin for viability assessment.

Technetium-99m–based agents have the potential to assess right ventricular perfusion, size and function. Right ventricular defects have been sought and often found after inferior infarctions on stress sestamibi studies (*146*). Sestamibi imaging demonstrated right heart enlargement and dysfunction in a case report of an elderly man evaluated for chest pain and found to have multiple pulmonary emboli with pulmonary hypertension (*147*). Other researchers have added to the series to demonstrate the value of the gated perfusion method for the identification of right ventricular disease (*148*). The right ventricle is not included in circumferential profiles, polar projection maps or other quantitative aids.

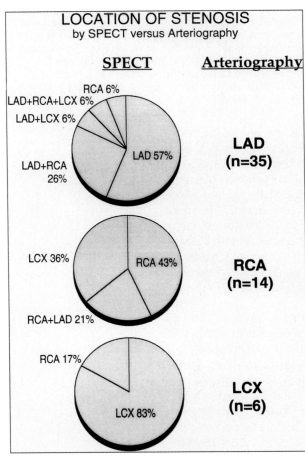

Figure 15 Reader defect localization compared with angiography. Here, pie diagrams show the scan localization of coronary artery disease compared with the actual angiographic distribution of diseased vessel(s). The involved vessel was correctly identified in 85% of studies, yet the scan incorrectly speculated on multivessel disease in 29%, and, in 15% of those identified as having single-vessel disease, the wrong vessel was identified. Most of the error came in confusion regarding right (RCA) and left circumflex (LCX) coronary arteries. LAD = left anterior descending coronary artery. (Reproduced, with permission, from Segall GM, Atwood JE, Botvinick EH, et al. Variability of normal coronary anatomy: implications for the interpretation of thallium SPECT myocardial perfusion images in single-vessel disease. *J Nucl Med* 1995;36:944–951.)

Special Circumstances

Women, large patients (*5,149*), those with LBBB (*150–157*), chronic obstructive pulmonary disease (*158*) and reduced left ventricular function (*159,160*) present special diagnostic challenges. These can be successfully managed with proper acquisition and interpretation methods, proper choice of radiopharmaceuticals and stress methods. As with all forms of stress testing, stress perfusion imaging may be problematic and is not generally recommended in asymptomatic patients who are at low risk for CAD (*161*).

DETECTION OF DISEASE IN INDIVIDUAL CORONARY ARTERIES

General Considerations

Coronary arteries and their branches supply specific regions of the left ventricular myocardium. Coronary angiography has demonstrated a general but variable anatomic relationship between the coronary arteries and related myocardial regions (Table 6D). These relationships were consolidated with the actual study of patients with single-vessel CAD by MPS with stress (*162*) and with balloon coronary occlusion (*163,164*) (Figs. 15,16). General guidelines have been developed for assignment of myocardial regions to specific coronary arteries. It is therefore possible to infer the presence of disease in a given coronary artery by noting the location of a perfusion defect on planar or tomographic perfusion images. These relationships vary among individual patients based on coronary dominance, in which the left anterior descending coronary artery (LAD) or right coronary artery (RCA) is dominant if it perfuses the posterior septum. Abnormalities of the anterior wall, anteroseptum and apex usually involve LAD disease, whereas those in the posteroseptum and inferior walls, most commonly at the base, relate to RCA disease. Those in the lateral or inferolateral walls indicate left circumflex coronary artery (LCX) disease. These coronary territories are thoroughly dealt with in *Self-Study Program III. Cardiology. Topic 5: Myocardial Perfusion Scintigraphy. Technical Aspects.*

The Planar Method

The mean sensitivities (*46,60,68,74,80,165,166*) of planar imaging interpreted visually for identification of disease in the LAD, LCX and RCA have been shown to be 69%, 37% and 65%, respectively, with mean specificities of 94%, 95% and 85% (Table 6B). The mean sensitivity and specificity of the method for detection of disease in any single coronary artery were reported to be 59% and 91%, respectively. It is of note that the sensitivity for LCX disease detection with planar ^{201}Tl imaging is lower than that for the detection of other individual diseased coronary arteries in patients with single- or multivessel disease. The imperfection of MPS in detecting all involved vessels and the lower sensitivity of planar compared with SPECT perfusion imaging for detection of disease in individual coronary arteries may be explained by 1 or more of the factors described in Table 9.

Overlap of vascular regions may be particularly responsible for the lower sensitivity of ^{201}Tl scintigraphy in the detection of LCX disease. The territory of the LCX is represented by the lateral wall in the 45° left anterior oblique (LAO) view, with significant overlap of proximal and distal portions as well as anterolateral and posterolateral regions. Alternatively, sensitivity in this area may relate to the location of the LCX region, which is deep within the chest and therefore subject to greater attenuation than other regions. It should also be noted that these results date from the early qualitative, subjective application of the method, predating the understanding of the subtleties of planar ^{201}Tl image. Quantitative analysis of planar ^{201}Tl images has improved identification of disease in individual coronary arteries. The literature notes sensitivities and specificities of 77% and 74% for LAD, 50% and 85% for the LCX and 91% and 59% for the RCA by quantitative planar methods (*51,52*). The sensitivity and specificity of the quantitative analyzed planar images for identification of disease in any single coronary artery are 74% and 73%, respectively. This improved sensitivity has been attributed to background subtraction and analysis of the regional washout rate. The use of background subtraction, inherent in all quantitative methods, may enhance ^{201}Tl perfusion defects in images that would otherwise be considered negative or equivocal by visual analysis. The regional washout rate is the net difference between myocardial input and output. This parameter has been found to relate directly to regional perfusion. Slow regional ^{201}Tl washout has been applied as an objective index of regional hypoperfusion in a relatively less affected myocardial region in patients with multivessel coronary disease and adjacent regions of ischemia.

The SPECT Method

An objective advantage of SPECT imaging relates to its ability to visualize and separate regions of vascular distribution, most prominently the posterior and anterior septum supplied generally by the RCA and LAD, the anterolateral region supplied by diagonal branches of the LAD and improved sensitivity for diagnosis of LCX disease (Table 6A–D). Further improvement of sensitivity for detection of disease in individual coronary arteries has been reported using the SPECT technique (*165,167*). This was achieved while maintaining specificity and reproducibility. The multicenter study discussed previously, that compared the sensitivity and specificity of [99mTc] sestamibi with that of ^{201}Tl stress MPS, revealed a uniformly high sensitivity of both agents for the diagnosis of 1-, 2- or 3-vessel disease by SPECT methodology (*114,118,139*). This is in contrast to the differential sensitivity determined in other planar and SPECT studies and with other noninvasive imaging methods, which increase sensitivity with increasing vascular involvement.

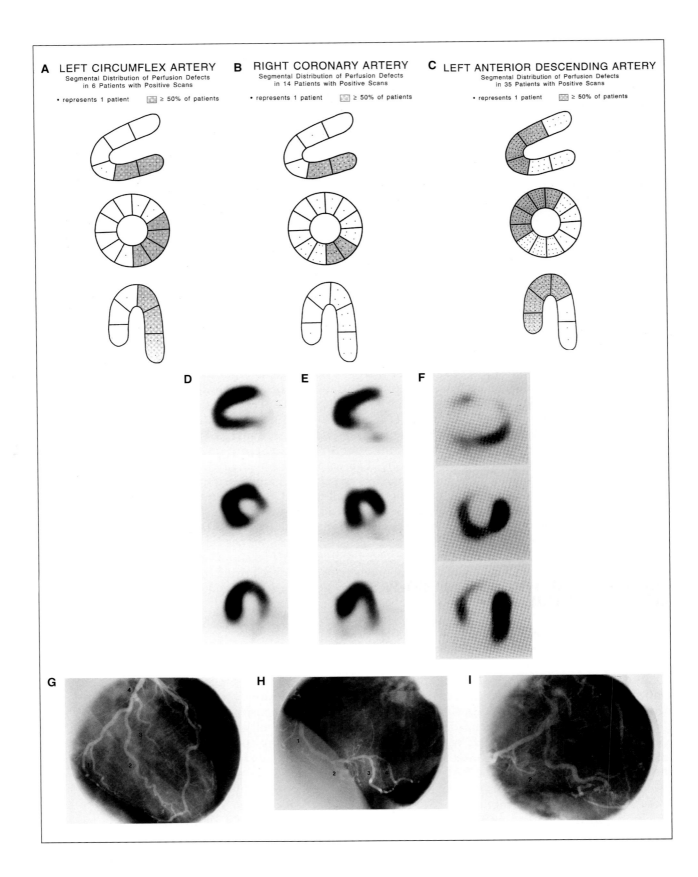

A LEFT CIRCUMFLEX ARTERY
Segmental Distribution of Perfusion Defects
in 6 Patients with Positive Scans

• represents 1 patient   ≥ 50% of patients

B RIGHT CORONARY ARTERY
Segmental Distribution of Perfusion Defects
in 14 Patients with Positive Scans

• represents 1 patient   ≥ 50% of patients

C LEFT ANTERIOR DESCENDING ARTERY
Segmental Distribution of Perfusion Defects
in 35 Patients with Positive Scans

• represents 1 patient   ≥ 50% of patients

Respective sensitivities and specificities of visually analyzed SPECT images are 75% and 85% for the LAD, 54% and 97% for the LCX, 88% and 84% for the RCA and 80% and 79% for any coronary artery (119,120). Respective sensitivities and specificities of quantitatively analyzed SPECT ^{201}Tl images are 80% and 83% for the LAD, 72% and 84% for the LCX, 83% and 84% for the RCA and 79% and 84% for any coronary artery (117,119,120,123,131–134). With tomographic imaging, improved sensitivity is noted particularly for detection of disease in the LCX, as shown by pooled literature results and direct comparison of SPECT and planar quan- titative imaging methods in the same patient population (168). This improved sensitivity may be related to the improved defect contrast and decreased overlap between myocardial regions that result from SPECT imaging. Current reported sensitivities for CAD diagnosis are generally ~90%, with per-vessel sensitivities in the range of 75%–80%! These values are somewhat higher with SPECT ^{99m}Tc-based agents. Four early studies (112,140,169,170) compared exercise SPECT ^{201}Tl with SPECT ^{99m}Tc sestamibi MPS and demonstrated increased sensitivity (83% versus 90%) and specificity (80% versus 93%) with SPECT ^{99m}Tc sestamibi. Such values are approached by no other method or modality.

Table 9

REASONS FOR THE UNDERESTIMATION OF DISEASE ON STRESS PERFUSION SCINTIGRAPHY

1. In studies with multiple adjacent areas of hypoperfusion, such as in patients who have multivessel disease, only the most hypoperfused regions may appear normal, because of the relative nature of myocardial perfusion defect analysis.

2. Because of the relative nature of the method, the presence of a single dense defect, such as with prior infarction, may make other less severe abnormalities difficult to appreciate.

3. In patients with multivessel disease, exercise may be terminated because of the development of limiting symptoms and associated ischemia in 1 region before another region becomes ischemic.

4. Stress may fail to reach the ischemic threshold, the double product at the onset of ischemia, with relatively low heart rate and systolic blood pressure and so fail to identify even a single stenotic vessel.

5. Given the limited linearity of flow related to all available perfusion agents, lesion stenosis may be at the limits of recognition by the method. Of course, such studies nonetheless relate to an excellent prognosis.

6. Coronary narrowings of 50%, which are considered significant by angiography, may not be hemodynamically significant. Thus, myocardial regions subtended by these vessels do not become ischemic during exercise.

7. The assignment of myocardial regions to coronary arteries is not perfect, because of significant variability among individuals and because of an overlap in territories of perfusion (169–173).

8. Overlap of various myocardial regions that is inherent in the planar imaging technique may obscure small defects in a given coronary territory and thus lower the regional sensitivity.

9. The role of collateral circulation in preventing ischemia in the distribution of a significant coronary region is variable and unpredictable.

PERFUSION AND FUNCTION: FIRST-PASS AND GATED STUDIES

The strong relationship between LVEF and mortality can be appreciated in the evaluation of postinfarction patients (see *Self-Study Program III. Cardiology. Topic*

Figure 16 Single-vessel disease: myocardial perfusion scintigraphy examples. (A), (B) and (C) are diagrams of the spectrum of the distribution of perfusion defects in the left circumflex (LCX) and right and left anterior descending coronary arteries (RCA and LAD, respectively) in this study of image patterns in patients with single-vessel disease. The patterns resemble those generally related to disease in these beds. However, right coronary disease often affects the inferior and posterior septal regions and less often the inferolateral wall, a classic distribution of circumflex disease. (D) Midventricular slices from the SPECT study with vertical long-, short- and horizontal long-axis slices displayed from above down, performed in a 54-yr-old man with isolated LCX disease. (E) Similar SPECT slices in a 44-yr-old man with severe single-vessel RCA stenosis. (F) Representative slices from a 72-yr-old man with lone severe LAD disease. Selected frames from the related coronary angiograms in these patients are shown in G, H and I. (G) Moderate LCX stenosis in a left anterior oblique view. (H) Tight RCA lesion. (I) LAD lesion. (Reproduced, with permission, from Segall GM, Atwood JE, Botvinick EH, et al. Variability of normal coronary anatomy: implications for the interpretation of thallium SPECT myocardial perfusion images in single-vessel disease. *J Nucl Med* 1995;36:944–951.)

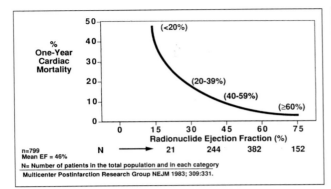

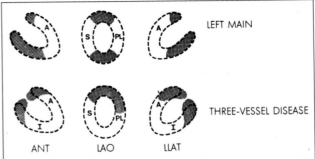

Figure 17 The prognostic value of left ventricular ejection fraction (LVEF). The 1-yr cardiac mortality versus the pre-discharge LVEF calculated by blood pool scintigraphy and EF after acute myocardial infarction. An LVEF <40% related to a major decrement in survival. (Reproduced, with permission, from the Multicenter Postinfarction Research Group. Risk stratification and survival after myocardial infarction. *N Engl J Med* 1983;309:331–336.)

Figure 18 Scintigraphy in left main and 3-vessel coronary disease. In this diagrammatic repesentation, the shaded areas represent relatively normal radiotracer uptake and the clear areas represent perfusion defects in these planar schematic anterior (ANT), left anterior oblique (LAO) and left lateral (LLAT) projections. The top panel illustrates a defect in the anterior (A) wall, septum (S) and posterolateral wall (PL). These abnormalities suggest a left main distribution. The bottom panel illustrates accumulation of activity at the base of the heart, with diminished perfusion of A, S, PL and inferior (I) walls, suggesting 3-vessel disease. (Reproduced, with permission, from Dash H, Massie BM, Botvinick EH, Brundage BH. The noninvasive identification of left main and three-vessel coronary artery disease by myocardial stress perfusion scintigraphy and treadmill exercise electrocardiography. *Circulation* 1979;60:276–284.)

1: Physical and Technical Aspects of Nuclear Cardiology) (Fig. 17). Prognosis is especially poor when LVEF falls below 30%. However, two-thirds of these postinfarction patients have LVEF >45% and so, as a group, have a low 1-yr mortality (*171*). The Duke Data Base (*172*) and several longitudinal population studies demonstrated the direct curvilinear relationship between depression of the LVEF and survival, with an almost exponential curve describing a rapidly increasing death rate as LVEF falls below 35%.

MPS is the only noninvasive method that permits the evaluation of both perfusion and function in a single study (*173,174*). This may be done in 2 ways when supported by commercial hardware and software. First-pass evaluation (*175*), based on the analysis of the time radioactivity curve generated after the bolus administration of the radionuclide, is performed at the time of injection. Gating, based on the timed acquisition of image data after myocardial localization of the agent, is performed with acquisition of the perfusion data at a time remote from radionuclide administration. Both yield regional wall motion and an objective, reproducible LVEF. First-pass evaluation presents only limited views but provides an accurate right ventricular ejection fraction (RVEF) and presents temporal advantages, with the generation of data at the time of radionuclide administration and at peak stress. Both may be performed in association with rest and stress acquisitions. When framed, first-pass analysis can be applied to generate a scintiventriculogram, but this depends on the presence of a regular rhythm, which is also required when gated studies are acquired in frame mode. When the rhythm is irregular, the variable number of accepted beats in each frame yields variable counts per frame and variable regional myocardial intensities, corrupting the SPECT perfusion data. This may be overcome when acquisition time is varied to accommodate equal numbers of cycles or, if possible, counts per frame. With expanding computer capabilities, list-mode acquisition of gated studies will permit postacquisition processing as with first-pass studies. This could provide a separate gated study for the analysis of functional data and an ungated study to provide uncorrupted perfusion data.

Although gated studies are performed with a variety of algorithms on standard equipment, first-pass data needs rapid acquisition on a state-of-the-art camera supporting rapid count rates. The first-pass protocol is also more demanding and requires a well-informed, steady and cooperative patient and a well-coordinated team to administer the bolus radionuclide injection at the appropriate time and with the best patient position. A significant failure rate still may be expected. Because of the "partial volume effect," the varying intensity through the cardiac cycle seen on gated images reflects myocardial thickening as well as wall motion. Both first-pass and gated methods are applied regularly using the technetium-based radiopharmaceuticals and demonstrate good reproducibility (175–177). Gated SPECT ^{201}Tl imaging is also of value but less thoroughly studied. Three years ago, gating was performed at only 10% of nuclear medicine imaging centers. Now 95% do so.

The first-pass approach is a proven method for the calculation of LVEF (178). The values of LVEF extracted at first-pass and gated imaging of MPS are accurate (111,178–183) and relate to those evident at the time of image acquisition, which is, certainly with gated studies, delayed from that of administration and often well into the recovery period. Functional parameters measured, then, generally indicate resting values, except when stress-induced dysfunction ("stunning") presents late into recovery.

Gated LVEF may be derived by a number of validated algorithms, each well correlated with established methods. A curve fit method is used to objectively and reproducibly find endocardial and epicardial boundaries and generally does so accurately, even in the setting of dense defects (179,184–186).

The gated method has been applied successfully to both ^{99m}Tc and ^{201}Tl SPECT studies (187–193) and, most recently, to those acquired with tetrofosmin. However, it is most widely successful when applied to high-counts studies, making gating of a high-dose ^{99m}Tc-based study most preferred. A recent study documented the inferior image quality of gated ^{201}Tl-based studies (193). Here, 33 patients with previous MIs were studied with 15-min gated SPECT acquisition performed 30–40 min after the administration of 22–30 mCi ^{99m}Tc sestamibi. On another day, gated ^{201}Tl SPECT was acquired for 15 min at 4-hr after a rest 3.5-mCi injection. The average count density in midventricular slices was 3.47 times as great for ^{99m}Tc-based images, with interobserver agreement on wall motion evaluation at .73 for sestamibi and .66 for ^{201}Tl. Two ^{201}Tl-based studies but no ^{99m}Tc-based studies were judged unreadable, and ^{201}Tl image quality was significantly poorer than that of ^{99m}Tc sestamibi. Although gating may be applied to planar studies, the intensity of the overlying wall likely influences apparent cavitary size more than does ventricular function. Although the LVEF calculated from gated planar images may correlate with other methods (189), this is probably a fortuitous effect of related physical factors but does not relate to actual measures of ventricular cavity size or prognostic measures reliably related to it.

The method also has been successfully applied in the identification of perfused but dysfunctional myocardium in the assessment of regional viability, with serial gated rest and stress studies to identify the presence of "stunned" myocardium. "Stunning" may be a more frequently appreciated circumstance observed earlier after stress, with gated ^{201}Tl imaging (179,190,191). Others have suggested that the serial measurement of LVEF at rest and after stress appeared related to the extent of MIR (192). A poststress fall in LVEF on gated sestamibi SPECT images was said to relate to the extent of stress-related "stunning" and predicted a poor prognosis (191).

Although early studies showed little advantage for first-pass function analysis, subsequent evaluation suggests an added diagnostic value in LVEF evaluation by both methods. Sciagraa et al. (194) studied the contribution of first-pass stress LVEF to CAD diagnosis. Although both perfusion imaging and quantitative first-pass radioangiographic evidence of induced ventricular dysfunction were accurate for the detection of CAD, perfusion imaging was far more sensitive, and the first-pass evaluation appeared to add little in this study of 30 patients. Similarly, although the gated evaluation of ventricular function sometimes aided ischemia diagnosis, the perfusion marker was the most valuable diagnostic tool (193,195). Other researchers found function evaluation to aid diagnosis. Borges-Neto et al. (196,197) performed simultaneous perfusion and first-pass function studies with stress ^{99m}Tc sestamibi in 54 patients with severe, multivessel coronary disease. The composite perfusion and function evaluation improved prediction of the extent of CAD beyond history, ECG findings and even perfusion image information alone. Palmas et al. (198) studied 70 consecutive patients and found that the addition of simultaneous SPECT perfusion imaging and first-pass evaluation of systolic left ventricular function to the results of the treadmill exercise test added significantly to the ability to diagnose the presence and predict the extent of CAD. Some recent studies demonstrate the potential advantage of gated SPECT images for the diagnosis of CAD (147,149,199–201).

The addition of functional data will probably play an important role in prognosis as well (202) and add importantly to the evaluation of regional myocardial viability. As in other efforts, LVEF and volumes appear to have independent clinical importance and prognostic value (203–206).

In addition, the method can be employed to aid image interpretation and the avoidance of errors based in attenuation artifact. It can play an important role in the differentiation of fixed defects resulting from prior infarction and those resulting from attenuation artifact. Here, fixed defects that appear to contract have been shown to most likely represent attenuation artifact (207). Similarly, wall motion and thickening on gated SPECT provide an important indicator of regional viability and, with the perfusion pattern, of an ischemic or nonischemic cardiomyopathy (208).

The method also has been shown to increase overall interpretive security without loss of accuracy, reducing the number of borderline readings (209). When left ventricular wall motion and thickening are normal in the setting of a clearly abnormal stress perfusion image, it suggests defect reversibility, making the rest or redistribution study unnecessary (179). Stress-related artifact may behave similarly, however.

Differences between first-pass and postlocalization gated function evaluation on MPS are reviewed in *Self-Study Program III. Cardiology. Topic 5: Myocardial Perfusion Scintigraphy. Technical Aspects.*

IDENTIFICATION OF SEVERE AND EXTENSIVE (HIGH-RISK) CORONARY ARTERY DISEASE

Delineation of the Issue

Stress MPS is now most generally applied for risk stratification in terms of its identification of the extent of MIR (Tables 10,11). Here, the defect extent, measured as the number of myocardial segments involved or the percentage involvement of each coronary artery region or of the total left ventricle, and the severity of that involvement are important prognostic factors. The presence of "balanced triple-vessel disease" presenting as a normal image with a markedly abnormal stress test and severe, widespread angiographic stenosis, although a popular focus of concern for critics of the method, was a greater possibility with the planar method. Here "washout analysis" appeared to be of benefit (see *Self-Study Program III. Cardiology. Topic 5: Myocardial Perfusion Scintigraphy. Technical Aspects*).

This concern is not supported by evidence from the SPECT method, because patients with severe widespread CAD demonstrate abnormal scans in the overwhelming number of cases, whereas occasional negative scans relate to an excellent prognosis. A disparity of this kind between the stress ECG and image is quite rare and may occur in association with a spectrum of coronary involvement.

Specific high-risk lesions, including left main and severe 3-vessel disease, have demonstrated increased risk, with patient benefit from coronary revascularization, especially in the presence of left ventricular dysfunction and reduced LVEF (*36,210*). Those who consider risk from a more anatomic point of view suggest that an important goal of the noninvasive assessment of patients with CAD should be the correct identification of those with extensive high-risk left main and triple-vessel CAD. Methods to determine the severity and/or extent of CAD are presented in Table 10. Indicators of scintigraphic evidence of extensive MIR and poor prognosis from stress–redistribution ^{201}Tl scintigrams and perfusion imaging in general are listed in Table 11 and generally have been shown to be equal or superior to anatomy for coronary risk stratification (*211–213*).

Identification of Left Main and Triple-Vessel Disease

Using the scheme described previously, it is possible to determine abnormalities involving the distribution of the left main coronary artery by presenting an abnormality visually similar to the combined territories of

---

Table 10

METHODS TO DETERMINE EXTENT OF MYOCARDIUM AT RISK (EXTENT OF CORONARY INVOLVEMENT)

1. The total size (extent) and intensity (severity) of defects representing ischemic and infarcted myocardium (often summarized in a segmental score)*

2. The number of diseased vessels as suggested by the number of coronary territories with perfusion defects or washout abnormalities*

3. The fixed or reversible nature of defects*

4. Diffuse slow washout rate of thallium-201 (^{201}Tl) (especially in planar images) with adequate exercise, as an index of extensive myocardial ischemia

5. In the presence of coronary artery disease (CAD), increased pulmonary capillary wedge and prolonged pulmonary transit as evidenced by increased ^{201}Tl extraction and lung uptake of [201]Tl (*8,78,219*)

6. In the presence of CAD, transient postexercise (stress) ischemic dilatation of the left ventricle (*8,220,221*)*

7. In the presence of CAD, basal uptake of radiotracer, indicating extensive distal myocardial involvement by ischemia and/or scar (*8*)*

8. Extensive, stress-induced wall motion abnormalities and/or reduced left ventricular ejection fraction*

9. Reduced left ventricular ejection fraction in the presence of extensive, severe CAD with limited fixed or extensive reversible defects*

---

*These same parameters have been related to the prognostic value of myocardial perfusion scintigraphy performed with any current agent, although all apply to imaging with [201]Tl.

Table 11

SCINTIGRAPHIC EVIDENCE OF EXTENSIVE MYOCARDIUM AT ISCHEMIC RISK AND POOR PROGNOSIS BASED ON GATED SINGLE-PHOTON PERFUSION IMAGING

1. Extensive, dense reversible perfusion defect

2. Modest or severe perfusion defects at a low level of stress or in the presence of extensive fixed perfusion defects

3. Perfusion defects outside the infarct zone in patients with prior infarction

4. Stress-induced lung uptake, cavitary dilation and basal uptake in the presence of coronary disease

5. Extensive washout abnormalities with adequate exercise, even in the presence of a modest perfusion defect

6. Extensive, stress-induced wall motion abnormalities and/or reduced left ventricular ejection fraction (LVEF)

7. Reduced LVEF in the presence of extensive, severe coronary artery disease with limited fixed or extensive reversible defects

8. Postexercise reduction in wall motion and LVEF, especially with perfusion defects

the LAD and LCX and the distribution of all 3 coronary arteries (Figs. 18–20) (Tables 10,11). In addition, the level of the lesion, whether proximal, middle or distal in the vessel, could be determined on SPECT study. Several reports have demonstrated that, with this approach, the sensitivity (as high as 75%) of conventional planar visual analysis for correct identification of extensive coronary disease is superior to other exercise-monitored parameters but is still generally lower than that desired. SPECT adds to this ability (*47,74,165,166,196,214–220*). This sensitivity has been attributed to the limitations of spatially relative perfusion defect analysis in revealing all hypoperfused myocardial regions in patients with multivessel CAD. It may be related as well as to the same

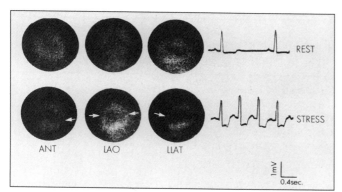

Figure 19 Left main pattern. Shown are planar perfusion scintigrams and the stress electrocardiogram (ECG) from a patient with triple-vessel disease. The stress ECG is markedly positive, with deep horizontal ST depression occurring early in exercise. The scintigram presents a left main pattern of abnormalities with defects in the apex, anterior wall, septum and posterolateral wall (arrows). The inferior wall appears relatively well perfused, despite a high-grade right coronary artery lesion. Although the pattern of myocardial involvement was similar and there was severe triple-vessel disease, there was no left main lesion. Although left main disease bears a prognosis of its own, scintigraphic study has demonstrated that prognosis relates best to the extent of myocardium at ischemic risk. ANT = anterior; LAO = left anterior oblique; LLAT = lateral projections. (Reproduced, with permission, from Dash H, Massie BM, Botvinick EH, Brundage BH. The noninvasive identification of left main and three-vessel coronary artery disease by myocardial stress perfusion scintigraphy and treadmill exercise electrocardiography. *Circulation* 1979;60:276–284.)

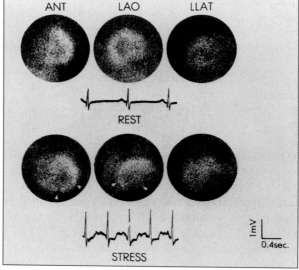

Figure 20 Three-vessel disease pattern. Planar perfusion scintigrams and the stress electrocardiogram (ECG) from a patient with triple-vessel disease. The stress ECG is positive with 1.5-mm horizontal ST depression occurring early in exercise. The scintigram presents a pattern of abnormalities with defects in all 3 vascular areas, anterior, apical, inferior and lateral defects (arrow heads). ANT = anterior; LAO = left anterior oblique; LLAT = left lateral projections. (Reproduced, with permission, from Dash H, Massie BM, Botvinick EH, Brundage BH. The noninvasive identification of left main and three-vessel coronary artery disease by myocardial stress perfusion scintigraphy and treadmill exercise electrocardiography. *Circulation* 1979;60:276–284.)

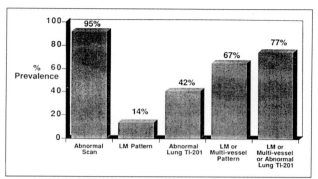

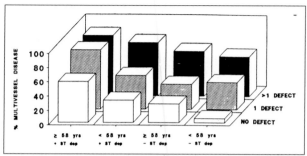

Figure 21 The scintigraphic diagnosis of left main (LM) and multivessel disease. The incidence of various planar image findings among 43 patients with at least 50% stenosis of the left main coronary artery who underwent symptom-limited exercise thallium-201 stress testing. Here, an LM scattered pattern required a uniform decrease in septal and lateral wall activity on the 45° left anterior oblique projection. A multivessel disease diagnosis required perfusion defects in more than 1 coronary vascular area. Although a LM pattern was unusual, many had multivessel patterns. However, balanced reduction in septal and lateral wall perfusion need not be present even in LM disease. SPECT now gives a better chance to recognize regional coronary artery disease but often still fails to identify the full anatomic involvement. Recent work suggests that the extent of myocardium at ischemic risk, rather than the apparent anatomic involvement, is the best prognostic indicator. (Reprinted, with permission, from Nygaard TW, Gibson RS, Ryan JM, et al. Prevalence of high-risk thallium-201 scintigraphic findings in left main coronary artery stenosis: comparison with patients with multiple and single-vessel coronary artery disease. *Am J Cardiol* 1984;53:462–469.)

Figure 22 The additive prognostic value of clinical, stress electrocardiography and scintigraphic variables. Shown graphically is the combined effect of age (>58 yr), ischemic ST depression (+ST DEP) and numbers of perfusion defects on the likelihood of multivessel coronary artery disease in 383 consecutive patients who underwent exercise thallium-201 myocardial perfusion scintigraphy and angiography. When all 3 variables were present, multivessel disease was at its highest incidence. Although the relationship with anatomy persists, current quantitative SPECT studies demonstrate a strong independent prognostic value of image defect size. Unusual in this study is the frequent finding of multivessel disease among some subgroups with normal images. However, these were largely seen in small select populations with abnormal stress tests, and images were planar. The numbers in each group are not shown. (Reprinted, with permission, from Pollock SG, Abbott RD, Boucher CA, et al. A model to predict multivessel coronary artery disease from the exercise thallium-201 stress test. *Am J Med* 1991;90:345–352.)

factors reviewed previously with regard to the identification of involved coronary arteries (Fig. 21).

A planar imaging study by Pollock et al. (*221*) (Fig. 22) demonstrates the additive value of tests performed in parallel, where exercise-induced ST depression and the number of reversible ^{201}Tl perfusion defects provide additive ability for prediction of multivessel disease, to the factor of age in a group of patients with a high likelihood of CAD. SPECT with [99mTc]-based agents has added image resolution and the ability to better discern specific vascular regions (*222*) (Figs. 23–26).

A number of studies have demonstrated the advantage of combined scintigraphic and ECG findings for the identification of high-risk coronary lesions (*220–222*). The analysis of regional washout has been demonstrated to enhance the assessment of regional perfusion and hypoperfusion (*219*). The use of the combined criteria of exercise defects and abnormal regional ^{201}Tl washout improved the sensitivity of visual planar ^{201}Tl image analysis for correct identification of patients with left main and triple-vessel coronary disease (from 16% to 63%) without significant loss of specificity (*222*). Conversely, a normal stress MPS, even in the presence of a markedly positive stress test or in the presence of known CAD (*223*), is generally expected to relate to limited CAD and to a benign prognosis (*224*) (Table 6F).

Without consideration of stress test findings, SPECT imaging adds significantly to the identification of involved individual coronary beds and so to the

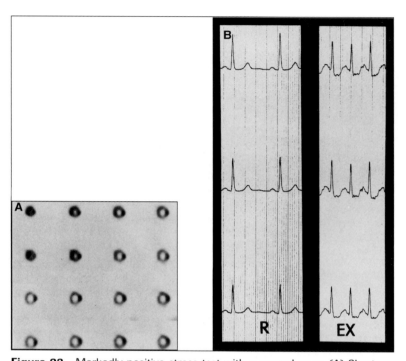

Figure 23 Markedly positive stress test with a normal scan. (A) Short-axis slices, from apex (top left) to base (bottom right), from the normal thallium-201 SPECT perfusion study in a 69-yr-old woman with atypical chest pain and a markedly positive exercise electrocardiogram. Immediate postexercise images are shown in the first and third row, with matching slices acquired with 4-hr delay in alternate rows below. The patient exercised 5.2 min to a heart rate of 155 beats/min. (B) In the same patient, leads V4–V6 at rest (R) and at peak exercise (EX) are shown. Coronary angiography was normal. The image pattern demonstrates a "hot" spot in the lateral wall, a technical phenomenon explained elsewhere. (Reproduced, with permission, from Krishnan R, Lu J, Dae MW, Botvinick EH. Does myocardial perfusion scintigraphy demonstrate clinical utility in patients with markedly positive exercise tests? An assessment of the method in a high-risk subset. *Am Heart J* 1993;127:804–815.)

identification of multivessel disease with preserved specificity and a widely reported sensitivity of 70% (*119,120, 123,133,135,222*). The incremental value of MPS for the detection of CAD and high-risk coronary anatomy as 3-vessel or left main CAD, as well as prognosis, has been documented (*11, 12,225,226*) (Table 12). However, lung uptake and even cavitary dilation, which add to our ability to identify extensive coronary involvement, may be better appreciated on planar imaging (Fig. 27). Patterson et al. (*227*) analyzed the ability of stress testing to identify left main and triple-vessel disease after infarction.

Diffuse Slow Washout of Thallium-201

Theoretically, when CAD is extensive and of relatively uniform severity, regional myocardial hypoperfusion may be balanced during stress, precluding the development of spatially relative perfusion defects. Assessment of the objective myocardial ^{201}Tl washout rate may provide diagnostic assistance in these unusual cases, which are more evident on planar imaging. The decay-corrected loss of regional intensity over time, the "washout rate," which is low in the setting of relative underperfusion (*228*), has been most valuable when applied to exercise imaging and less so in association with pharmacologic stress (*229*). Bateman et al. (*230*) found a 1% incidence (13 patients) of diffuse slow washout in the absence of evident perfusion defects among quantitatively analyzed planar MPS in 1265 consecutive patients. Nine of these 13 (69%) had left main or triple-vessel disease. In practice, it is important to keep in mind that the incidence of the diffuse ^{201}Tl slow washout pattern indicating extensive ischemia is low and that several factors unrelated to regional perfusion, such as low achieved heart rate, may cause diffuse slow ^{201}Tl washout in the absence of CAD. The occurrence of diffuse ischemia in the setting of an otherwise normal stress image appears to be vanishingly small when the SPECT method is applied and very unusual in the absence of other ischemic indicators. For this reason, washout analysis has been of little added value when the sensitive SPECT method is applied. In fact, patients with CAD and even multivessel disease have been shown to have a good prognosis in the presence of a normal stress MPS (*223*). For these reasons, the method is not generally applied well in studies acquired with coronary dilators, adenosine and dipyridamole. Yet, most recently, Teragawa et al. (*231*) have demonstrated the value of regional ^{201}Tl washout on SPECT short-axis slices to determine the severity of coronary stenoses after adenosine pharmacologic stress testing.

Supplementary or Nonperfusion Indicators of High-Risk Coronary Artery Disease

Canhasi et al. (8) studied planar MPS in 97 patients with CAD and coronary angiography. They found that the presence of associated supplementary nonperfusion indicators of coronary involvement and extensive myocardial underperfusion complemented the perfusion pattern and increased the ability of the method to identify extensive, anatomic high-risk CAD, without reducing specificity. These nonperfusion indicators included: cavitary dilation, lung uptake and basal uptake. The latter, related to increased radiotracer activity at the left ventricular base, indicates a relative scarcity of distal perfusion and is the least known of the 3. By a similar mechanism, a relative increase in right compared with left ventricular activity on stress MPS has been reported to be a sign of extensive induced hypoperfusion or ischemia (232).

Increased Pulmonary (Lung) Uptake of Thallium-201. An increase in pulmonary ^{201}Tl activity, >52% of the activity of the adjacent anterior left ventricular wall, may be noted on anterior

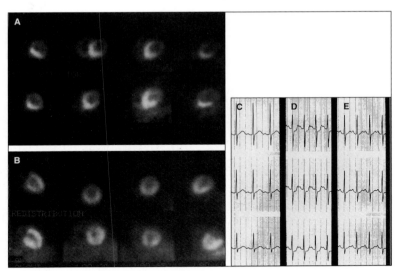

Figure 24   Markedly positive stress test with a high-risk scan. (A) Shown, left to right, are enhanced thallium planar perfusion images in anterior, 30°, 45° and 60° left anterior oblique (LAO) projections acquired immediately after exercise (top) and with a 4-hr delay (bottom) in a 72-yr-old woman with worsening angina. Gross, partially reversible defects evident in apical, anterior, inferior and lateral walls could not be explained by attenuation effects and were related to deep ST depression, early, 5.5 min into exercise at a peak achieved heart rate of 147 beats/min and peak blood pressure of 170/90 mm Hg (double product = 24,990). Angiography revealed severe triple-vessel coronary artery disease. (B) Shown in the same format are the normal exercise planar images acquired when this same patient presented with neck pain soon after coronary artery bypass graft (CABG). The double product was 23,580, not significantly different than previously, at 6.1 min. The stress electrocardiogram was normal and 4-yr follow-up was benign. Shown are precordial leads V4–V6, at rest (C), stress before CABG (D) and at stress after CABG (E). (Reproduced, with permission, from Krishnan R, Lu J, Dae MW, Botvinick EH. Does myocardial perfusion scintigraphy demonstrate clinical utility in patients with markedly positive exercise tests? An assessment of the method in a high-risk subset. *Am Heart J* 1993;127:804–815.)

planar images in patients with CAD. Both experimental studies and clinical evidence suggest that this increased pulmonary ^{201}Tl activity is related to the development of left ventricular dysfunction and elevated pulmonary venous pressure with exercise, with secondary slow pulmonary transit and increasing pulmonary ^{201}Tl extraction (8,76,233,234). Two methods have been developed to objectify the assessment of pulmonary uptake of ^{201}Tl. In the method of Kushner et al. (235) the degree of stress-related pulmonary ^{201}Tl activity is expressed as the quantitative fraction of the adjacent myocardial value. Another approach, described by Levy et al. (236), quantified the percentage of pulmonary ^{201}Tl washout from immediate postexercise and 4-hr redistribution anterior view images and related this measure to both the anatomic extent and functional severity of disease. With both techniques, abnormal values have been observed in greater frequency in patients with extensive multivessel CAD. Several studies demonstrated lung uptake in rest–redistribution ^{201}Tl images to be an important prognostic indicator and predictor of adverse outcome (211,221,237,266) (Figs. 27–29).

However, increased pulmonary capillary wedge pressure and increased pulmonary uptake of ^{201}Tl may be caused by conditions other than extensive and

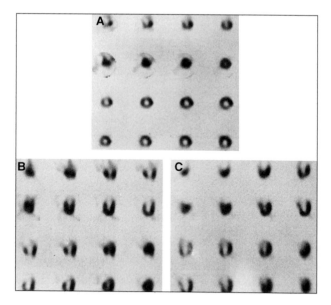

Figure 25 Markedly positive stress test and image. (A) Shown in alternating rows at stress above rest are short-axis slices from apex (upper left) to base (lower right); (B) horizontal long-axis slices from inferior (upper left) to anterior (lower right); and (C) vertical long-axis slices from septum, upper left, to the lateral wall, lower right, of the exercise thallium-201 SPECT study acquired in an asymptomatic 76-yr-old man with deep, early ST abnormalities. Gross reversible defects are evident in multiple vascular areas that correlated with extensive triple-vessel disease. (Reproduced, with permission, from Krishnan R, Lu J, Dae MW, Botvinick EH. Does myocardial perfusion scintigraphy demonstrate clinical utility in patients with markedly positive exercise tests? An assessment of the method in a high-risk subset. *Am Heart J* 1993;127:804–815.)

severe CAD that prolong pulmonary radionuclide transit. These include mitral valve regurgitation, mitral stenosis, decreased left ventricular compliance and nonischemic cardiomyopathy with left ventricular dysfunction. It is therefore important to apply caution in interpreting increased pulmonary uptake of ^{201}Tl as an index of extensive CAD when it occurs in isolation (without myocardial perfusion defects) or in patients with one of the previously mentioned conditions. Lung uptake has not been seen often, nor correlated well when seen, with extensive CAD imaged with ^{99m}Tc agents, possibly because of agent kinetics and the late poststress imaging time.

Transient Cavitary Dilatation. Some patients with CAD have a pattern of transient dilatation of the left ventricle on the immediate poststress planar images as compared with the 4-hr redistribution or rest images (*212,221,219*) (Fig. 30). This dilation must be present for at least 10–15 min after exercise to be visualized on the postexercise image. It often represents severe ischemia related to extensive CAD, causing transient ischemic dilation (TID) of the left ventricle after exercise. The angiographic correlates of this finding were assessed in a large number of consecutive patients who underwent both stress–redistribution ^{201}Tl scintigraphy and coronary arteriography (*219,226, 238*). A TID ratio was determined by dividing the computer-derived left ventricular area of the immediate poststress anterior image by that of the 4-hr redistribution image. An abnormal transient dilation ratio had a sensitivity

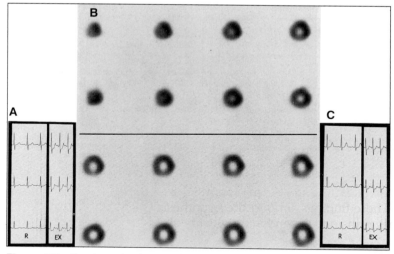

Figure 26 Persistently abnormal stress test after coronary artery bypass graft (CABG) (A) From above down, are electrocardiograph (ECG) leads V4–V6 at rest (R) and exercise (EX) in the patient studied before CABG in Figure 25, at 4.3 min of a Bruce protocol with a peak heart rate of 147 beats/min and blood pressure of 200/80. Successful CABG was performed with the subsequent acquisition of normal myocardial perfusion scintigraphy but continued abnormal exercise test, albeit at a higher workload (8 min) and double product (heart rate = 167 beats/min and blood pressure = 230/60). (B) Short-axis slices from this normal study in the same format as Figure 25. (C) Post-CABG R and EX ECGs in the same patient. Not infrequently, the stress ECG remains abnormal in spite of apparent excellent revascularization. (Reproduced, with permission, from Krishnan R, Lu J, Dae MW, Botvinick EH. Does myocardial perfusion scintigraphy demonstrate clinical utility in patients with markedly positive exercise tests? An assessment of the method in a high-risk subset. *Am Heart J* 1993;127:804–815.)

of 60% and specificity of 95% for identifying patients with multivessel critical stenosis and was more specific than other known image markers of severe and extensive CAD, such as the presence of multiple perfusion defects or washout abnormalities or both. The authors of one article relate the finding to proximal LAD disease (*238*). In another study of 512 patients who had pharmacologic stress testing, transient cavitary dilation was related to a higher incidence of MI, whereas fixed dilation related to a higher death rate and hospitalization for heart failure (*239,333*).

Although true left ventricular dilation indeed relates to severe CAD, it may be more apparent than real. That is, in many cases, dilation in planar images is projection dependent and appears to affect the inner rather than the outer image dimension (*212,213,219*). These findings, with their appearance 10–20 min after exercise, suggest not a real but an apparent dilation, related to ischemia in an overlying wall exposing the radionuclide-poor left ventricular cavity. With redistribution of relative perfusion, this overlying wall, seen *en face,* is no longer ischemic, transparent or related to apparent cavitary

Table 12
THE ADDED ADVANTAGES OF SCINTIGRAPHIC RISK (SUB)STRATIFICATION*

Angiography

No. of stenotic vessels	Event rate
1	7.0%
2	11.2%
3	16.8%

Stress scintigraphy defect type

Fixed	Reversible			
	Small	**Moderate**	**Large**	**Total**
Small	53 (2%)	25 (19%)	16 (19%)	94 (4%)
Moderate	40 (0%)	24 (8%)	15 (15%)	84 (6%)
Large	54 (15%)	27 (22%)	9 (44%)	90 (20%)
Total (Average)	147 (6%)	76 (15%)	45 (22%)	268 (11%)

*Data from a study in which patients undergoing myocardial perfusion scintigraphy had coronary angiography and were followed for 1 yr without revascularization. There was a 2-fold risk stratification with angiography and a >20-fold risk stratification with myocardial perfusion scintigraphy. The scintigraphic event rate is shown in parentheses.

Adapted, with permission, from Kotler TS, Maddahi J, Berman DS, Diamond GS. Is thallium scintigraphy better than coronary angiography for prognosis? *Circulation* 1986;74(suppl II):II-512.

dilation. The converse of this phenomenon could be the absence of an apparent cavity in LVH (*240,241*). Although pulmonary uptake and transient cavitary dilation have both been associated with advanced CAD, Hansen et al. (*242*) found a weak correlation, suggesting their relationship with different pathophysiologic responses to exercise-induced ischemia. These findings support the hypothesis that transient cavitary dilation represents transient subendocardial ischemia rather than true physical ventricular dilation.

Alternatively, the cavity may appear to dilate as a result of altered regional wall motion and a partial volume effect. Here, reduced wall excursion fails to fully fill pixels and gray shades or color are diluted to fill the pixel with lower intensity (counts). In this way, reduced wall motion and ventricular dilatation may themselves relate to perfusion image defects. This phenomenon undoubtedly plays a role in the presentation and appearance of all perfusion images, both planar and SPECT. It has a more specific role in explaining the variable intensities presented by gated SPECT perfusion images as they change cavitary size and wall thickness through the cardiac cycle. It is also important to consider when interpreting apparent defects in a dilated ventricle and, in the interpretation of images in patients with dilated noncoronary cardiomyopathies, may help explain some of the apparent segmental perfusion defects (*243,244*).

Transient left ventricular dilation appears to have similar significance when seen in association with pharmacologic stress (*54*). Evident dilation and

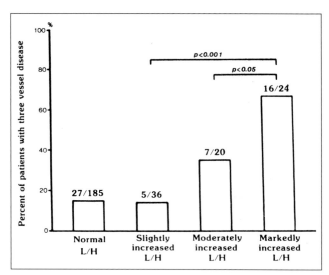

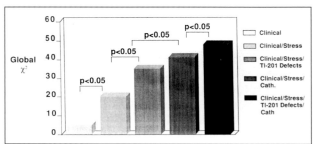

Figure 27 Lung uptake as an indicator of extensive coronary disease. Percentage of patients with 3-vessel disease among 265 patients with known coronary artery disease, based on their related normal, slightly increased, moderately increased and markedly increased lung-to-heart (L/H) thallium-201 ratios. (Reprinted, with permission, from Kurata C, Tawarahara K, Taguchi T, et al. Lung thallium-201 uptake during exercise emission computed tomography. *J Nucl Med* 1991;32:417–423.)

Figure 28 The added prognostic value of stress testing, planar imaging and angiography. Shown is the incremental prognostic value of stress test variables (stress) beyond that of clinical data (clinical). The number of reversible thallium-201 defects adds to clinical and stress test data. In this study, prognostic information provided by coronary angiography (Cath), when combined with clinical and stress test findings, added insignificant prognostic value beyond that of myocardial perfusion scintigraphy (MPS), but perfusion image findings added yet further prognostic information even in the presence of angiographic findings. Clinical, stress test and MPS provided more than 80% of all prognostic information. (Reprinted, with permission, from Pollock SG, Abbott RD, Boucher CA, et al. Independent and incremental prognostic value of tests performed in hierarchical order to evaluate patients with suspected coronary artery disease. Validation of models based on these tests. *Circulation* 1992;85:237–248.)

photopenia would be expected to occur less frequently with sestamibi because of the imaging delay after stress, with related resolution of ischemia and associated findings. However, when evident, left ventricular dilation is probably clinically important. A certain amount of evident dilation, up to ~30% of the cavitary diameter, is permitted as a normal variant when interpreting images generated from the dual-isotope sequential rest ^{201}Tl/stress ^{99m}Tc sestamibi (tetrofosmin) protocol. Here, the better-resolved ^{99m}Tc walls are characterized by less scatter and appear thinner than those imaged with ^{201}Tl, and the cavity, by default, appears larger. In all cases, especially with the sensitive SPECT method, the significance of cavitary dilation in the absence of perfusion defects must be approached carefully, as this combination suggests a higher incidence of noncoronary causes and technical artifacts.

Dense Cavitary Photopenia

Another finding related to severe ischemia or dense scar and aneurysm formation is dense cavitary photopenia (*245*). When initially observed and upon learning its name, a first impression suggests that the finding relates to the presence of a left ventricular thrombus, displacing cavitary activity. However, after ^{201}Tl (and ^{99m}Tc) extraction, the blood pool contains <1% of the injected dose. In fact, evidence of cavitary photopenia indicates ischemia or scar in the overlying wall on planar perfusion images. Here, a dense overlying perfusion abnormality, viewed *en face*, provides a localized window on the ^{201}Tl-poor blood pool. The overlying defect presents the appearance of a regional decrease in "cavitary" radioactivity as a result of the varying intensity of uptake in the overlying myocardium (*219*). When this finding is associated with a localized left ventricular aneurysm, related diverging walls often can be seen in the distal left ventricle of ungated images. Of note is the occasional normalization of these findings at rest, indicating the stress induction of not only dense and extensive ischemia but also of related severe left ventricular dysfunction (246). The converse of this phenomenon, the lack of an apparent "left ventricular cavity," obscured by a thick wall, dense with ^{201}Tl and equal in intensity when seen *en face* to the walls imaged in tangent in the same projection, strongly suggests hypertrophy on planar images (5,41,161,170,171). Prominence of the right ventricular wall, especially in rest–redistribution images, also has been demonstrated to be a good indication of right ventricular hypertrophy (247) (Fig. 31). This general difference between the intensity of planar walls imaged in tangent and walls imaged *en face* relates to radionuclide content and makes for greater or lesser visibility of what appears to be and is mistakenly called the "left ventricular cavity." Such "cavitary" visualization is increased with ongoing ischemia and reduced with hypertrophy.

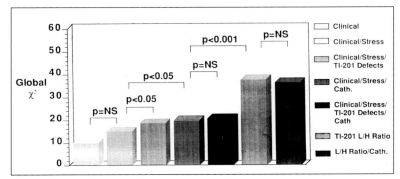

Figure 29 Added prognostic value considering lung uptake. In this data analysis, the impact of lung uptake is included. Here, exercise test (Stress) findings did not add prognostic information to clinical data, but thallium-201 (^{201}Tl) defects did. Angiography (Cath) added nothing further to image prognosis, and angiography added no additional prognostic value to myocardial perfusion scintigraphy. The lung-to-heart ^{201}Tl ratio (L/H) greatly improved prognostic value, which exceeded that of ^{201}Tl defects and was not augmented by the findings on angiography. (Reprinted, with permission, from Pollock SG, Abbott RD, Boucher CA, et al. Independent and incremental prognostic value of tests performed in hierarchical order to evaluate patients with suspected coronary artery disease. Validation of models based on these tests. *Circulation* 1992;85:237–248.)

Some researchers have sought to calculate the LVEF from the apparent varying size of the ventricular cavity on gated planar images. However, gating planar images may yield erroneous results, because the apparent cavity size probably relates more to overlying myocardial wall thickness than to cavitary dimensions. Methods that calculate ejection fraction from "counts" generated by inverting such planar image intensities must be prone to similar difficulties (189), because the parameter measured is most directly related to the intensity of the myocardium overlying the ventricular cavity at any stage of the cardiac cycle, a measure of its perfused mass and not of cavitary counts. Nonetheless, wall thickening and its related degree of apparent transparency and counts may parallel ventricular function, especially when the characteristics of the overlying wall are similar to those of the entire ventricle when it is normal or diffusely diseased.

Although lung uptake is sometimes difficult to appreciate on SPECT imaging, cavitary dilatation and evident "photopenia" are appreciated well without much of the ambiguity contributed by the overlying walls (8,219,245,248). Photopenia is probably evident on SPECT studies as a result of the imperfectly tomographic nature of this limited angle acquisition. As a result, the ventricular cavity seen on SPECT, which should be essentially without intensity because of the small amount of radionuclide in the blood at the time of imaging, is probably "contaminated" by a sample of the intensity of the overlying wall. This is augmented in systole by wall motion, which may invade the cavitary plane of reconstruction. Scarred or ischemic walls will have less radionuclide and will contract and contaminate the reconstruction plane less, permitting the reflection of true low cavitary intensity and producing the effect of "cavitary photopenia."

Cavitary photopenia is a marker for relatively reduced perfusion in the overlying wall on SPECT slices. Here, the cavity/myocardial intensity or count ratio

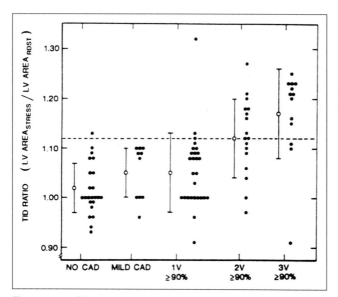

Figure 30 The importance of cavitary dilation on thallium-201 studies. The relationship between the transient (ischemic) dilation ratio (TID) and the presence, extent and severity of coronary artery disease. The horizontal line represents the upper limit of normal TID. These values have been recalculated for the dual-isotope protocol, although the principle persists. LV = left ventricular; RDST = redistribution; 1V, 2V, 3V = 1-, 2- and 3-vessel disease with ≥90% stenosis. (Reprinted, with permission, from Weiss AT, Berman DS, Lew AS, et al. Transient ischemic dilation of the left ventricle on stress thallium-201 scintigraphy: a marker of severe and extensive coronary artery disease. *J Am Coll Cardiol* 1987;9:752–760.)

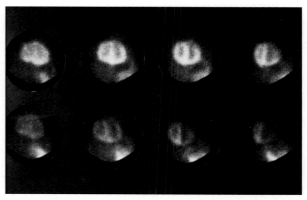

Figure 31 Increased uptake in the right ventricle (RV) with right ventricular hypertrophy (RVH). Shown are planar stress (top) and rest (bottom) thallium-201 perfusion images acquired in multiple projections in a patient with severe pulmonary hypertension, RVH and atypical chest pain. The prominent RV uptake is evident in the absence of clear left ventricular abnormalities and excellent biventricular washout.

may be taken as a marker for left ventricular dysfunction on rest [99mTc] sestamibi studies (*249*). This is a natural extrapolation, relating abnormalities of rest perfusion to rest dysfunction. Remember, however, that relative underperfusion may be more evident at stress. Variations in cavitary intensity have similar implications when seen in association with stress-induced underperfusion and related dysfunction in the presence of normal rest function (*219,245,246*).

PERFUSION IMAGE QUANTIFICATION

Overview

Perfusion images present a quantifiable continuum related to disease likelihood, prognosis and viability (*250*). The full value of the method is only now being revealed with its application as a quantitative parameter of coronary risk (*115,128,211,215,217,221*) (Figs. 32–36).

Quantitative methods utilize the digital nature of scintigraphic data and represent a major advantage of MPS. The reading of artifacts, most often the result of attenuation and motion, is likely the most common error in image interpretation. To take full advantage of the graded, quantitative image response, all defects scored must be analyzed to exclude artifacts. Readers must be obsessive in excluding these possibilities by using the numerous tools (polar maps, projection

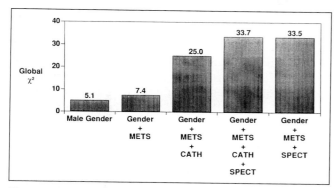

Figure 32 Incremental prognostic value of SPECT thallium-201 (^{201}Tl). Knowledge of sex, exercise (METS) and SPECT ^{201}Tl variables provided maximum prognostic value, virtually unaltered by the addition of angiographic findings (CATH). (Reprinted, with permission, from Iskandrian AS, Chae SC, Heo J, et al. Independent and incremental prognostic value of exercise single-photon emission computed tomographic (SPECT) thallium imaging in coronary disease. *J Am Coll Cardiol* 1993;22:665–670.)

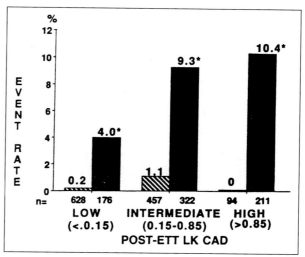

Figure 33 Pretest probability of coronary artery disease (CAD) and the incremental prognostic value of myocardial perfusion scintigraphy. Shown are the frequencies of hard (death and infarction) and soft (revascularization) events over the follow-up period in patients with low, intermediate or high postexercise treadmill test likelihood of coronary artery disease (POST-ETT LK CAD). Stratification is good in all groups. Solid bars = abnormal scan results; hatched bars = normal scan results. *$P < 0.05$. (Reprinted, with permission, from Berman DS, Hachamovitch R, Kiat H, et al. Incremental value of prognostic testing in patients with known or suspected ischemic heart disease: a basis for optimal utilization of exercise technetium-99m sestamibi myocardial perfusion single-photon emission computed tomography. *J Am Coll Cardiol* 1995;26:639–647.)

images, gated data and dynamic, color-coded 3-dimensional displays) (Fig. 37) and methods (prone imaging) available to optimize diagnostic specificity without jeopardizing sensitivity and to gain accurate quantitation. Direct interpretation of 3-dimensional displays of perfusion image data has been shown to be accurate (*251*).

Specific Quantitative Methods

Several methods for semiquantitative analysis of planar ^{201}Tl images have been reported. The initial method simply performed visual interpretation and segmental scoring of processed ^{201}Tl images (*7,85,86,252*). Computer analysis of planar images proved more accurate when combined with the interpretation of experienced observers (*115*). Circumferential profile analysis samples the intensity of the myocardium in planar images or in short-axis SPECT slices at brief angular intervals and records the most intense cross-sectional pixel. These values, recorded for rest and stress SPECT images and complemented by apical values extracted from the midventricular vertical long-axis slice, may be plotted as a bullseye or polar (coordinate) map, which compresses the left ventricular tomographic data with some distortion, much as does a polar map of the Earth. Here, values for the left ventricular apex are plotted in the center of a circular display, with basal segments at the periphery, with the anterior

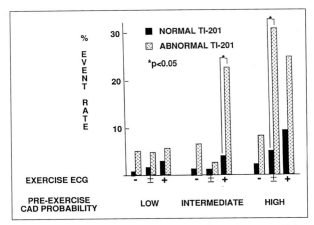

Figure 34 Incremental prognostic value of myocardial perfusion scintigraphy (MPS) according to the results of the stress electrocardiogram (ECG). Shown are event rates (death, myocardial infarction, late revascularization) in patients grouped according to the findings on the exercise ECG and pre-exercise test coronary artery disease likelihood. + = positive; − = negative or normal; ± = uninterpretable or equivocal. Planar MPS provided clinically meaningful risk stratification beyond ECG data in every subgroup, but the yield was low and cost effectiveness was questionable within the low-likelihood group. The best substratification came when MPS was applied in those in intermediate- and high-likelihood groups. (Reprinted, with permission, from Ladenheim M, Kotler T, Pollock B, et al. Incremental prognostic power of clinical history, exercise electrocardiography and myocardial perfusion scintigraphy in suspected coronary artery disease. *Am J Cardiol* 1987;59:270–277.)

wall projected superiorly, the inferior wall below, the septum to the reader's left and the lateral wall to the right. These and other commonly employed quantitative techniques have utilized objective criteria for detection of perfusion defects based on comparison of image data with results from a normal database (*52,253–256*). Such polar maps have been generated for males and females based on ^{201}Tl and ^{99m}Tc sestamibi studies. Maps and normal databases will be available for ^{99m}Tc tetrofosmin. Gender-specific normal data sets are important for risk stratification and necessary to account for soft tissue patterns of attenuation. Gross intramyocardial radionuclide distribution patterns are similar, with slight exceptions, possibly the result of the linearity of radiotracer distribution with regional flow or perhaps the ability of the tracer to differentiate viable tissue from scar. However, background varies and could influence myocardial intensity, as does the attenuation coefficient and the related degree of attenuation for each radionuclide. In addition, the diagnostic accuracy of planar images has benefited from the analysis and application of regional "washout rates" (*219*).

Polar maps compare image data with normal databases at rest and with stress. Because of the broad range of normal, this may yield normal polar patterns at opposite ranges of the normal spectrum, overlooking the abnormality evident in the difference between these images, often generated as a "difference bullseye." Nor does this method always present an accurate assessment of sequential changes. For this reason, most research studies have applied the analysis of the relative intensity of 20 myocardial segments developed and applied by the Cedars Sinai Group (*32*), 6 in each of 3 distal, mid- and basal short-axis slices and 2 from the apex in the vertical long axis. The greater the number of segments, the more likely that normal segments will be found to be abnormal as a result of the statistical chance of finding at least 1 segment outside its normal limits, and thus the lower the related specificity. For this reason, the interpretation of the 20-segment model requires segmental values to be abnormal in 2 contiguous segments, and a threshold score of abnormal has been established in patient populations (*107*). This SPECT scoring method is quite popular and has been well validated as an easily automated measure of coronary-related risk (*128*). It compares well with the polar map measure of defect size (*257,258*). Each segment is given an intensity score (0–4), and the sum is used to determine severity score, a value related strongly in the literature to coronary risk (*135,183,185,250*). Here, summed stress severity scores are grouped as mild (5–8), moderate (8–13) or severe (>13) defects, with moderate and severe defect scores related to significant risk of "hard" coronary events in several studies. Here, artifacts can be appreciated and segmental activity compared blindly and sequentially. Reproducibility is established in a control population. Defect size,

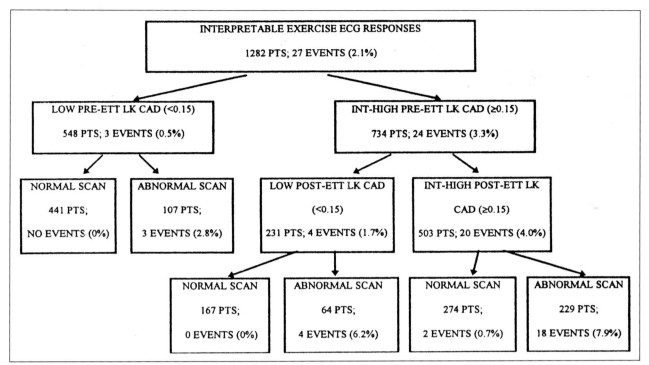

Figure 35 Incremental prognostic value of myocardial perfusion scintigraphy (MPS) and interpretable stress electrocardio-grams (ECG). Shown are outcomes in patients with interpretable exercise ECG based on gross scintigraphic findings. MPS provided clinically meaningful risk stratification beyond ECG data in every subgroup, but the yield was low and cost effective-ness questionable within the low-likelihood group. EVENTS = frequency of hard events; INT-HIGH = intermediate-to-high; PRE-ETT(POST-ETT) LK CAD = pre(post)exercise treadmill test likelihood of coronary artery disease; PTS = patients. (Reprinted, with permission, from Berman DS, Hachamovitch R, Kiat H, et al. Incremental value of prognostic testing in patients with known or suspected ischemic heart disease: a basis for optimal utilization of exercise technetium-99m sestamibi myocardial perfusion single-photon emission computed tomography. *J Am Coll Cardiol* 1995;26:639–647.)

related to a volumetric analysis of left ventricular involvement, also compared well with the 20-segment score (*259*). Objective, quantitative methods have been applied widely in the literature as the basis for the demonstrated great ability of SPECT perfusion image risk stratification in CAD. Differences in serial images mark the effectiveness of the intervention. However, the specific method to apply in serial studies has not yet been fully resolved (see *Self-Study Program III. Cardiology. Topic 5: Myocardial Perfusion Scintigraphy. Technical Aspects*).

The Value of Quantitation

Quantitative analysis of ^{201}Tl scintigrams reduces inter- and intraobserver variability, permits objective and reproducible serial study and serves as an objective guide to image interpretation and as an aid to the uninitiated and less experienced. However, these methods are blind to artifacts and, in expert hands and in the literature, their effect on the overall sensitivity and specificity of ^{201}Tl testing has not been dramatic. This is well demonstrated by results of reports comparing visual and quantitative analysis in the same patient population (*55*). If the effect of quantitation of images on sensitivity and specificity of ^{201}Tl testing is assessed by comparing mean literature results obtained in different patient populations, there appears to be a trend toward increased sensitivity and decreased specificity.

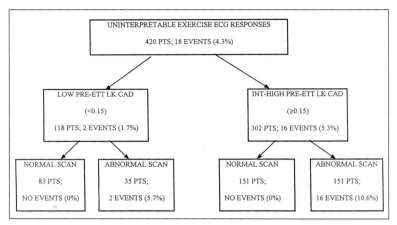

Figure 36 Incremental prognostic value of myocardial perfusion scintigraphy (MPS) in uninterpretable stress electrocardiogram (ECG). Shown are outcomes in patients with uninterpretable exercise ECG. MPS provided clinically meaningful risk stratification in every likelihood subgroup among these patients in whom the stress ECG was not helpful. EVENTS = frequency of hard events; INT-HIGH = intermediate-to-high; PRE-ETT(POST-ETT) LK CAD = pre(post)exercise treadmill test likelihood of coronary artery disease; PTS = patients. (Reprinted, with permission, from Berman DS, Hachamovitch R, Kiat H, et al. Incremental value of prognostic testing in patients with known or suspected ischemic heart disease: a basis for optimal utilization of exercise technetium-99m sestamibi myocardial perfusion single-photon emission computed tomography. *J Am Coll Cardiol* 1995;26:639–647.)

The mean sensitivity and specificity in the literature for quantitative planar ^{201}Tl imaging in a total of 800 patients are 89% and 68%, respectively (*51,55, 253–256,260*). The lower specificity and higher sensitivity, however, are most likely the result of the increased referral bias encountered in more recent publications that relied on quantitative analysis and may relate as well to the possible inclusion of artifacts. Kang et al. (*261*) demonstrated the value of quantitative methods for measurement of infarct size and their correlation with left ventricular function.

Overall, quantitative SPECT methods have added objectivity and anatomic resolution to the perfusion imaging method, contributing to wider success in its application and acceptance (*66, 111–118,125*). Quantitative SPECT analysis has demonstrated superiority for risk stratification, in which more patients were correctly assigned to high- and low-risk subgroups than to the intermediate-risk group, which was significantly larger when applying qualitative methods (*262*). Several studies testify to the added prognostic value of MPS; when quantitative methods are applied, risk categories are drawn more clearly (*262*).

Although polar maps add objectivity and aid quantitation, care must be applied in their application. Total reliance on such methods is an error often made by the inexperienced. Although serving as an important interpretive aid that calls attention to areas of potential abnormality, polar maps should never replace the ability and judgment of the skilled interpreter. Artifacts may be generated and responsible for polar map defects, and subtleties may sometimes be missed, although evident on SPECT slices and of potential clinical importance. On the other hand, such subtleties are sometimes better ignored.

PERFUSION IMAGE REPRODUCIBILITY

Visual Analysis

Although demonstrated early to be quite good (*53,68,165,167,263,264*), the intra- and interobserver variability of the visual analysis of MPS probably contributes to the varying sensitivities and specificities of visually interpreted planar images that are reported from different centers. The intraobserver variability of visual analysis has been shown to range from 4% to 11%, with the interobserver variability ranging from 3% to 16% (*53,87,225,226*), not markedly different from the variability noted in other well-established imaging studies, such as angiography. In spite of its increased complexity, SPECT imaging has also demonstrated a high level of reproducibility, with interobserver variability at ~10% and intraobserver variability <5% (*162,265*). A multicenter trial (*118,139*) of planar

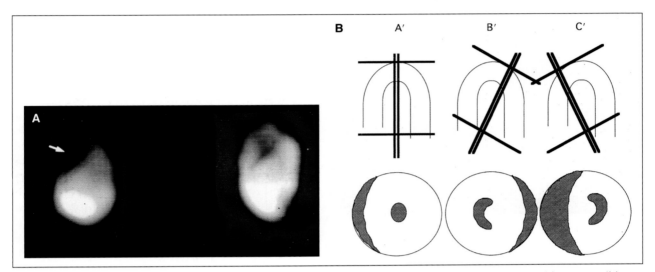

Figure 37 Three-dimensional reconstruction. (A) Volume-rendered SPECT reconstructions with an evident reversible basal-septal defect. Perfusion defects in this location are rare and are most frequently seen after bypass surgery or in the presence of well collateralized LAD disease. More commonly, they are technical in origin, related to a processing error with variation in placement of the long-axis on rest and stress studies, as shown in (B), with the resultant appearance of redistribution in slices at the septal base. A', B' and C' diagram the effects of an altered long axis on the resultant data and related polar map, in which A' is the normal orientation and B' and C' are angulated to produce basal lateral and septal "defects." Three-dimensional reconstruction permits evaluation of the full ventricle at all angles, and any difficulty in comparing slices is removed. Note the stress-induced apical dilation in A. (Reprinted, with permission, from Starksen NF, O'Connell JW, Dae MW, Botvinick EH. Basal interventricular septal thallium-201 defects: real or artifact? *Clin Nucl Med* 1993;18:291.)

and SPECT imaging methods was conducted at 22 centers in the United States and Canada and demonstrated a 92% agreement in the interpretation of 4622 segments analyzed by 2 methods, a 2-day stress–rest ^{99m}Tc sestamibi and a stress–redistribution ^{201}Tl protocol. There was a 94% agreement between the methods in interpretation of 4358 segments read as normal or abnormal. Mahmarian et al. (*266*) demonstrated the upper limit of technical variability and reproducibility of adenosine ^{99m}Tc sestamibi SPECT to be a defect change of 8%. Therefore, a change in SPECT defect size on serial study of 9% exceeds the 95% confidence interval and represents a real change beyond technical variability. Such quantitation with clear evaluation of reproducibility limits makes application of the method valuable for the assessment of the effects of treatment (*282–284,297*).

SPECT reproducibility has been well documented in repeated readings of the same studies and in the interpretation of serial studies performed at intervals of 1 yr among images with defect size ranging from 0% to 73%, with a correlation coefficient of 0.94% and mean absolute deviation of 4.5% (*135,267*). As an automated method, SPECT processing is highly reproducible. The variability in image processing, not interpretation, was found to represent roughly 40% of the small overall error in serial study (*268*). Parameters of both left ventricular size and function generated from gated SPECT data are also quite repeatable and reproducible (*269*).

Quantitation

The several objective, quantitative and often automated methods of perfusion image analysis, as segmental scores, circumferential profiles and polar maps,

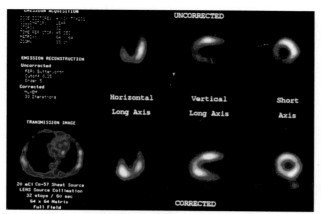

Figure 38 Attenuation correction. SPECT thallium-201 slices from a normal individual acquired after stress in selected horizontal, vertical and short-axis slices. (Top) Uncorrected slices with gross inferior and posterior septal attenuation. (Bottom) Same slices are presented after attenuation correction. (Reprinted, with permission, from ADAC, Inc., Milpitas, CA, and from Botvinick E, Dae M, O'Connell JW, Ortendahl D, Hattner RS. The scintigraphic evaluation of the cardiovascular system. In: Parmley WW, Chatterjee K, eds. *Cardiology.* Philadelphia, PA: J.B. Lippincott; 1991.)

have been developed to overcome the initially qualitative, subjective nature of this imaging method. Reproducibility of MPS is excellent and compares well with other imaging methods. This is true when applying visual interpretation, is significantly improved with application of quantitative methods (*270*) and is improved further with use of technetium-based radiotracers (*271*). Although visual image interpretation has been successfully applied and is quite reproducible among readers with a range of experience (*272*), quantitation adds objectivity and reproducibility to the process, an advantage of this imaging method over others. Its low variability, relative objectivity and good reproducibility has made MPS the principle quantitative and noninvasive physiologic tool employed when seeking clinical evidence of the effects of coronary interventions or the cause of recurrent symptoms after revascularization. To reduce the necessary population size to prove a favorable clinical end point, MPS has been used as a surrogate end point to reduce patient numbers needed to demonstrate efficacy in thrombolytic trials (*273–279*), in the serial evaluation of the effects of agents on coronary flow and their ability to affect ischemia (*280,281*) and in the development of new anti-ischemic devices. MPS is part of the research protocols of several multicenter trials conducted around the world, testing the effects of agents that, by different mechanisms, seek to provide medical coronary revascularization (*282–284*).

The 3-dimensional display of perfusion SPECT has been found to yield highly reproducible readings when serving as the basis for evaluation of serial perfusion changes (*285*).

IMAGE INTERPRETATION

Overview

The value of perfusion scintigraphy has been strongly validated for both diagnosis and prognosis. However, the application of planar methods, compounded by the inexperience of early workers, brought ambiguities and errors in image interpretation. These were often the result of patterns created by overlying activity; the presence of image artifacts related to patient motion, attenuation or other technical factors; or normal image findings interpreted as perfusion defects. Initially, technical and interpretive difficulties suggested little advantage of the SPECT method, and some were reluctant to abandon planar imaging. Increased experience, the advent of [99mTc]-based radionuclides, improvements in and experience with SPECT imaging, prone imaging or imaging with an altered patient position and the advantages of gating have reduced these problems and increased the accuracy and security with which images are read, particularly in heavy patients and women. Attenuation correction promises yet more progress (Fig. 38) (see *Self-Study*

Program III. Cardiology. Topic 1: Physical and Technical Aspects of Nuclear Cardiology). It is tempting to interpret images based on the findings of polar maps, circumferential profiles and other processed displays. However, artifacts will be overlooked, and it would be a mistake to simply base image reading on such displays. The reader also must understand the origin of the image data.

The Tools Required

The exercise of image interpretation should be quite active and analytic and should employ all ancillary images and objective tools for identification of the cause of any apparent image defect. These should include dynamic projection data (*286*), axes of reconstruction, "linograms," "sinograms" and "blurograms." Center-of-rotation and field homogeneity data, as well as methods to realign projection images in the presence of vertical and shifting lateral motion, should be available, as should a full choice of color scales, image enhancement capabilities and a multifaceted adaptable display. Images should be enhanced when intensity normalization is required, but enhancement is not generally needed when the gray shades or colors are represented and the highest image intensity is in the myocardium. In addition, polar maps should be consulted, and other quantitative methods, such as circumferential profiles and washout analysis, should be available to apply as appropriate. The data should be reviewed before the patient leaves the imaging suite, so that other acquisitions, in prone or varied projections, may be requested, if needed, and postreinjection and/or delayed images may be scheduled. The benefit of prone imaging for resolving the cause of inferior and many anterior defects and for the stabilization of patient motion is well established (*287*) but still not fully appreciated. Attenuation correction is, at this time, best addressed with a careful analytic approach to image interpretation. The application of automated attenuation-correction algorithms should be approached with care. They are costly and have varying abilities, and their potential to fully correct for attenuation without the introduction of artifacts is as yet not established.

The Method

The Objective. Most patients come be imaged as a result of some ambiguity or insecurity of diagnosis or risk stratification. The objective of interpretation should be to overcome any ambiguities and to give a definitive normal or abnormal reading. This should be possible in the great majority of cases. Beyond this, areas of abnormality should be listed, related to vascular regions and the abnormalities quantified. This is critically important if the results are to affect patient management decisions appropriately. Such quantitation is most often done verbally with applied adjectives. However, with the firming of the data and the proliferation of supportive software and displays, the use of polar scores and regional and total stress, rest and difference ventricular defect scores is growing. These values are now being calculated in an automated manner and related to outcome based on values in the literature in limited available software packages. They will be more often reported with the development, proliferation and application of similar commercial software. However, they again may err and should only be applied as a guide to management based in clinical judgment and never applied by rote. The practice of medicine may be guided by numbers but never replaced by them!

The Activity. The first task of the image reader is to determine whether the study is normal or abnormal. Because normalization of an abnormal image by image artifacts is rare, the finding of a normal image virtually excludes artifact. One exception is the apparent normalization of an underperfused inferior wall because of the presence and effect of intense adjacent scattered subdiaphragmatic activity. Imagine the finding of an image so clearly normal and without high adjacent background that it would be accepted readily as such by a large, informed and critical audience if viewed as the first slide, a normal example, in a presentation of "Perfusion Imaging: State of the Art" at the national meeting of the Society of Nuclear Medicine (SNM), the American College of Cardiology (ACC) or the Radiological Society of North America (RSNA). With the exception of such "SNM, ACC or RSNA normal studies," all others with real or apparent defects, heterogeneity of unclear origin or unusually high paracardiac background must undergo careful and critical analysis.

Generally, the clinical presentation and stress test result do not play a part in the image analysis but, with the image findings, formulate the full clinical import and perspective of the study. The polar map and increased regional contrast of color-enhanced images will point to regional heterogeneity that may be of any cause and needs attention and analysis. Such regions must not be accepted as abnormal at face value but should be evaluated for patterns consistent with those of segmental coronary underperfusion.

With the presentation of an apparently or possibly abnormal image, a cause in artifacts must first be sought. Attenuation and motion are most common. Defects in areas associated with possible attenuation (the inferior wall in males, the anterior wall in females) should be carefully scrutinized. Other areas, including the lateral wall, should be examined and correlated with the size and mass of the patient and with evidence of attenuation on projection images. Improvement in the rest study generally suggests a true perfusion defect but could relate to shifting soft-tissue artifacts or other cause. These can often be identified on comparison of rest and stress projection sets and resolved with a new, well-positioned acquisition. Prone imaging may resolve diaphragmatic or breast attenuation and stabilize a restless patient. Rarely, sedation during imaging may be appropriate. An anterior defect sparing the apex and anteroseptum is most likely attenuation in origin. Most commonly, defects at the base of the anterior septum are also artifacts, even when apparently reversible, and are made most commonly by misalignment or applying inconsistent axes to a normal rest and a somewhat smaller stress image contour (288). An exception is the rare relationship of such findings to incomplete revascularization after bypass surgery, in which defects subtending limited and seemingly nonsegmental (noncoronary) myocardial regions may be associated with relatively underperfused coronary segments. Defects at the base of the inferior and lateral walls in large patients may also relate to attenuation. The interpretation of fixed defects of questionable origin may be aided by analysis of related systolic wall motion and "thickening" on gated study. The normal apical slit may be confused with an apical perfusion defect. An isolated linear apical defect is not consistent with CAD, which generally extends to the adjacent anterior, septal, lateral or inferior walls. Especially in the dual-isotope ^{201}Tl rest/^{99m}Tc sestamibi or tetrofosmin stress protocol, the normal apical slit may be seen best in the better-resolved stress-related image. Also, with this protocol, differences in attenuation coefficients commonly produce "normalization" in stress images of apparent defects (probably based in attenuation) at rest.

Eventually, image interpretation will be performed with the aid of neural networks and expert systems, a computerized approach to image reading based on logical rules developed from an optimal and organized approach to reading. Such aids will be of greatest value to those with least experience but should provide support for interpretation by even the most experienced readers (*289*).

First-Pass and Gated Images. A number of validated curve fit methods may be used to objectively, reproducibly and, in cases, automatically find endocardial and epicardial boundaries for LVEF calculation (*179,184–186*) (see *Self-Study Program III. Cardiology. Topic 1: Physical and Technical Aspects of Nuclear Cardiology*). Gating of the SPECT perfusion image is quite accurate for the objective quantitation of regional wall motion, wall thickening and LVEF (*108,177–183*). Gating has been successfully applied to both ^{99m}Tc and ^{201}Tl SPECT studies (*178,187,188*).

Support is accumulating to demonstrate that the evaluation of left ventricular function is a valuable complement to perfusion data for both CAD diagnosis and risk stratification (*194–202*). The combination of first-pass function evaluation during stress with perfusion data seems especially valuable for prediction of outcome (*290*). The combined evaluation of perfusion and function also has been applied successfully in the assessment of regional viability (*179,190*), helps differentiate perfusion defects from attenuation artifact and adds to interpretive security (*207–209*).

Attenuation Correction. Attenuation correction has been introduced in several forms (see *Self-Study Program III. Cardiology. Topic 1: Physical and Technical Aspects of Nuclear Cardiology*). However, it is not yet established as a standard interpretive clinical tool. Although it works well in some circumstances and limited studies have demonstrated its value in increasing specificity without sacrificing sensitivity, at times "attenuation correction" may remove a defect based in abnormal perfusion (*291*). Attenuation-corrected images cannot be fully relied upon yet to resolve interpretive ambiguities. Development of a reliable program is being pursued actively and will be extremely valuable when established.

Attenuation correction was a greater aid to image interpretation among less experienced than among expert readers (*292*). Attenuation correction and scatter correction have again demonstrated the anatomic nature of reduced apical activity, the "apical slit" and the importance of respiratory motion (*293*).

The Report

The body of the report should include all necessary components, such as the indication for study; the protocol applied; the name, dose and time of radionuclide administration; and a summary of the stress test findings. For educational (and medicolegal) purposes, all steps taken in reaching a conclusion from the image data should be noted among "Image Findings." This may simply be a brief analysis of the origin of regions of reduced activity or a description of the findings on projection images, polar maps and prone images. In this way, the ordering physicians can educate themselves in the methods of reading or ignore them, but the reader still must analyze image findings. If errors in diagnosis are later uncovered, this section also informs the reader (and others) of their analysis and the path taken to the conclusion. This analysis may present clues to errors made, serve as a tool for reader education and improvement and should always present a firm basis for conclusions reached.

The "Conclusions" or "Impressions" of the final report should briefly and unambiguously address the clinical question. Words such as "possibly" or "suggests" and phrases such as "may indicate" or "might represent" should be avoided. The term "probably normal" should be used rarely and then only refer to a scan with prognostic value equal to that of a normal study but that requires careful analysis of apparent image artifacts or other technical factors before the reader can conclude that perfusion is normal. The referring physician must understand that this term implies no ambiguity or indefinite conclusion but is taken from the literature, in which such studies do, in fact, have the same prognoses as "normal" studies. The report must present the image findings in visual and anatomic terms, with presentation of size, intensity and reversibility of defects. These findings should be related to the form and intensity of the stress that provoked them. Evidence of the nonperfusion indicators of extensive disease, such as cavitary dilatation and lung uptake, should be noted, as must a statement about ventricular size and function, when the latter are available. Finally, the clinical importance of the findings must be stated and verbally transmitted to the ordering physician at the time of review and followed by the written report and, optimally, a print(s) of the images and derived displays and values, demonstrating and supporting the reported findings.

Mixing Imaging and Clinical Findings

Clinical information must be integrated in the assessment—but not in the primary interpretation—of perfusion images. Bayes's theorem indicates that the pretest disease likelihood must be considered in gauging the impact of subsequent test (imaging) results (294). In one classic paper, the authors analyzed clinical and demographic factors and correlated these with symptoms and the results of angiography to determine the "pretest" probability of CAD (102). Thus, factors such as age, gender, chest pain characteristics, risk factors, prior coronary history, events and revascularization procedures must be considered to place image findings in a clinical context.

Depending on the patient population, 20%–50% of patients will present with abnormal stress images but will not meet the criteria to be categorized as high risk. This could be called the intermediate risk group and includes patients with defects involving a single coronary artery excluding a major LAD region, such as as LCX, RCA or branch LAD (diagonal vessel) territory. An abnormality induced proximal to a bypass graft or involvement of a branch vessel after stent placement also should not bring aggressive intervention unless symptoms demand it. Although such patients once would have been referred immediately to catheterization with subsequent revascularization, current studies strongly suggest medical management in many such cases. Care must be taken in the generation of the image report, as the report probably will influence management.

Also critical to image interpretation, especially in its prognostic impact, are the parameters related to stress testing: workload, ECG changes, blood pressure and heart rate, as well as the symptoms evolved at testing. These serve to modulate image findings and act in a complementary role to aid CAD prognosis (11,215). ECG changes with coronary dilator stress are especially specific for high-grade coronary stenosis (295). The method of stress testing and the parameters of stress are extremely important for the interpretation of image findings and the determination of changes on serial stress testing and imaging (Fig. 39). Not all patients require imaging (Tables 13,14).

IMAGING THE EFFECTS OF MEDICAL THERAPY

Because of its objectivity and reproducibility, MPS may be applied to assess the effects of risk factor modification, the effects of anti-ischemic drugs and coronary interventions (296). Recent studies indicate that outcome can be improved with ischemia suppression but is not correlated well with symptomatic improvement. This makes the application of quantitative, reproducible MPS even more important for the evaluation of ischemia suppression by medical therapies (297). The method was applied to the evaluation of the effects of nitroglycerin patches (298) and demonstrated the ability of the method to reduce ischemic defect size, an effect that is most prominent in those with the largest defects before therapy. A reduction in defect size $\geq 9\%$ defined significant improvement in the study (266). MPS was used to document the decremental effects of propranolol on dobutamine-induced ischemia (299) and to measure the effects of nicotine patches on myocardial perfusion (300). Dakik et al. (301) used adenosine MPS to evaluate the effects of intensive combination medical therapy on the suppression of myocardial ischemia in high-risk MI survivors and the implications of this variable effectiveness on outcomes. Outcome correlated significantly with the effects of treatment on adenosine-induced defect size. Here, the event-free survival was 96% among those with evidence of reduced induced defects size <9%, compared with 65% among those with defect size >9% ($P < 0.009$). Sharir et al. (302) studied the effects of multiple medical therapy on dipyridamole defect size. In the Angioplasty Compared to Medicine (ACME) study (303), 270 patients with CAD were randomized to medical or revascularization therapy. Thallium-201 stress planar MPS was performed at baseline and after 6 mo of treatment. Outcome was significantly better among those whose defect normalized with either therapy than among those with persistent image evidence of ischemia (.92 versus .82; $P < 0.02$). These studies indicate that MPS can be used both to assess initial risk and track its amelioration with treatment. Like other studies to be discussed later, the ACME study suggests that the effect of therapy on stress MPS, regardless of the mechanism, is an important prognostic sign.

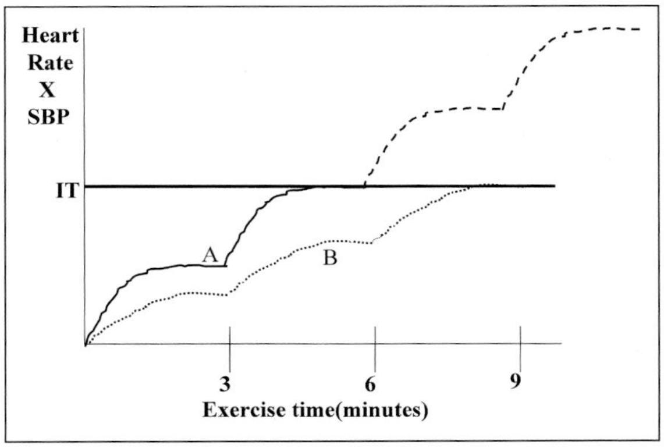

THE PROGNOSTIC VALUE OF SPECT PERFUSION SCINTIGRAPHY

Overview

In a summary statement relating ischemia to coronary risk, Rahimtoola noted, "For any severity and extent of

Figure 39 Stress test interpretation. (A) The curved solid line presents the baseline response to exercise in a coronary patient who developed chest pain, ST changes and perfusion defects at 6 min. (B) After treatment with beta blockers, the same patient achieved 9 min of the same protocol and stopped at the same double product, again with chest pain, ST changes and similar perfusion defects. Note that the increase in exercise time related simply to a slower rise in the double product (heart rate $\times$ systolic blood pressure [SBP]) to the same level related to the development of ischemic indicators, the ischemic threshold (IT). In the continuation of A (dashed line) the same patient achieved 12 min and reached a much higher double product before stopping with fatigue and shortness of breath in the absence of evidence of ischemia. The IT was elevated strongly, suggesting improved coronary blood supply. The patient did not reach his or her IT, because he or she was limited by more physiologic end points (normal individuals do not manifest ischemia at maximal effort but are limited by other symptoms) after total revascularization of extensive CAD.

Table 13

WHY NOT PERFORM STRESS MYOCARDIAL PERFUSION SCINTIGRAPHY (MPS) WITH ALL STRESS TESTS IN ALL PATIENTS?

MPS makes stress testing more expensive.

MPS makes stress test evaluation more complex.

MPS increases study time, equipment and personnel needed.

MPS increases costs.

MPS may add little to diagnostic or prognostic evaluation.

MPS may not be reliable in certain venues.

The method may be unavailable.

Table 14

GENERAL APPROACH TO MANAGEMENT DECISIONS BASED ON STRESS MYOCARDIAL PERFUSION SCINTIGRAPHY (MPS)

The search for ischemic myocardium is based on the preservation and restoration of left ventricular function.

The patient should be treated conservatively if myocardium at ischemic risk is not anticipated to result in death or significant disability.

CAD, and for any level of impaired left ventricular performance, survival rate is related to the presence, magnitude and frequency of ischemia" (*304*). MPS is the only noninvasive method that directly and reliably evaluates this complex parameter and quantitatively assesses left ventricular function. It remains the clinical modality most commonly used for evaluating MIR and patient prognosis in CAD.

Many clinical factors that have been associated with prognosis in CAD, including prior infarction, heart failure, arrhythmia, progressive angina, an abnormal ECG, an elevated cholesterol, diabetes mellitus, hypertension, smoking and age. Each contributes to the extent or rate of progression of 2 major factors related to risk: the state of resting left ventricular function, characterized as the LVEF (*172*), and the extent of MIR. The extent of coronary involvement also obviously relates to the extent of MIR and is well established as an important risk factor in CAD. When severe enough, as in the setting of left main or 3-vessel disease or in association with LVEF <35%, multivessel CAD has been related to a clear survival benefit from revascularization with coronary artery bypass graft surgery (CABG) (*36*). Although the presence of an abnormal stress test does not relate to a preferential benefit from revascularization compared with medical treatment, the presence of deep early ST depression or a low achieved workload has demonstrated a benefit from revascularization compared with medical therapy, regardless of the resting LVEF (*210*). Extensive or modest MIR on MPS with left ventricular dysfunction, presumably as a result of scar, present significant and well-documented risk. Although the possibility of improvement with revascularization is high, the MPS method is well established and such randomized studies will never be done.

The extent of MIR, the extent of scar and left ventricular systolic function relate in part to the extent of coronary involvement and play an important role in the scintigraphic diagnosis and prognosis of CAD. Each of these can now be well delineated on SPECT perfusion scintigraphy and contribute to the high diagnostic and prognostic value of the method, applicable to a wide variety of patients (Table 15). The ability of the method to assess wall motion and LVEF adds to its prognostic power, and the assessment of this specific added contribution is only now being investigated (*206*). In addition, because invasive management strategies for CAD, coronary angioplasty and CABG are associated with both risk and cost, rational selection of patients for these interventions requires knowledge of their risk without treatment. A major application of MPS involves risk stratification of patients with known or suspected CAD, including those patients who are post-MI (*257,302,304–307*) (Fig. 40).

A wealth of data has demonstrated that the amount of jeopardized

---

Table 15

CHARACTERISTICS OF PATIENTS WITH CHRONIC STABLE CORONARY DISEASE WHO ARE LIKELY TO BENEFIT FROM RISK STRATIFICATION WITH PERFUSION IMAGING

Intermediate risk of cardiac death or myocardial infarction

Intermediate-to-high likelihood of coronary artery disease

Uncomplicated infarction

Suspected ischemic cardiomyopathy—for diagnosis and viablity

Before vascular or other major noncardiac surgery

After angiography, to identify the "culprit" vessel or pathophysiology

After angioplasty or coronary artery bypass graft surgery—with failure of the procedure, possible remnant ischemia or with recurrent symptoms

For evaluation of the effects of medical therapy

Stabilized with unstable angina

Presenting to emergency department with ambiguous or low-likelihood coronary artery disease, especially if unable to exercise or if rest electrocardiography is abnormal

---

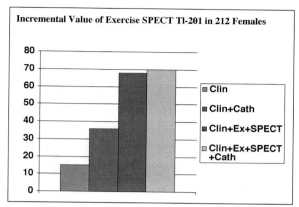

Figure 40 The added prognostic value of mycardial perfusion in women, measured in terms of the calculated χ^2, beyond that of clinical information (Clin), exercise testing (Ex) and cardiac catheterization (Cath) combined. In fact, in this large population of women, scintigraphy provided prognostic data as powerful as that provided by angiography. (Reprinted, with permission, from Pancholy SB, Fattah AA, Kamal AM, et al. Independent and incremental prognostic value of exercise thallium single-photon emission computed tomographic imaging in women. *J Nucl Cardiol* 1995;2:110–116.)

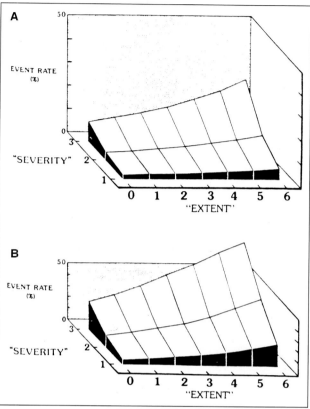

Figure 41 Relationship to prognosis. This 3-dimensional plot drawn from results generated in a large patient population shows the relationship between induced perfusion image defect extent (size, on the abscissa), severity (density, on the ordinate) and event rate (prognosis, on the vertical axis). Note the almost exponential relationship. The data are divided into 2 plots: (A) Patients who achieved 85% of predicted heart rate for age. (B) Patients who failed to reach that level. The suggestion is that defects of similar conformation have a much higher event rate and relate to a graver prognosis when acquired in association with lesser stress and test of the coronary flow reserve. The impact of image data must be related to the associated stress. (Reprinted, with permission, from Ladenheim ML, Pollack BH, Rozanski AM, et al. Extent and severity of myocardial reperfusion as predictors of prognosis in patients with suspected coronary artery disease. *J Am Coll Cardiol* 1986;7:464–471.)

myocardium or MIR on MPS is a (and possibly *the*) major factor in predicting future adverse events over a wide spectrum of patient populations and disease prevalence (*10,308,309*) (Figs. 41,42). In several studies, the method has been shown to present incremental prognostic value about risk in CAD beyond clinical and exercise parameters (*10,211,212,221*) (Figs. 22,28,29,41,43). The prognostic value of stress MPS appears equal to that of coronary angiography, and it has been shown to provide additional information (*213,215,310–313*) (Figs. 32, 44). The percentage of stenosis evident in the anatomic lesion has been found to relate poorly to the local CFR (*314,315*) and correlates poorly in animal studies with the extent of MIR (*163*). The MIR could be even more variable in patients in whom it would not only depend on the vascular territory, site, duration

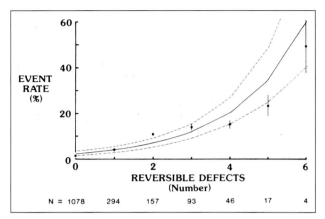

Figure 42 Incremental risk. The relationship between the number of reversible planar perfusion defects and the coronary event (cardiac death, nonfatal infarction or coronary bypass surgery >60 days after testing) rate is shown in >1600 patients with symptoms suggestive of coronary artery disease but no prior infarction. The relationship appears exponential where limited defects may have little implication, but large defects are clinically important ($r = 0.97$; $P < 0.001$). (Reprinted, with permission, from Ladenheim ML, Pollack BH, Rozanski AM, et al. Extent and severity of myocardial reperfusion as predictors of prognosis in patients with suspected coronary artery disease. *J Am Coll Cardiol* 1986;7:464–471.)

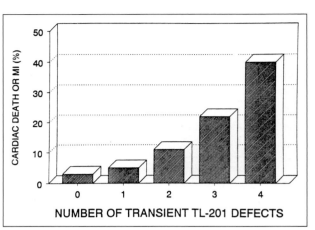

Figure 43 Prognostic value of reversible defects. The risk of cardiac death or nonfatal myocardial infarction (MI) is shown as a function of the number of segments with reversible thallium-201 defects. The risk of "hard" events increases exponentially with the number of reversible defects and the amount of myocardium at ischemic risk. (Reprinted, with permission, from Brown KA, Boucher CA, Okada RD, et al. Prognostic value of exercise Tl-201 imaging in patients presenting for evaluation of chest pain. *J Am Coll Cardiol* 1983;1:994–1001.)

and completeness of obstruction but also on the presence of collaterals, the cardioprotective effects of drugs and other factors (*164,316*). Because of this pathophysiologic relationship with MIR, there is increased confidence in the method, with greater weight placed on the results of MPS, which has greater influence on patient management and the decision to perform angiography (*48,126,127*) (Fig. 45). Because of its ability to measure the extent of MIR, MPS is well suited to serve as the "gatekeeper" for angiography, determining which patients will have it and which will be treated medically or go on to a noncardiac evaluation (*32,128,317–320*).

The Current Application of Myocardial Perfusion Scintigraphy to Coronary Disease Risk Stratification

MPS remains an excellent diagnostic method to determine the presence of CAD and the cause of symptoms. It continues to be applied as a "roadmap" to localize disease and the "culprit" lesion. However, its greatest strength and the feature that enhances these other applications is its ability to risk stratify for CAD. When applying MPS for this purpose, we do not specifically seek left main or multivessel disease. Instead, we seek to relate the image findings directly to prognosis—omitting the "middle man" of earlier days, the specific coronary anatomy. This application relates to the fact that angiographic anatomy bears a highly variable and unpredictable relationship to MIR (*163,164,316*), which MPS measures well. Although the anatomy itself gains importance as a management strategy is sought, the management decision is increasingly related to the MIR evident on the scan, not to the angiographic anatomic findings! A modern approach to the use of stress MPS for the prognostic evaluation of CAD should relate image findings to prognosis. The physician thinking of applying the method to risk

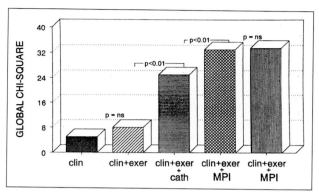

Figure 44 Incremental prognostic value of clinical, exercise and scintigraphic variables. The incremental prognostic values of clinical (clin), exercise electrocardiographic (exer), angiographic (cath) and perfusion imaging (MPI) variables are shown. Here, SPECT MPI data significantly increased the prognostic ability of clinical and exercise findings and had greater prognostic power than angiography, which added nothing to the value of MPI (far right). (Reprinted, with permission, from Iskandrian AS, Chae SC, Heo J, et al. Independent and incremental prognostic value of exercise single-photon emission computed tomographic (SPECT) thallium imaging in coronary disease. *J Am Coll Cardiol* 1993;22:665–670.)

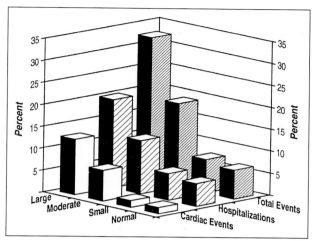

Figure 45 Relationship of perfusion defects to event and admission rate. The annual percentage of cardiac events (death and infarction) and cardiac-related hospital admissions in relation to defect size are shown. Results demonstrate a progressive increase in the percentage of both cardiac events and hospital admissions with increasing defect size. (Reprinted, with permission, from Heller GV, Herman SD, Travin MI, et al. Independent prognostic value of intravenous dipyridamole with technetium-99m sestamibi tomographic imaging in predicting cardiac events and cardiac-related hospital admissions. *J Am Coll Cardiol* 1995;26:1202–1208.)

stratifying his or her patient should ask the following questions:

1. Does the test result effectively risk stratify the patient group assessed?
2. Are test results predictive of patient outcome after other available clinical information is considered?
3. Does application of the test save cost relative to the use of other modalities?

These issues are best addressed by measuring:

1. The incremental statistical value of prognostic data, which is defined as the statistical difference in added prognostic information provided by MPS compared with other available data.
2. The incremental clinical value of prognostic data, which is defined as the added ability of MPS to substratify patients into low- and high-risk groups after risk stratification by clinical and/or exercise parameters. Such stratification would make MPS pivotal in patient management decisions, so that the low-risk group would need no further testing and the high-risk group would need aggressive intervention.
3. The incremental economic value of prognostic data, which is defined as the added cost benefit resulting when MPS data are applied for clinical management in specific patient groups or clinical settings, perhaps as a guide to the utility of more expensive methods, such as angiography.

Patient information must be considered in a clinical and economic hierarchy, beginning with patient characteristics and history (which are very inexpensive), followed by stress testing (still inexpensive to both patient and provider), MPS (moderately expensive) and cardiac catheterization and angiography (which are most expensive). Stress echocardiography appears somewhat less costly than stress MPS but in the same class of expense. Further, if one considers the time, personnel and effort required for dobutamine infusion, the cost of echo contrast, now used with increasing frequency to visualize the endocardium, and the cost of current equipment, this difference vanishes. More impressive is the reimbursement or cost to the payer for such studies. This is being reduced by Medicare and others, at once reducing their costs but also reducing financial incentives on the part of the provider! In this hierarchy, stress echocardiography stands at a similar cost level as MPS, with far less cost difference between these 2 than between either method and those less and more expensive methods that bracket them. Beyond this lies the greater "cost" of patient management, related procedures and the high cost of clinical error to the quality of life and survival of the patient! The end points of this new approach to cost assessment are prognostic rather than simply diagnostic and include an evaluation of cardiac death and nonfatal MI, as well as cost effectiveness measured as cost utility or quality adjusted life years and cost per life saved.

Testing for Diagnosis or Risk: An Important Difference

The probability that a patient referred for evaluation has significant CAD can be estimated using previously validated measures, such as the CADENZA computer program first described in 1983 by Diamond et al. (321). Remembering the concept of Bayesian analysis, test results and post-test disease likelihood relate to the presenting or pretest likelihood of disease. In order to keep erroneous diagnosis to a minimum and to most accurately and securely address management, patients are best grouped within narrow limits of low and high pretest likelihood, with a wide window for the insecure, intermediate likelihood group. Patients who are asymptomatic or have nonanginal symptoms have a low pre(stress)-test likelihood of CAD (<15%) and are unlikely to be reclassified as high likelihood, irrespective of test results. Similarly, patients with a high pretest likelihood of CAD (>85%) are unlikely to be reclassified as low likelihood on the basis of further testing. Unlike patients presenting with a very high or very low pretest likelihood, it is patients with intermediate CAD likelihood (15%–85%) who will most benefit from further testing. Here, barring equivocal image findings or inadequate testing, they will be reclassified most effectively with MPS, into low- or high-likelihood groups having either high or low probability of disease (3–5,17,20,322). However, although there may be individual exceptions, based on this classification and with concern only for diagnosis, the group with a low pretest disease likelihood and an interpretable rest ECG generally needs no further noninvasive evaluation, because no method has been shown to add to the diagnostic certainty in a cost-effective manner. Patients with a high pretest CAD likelihood would not benefit from further noninvasive testing with a diagnostic goal and, if further diagnostic evaluation is desired, should be referred to catheterization for the specific anatomic diagnosis.

Risk stratification provides a broader objective for testing in chronic CAD and is well suited to the scintigraphic method. MPS provides incremental information and substratifies risk in patients in all categories of pretest likelihood. Because of the relatively small number of high-risk patients among those with a low pretest disease likelihood in the presence of an interpretable rest ECG, the method is best applied for risk stratification in those with an intermediate or high CAD likelihood. Based on published guidelines (31) for the evaluation and management of CAD in unstable angina, thresholds of <1% and >4% hard event (cardiac death or nonfatal infarction) rate, based on the clinical or stress test profile of CAD, are defined as low-risk and high-risk groups, respectively (32,128,220,323). If these guidelines are strictly followed, then those with high risk should go directly to angiography, whereas patients with a low risk (<1% hard event rate/yr) clinical or stress test profile of CAD should be treated medically and with risk factor modification. Patients with an intermediate risk (>1 and <4% hard event rate/yr) clinical or stress test profile of CAD should be directed to conservative medical or aggressive angiographic management, based on the findings of noninvasive testing. If the scintigraphic method is capable, management should be delivered based on its ability to identify and differentiate between these subgroups. With an uninterpretable rest ECG, patients with a low pretest likelihood may also be benefited by stress MPS for both diagnosis and prognosis.

Incremental Statistical Value: Methodology for the Assessment of Prognostic Value

Incremental prognostic value implies that the information provided by testing is unique relative to that already available from known variables or is significantly less expensive to acquire. Statistical methods used to evaluate the incremental prognostic value of MPS studies include multivariate analysis (logistic regression or Cox proportional hazards analysis), ROC curve analysis and Kaplan-Meier survival analysis (324–328).

Incremental Clinical Value: Conceptual Basis and Application. Multivariate analysis determines which one(s) among a number of variables is (are) most closely associated with an outcome. The Cox proportional hazards model is a form of multivariate analysis in which the outcome of interest is both the event and the time to the occurrence of the event (324–328). In order to determine incremental value, the statistical model should be derived in a "stepwise" fashion. The amount of information present in the statistical models generated is expressed by the χ^2 figure. Unfortunately, this test statistic requires a large number of outcomes and large patient populations and cannot always be applied to patient subgroups (324,326,328). These limitations are overcome, in part, by the use of ROC curves (325,326), which represent the relation between a test's true-positive rate and false-positive rate, as the threshold for abnormality is changed. The plotted ROC curve subtends the largest area when the true-positive rate is 100% and the false-positive rate is 0%. The power of a model can be expressed as the area beneath this curve, a measure that reflects the discriminatory power of the test in question; here, the differentiation of high- from low-risk subgroups, independent of factors such as diagnostic threshold, the baseline event rate in the study sample or selection bias. Although rare stress echocardiographic studies claim a tight ROC curve, factors such as test reproducibility, varying definition of the normal response, clinical characteristics of the study group with a very low-likelihood study population and the documented high event rate among too many with negative test results belie such data (329). Other studies that claim a high diagnostic or prognostic value or cost effectiveness of the echocardiographic method (330) are not rooted in prospective clinical data or consecutive patient studies but are often based on old and/or selected data, analyzed with respect to statistical models or compared with controls from the literature (329–331). In all such studies, the selective nature of the patient population must be noted and considered as a factor contributing to the study results.

The Kaplan-Meier survival curve permits the determination of incremental prognostic value in a manner analogous to a clinical strategy. Generally, this statistical method is used to measure differences in survival rates between 2 patient cohorts (330–334). The advantages of this method include its ability to test varying thresholds for clinical or exercise variables, as well as the ability to analyze survival. The method lacks a single statistic that reflects the power of the test to risk stratify among patients (17,20,301).

Incremental Economic Value. The application of cost analysis, comparing strategies with and without MPS, is of particular importance and is increasingly reported in large series (18–20,104,128,182,227,308,318,324,332). Such analysis can distinguish between methods that yield information that improves cost effectiveness or cost utility and those that simply provide information. Important considerations in constructing or interpreting these analyses relate to the realistic nature of pricing, which should be based on the costs to the institution, the inclusion of associated costs of testing and the appropriate applied value of test accuracy. Unlike clinical risk assessment, economic analysis must compare not only the "hard" outcomes of death and nonfatal infarction but all related events of clinical relevance and expense. "Soft events," such as early revascularization, may themselves be influenced by image findings. For this reason, the incidence of revascularization is calculated for those procedures occurring 2–3 mo after MPS, seeking to exclude those procedures that may have been performed simply based on scan findings. Finally, the importance of the threshold for abnormality and the quantitative, reproducible nature of the study, in addition to testing accuracy, take on particular importance in cost analysis, because of their impact on the need for subsequent expensive invasive testing.

Prognostic Value of Perfusion Imaging

We still have no method that can offer a specific individual and accurate coronary prognosis. However, complemented by the findings on other tests, MPS has gone beyond other methods in its ability to substratify and subgroup risk in large populations. In this way, individual patients can be assigned a more specific risk in a smaller subgroup and better approach the individualization of risk stratification that we seek. Rather than advising a patient to have a given therapy because he or she belongs to a large risk group with an average chance of benefit, we would rather inform the patient that a given management is indicated because of his or her specific risk and opportunity to benefit from therapy. MPS moves us closer to such individual risk stratification and management.

As noted previously, risk is generally measured in terms of "hard" events, those that occur spontaneously, and not those influenced by and counted with a decision to intervene, such as revascularization. The Unstable Angina Guidelines of the Agency for Healthcare Policy and Research (15) define a low risk as a cardiac death rate <1%/yr, and a high risk is measured in deaths >4%/yr. Many studies have demonstrated the cost-effective risk stratification of chronic stable CAD with an intermediate-to-high disease likelihood and an intermediate risk of death or infarction (20,32). Although those with a low likelihood can also be risk stratified, this does not appear cost effective in all cases because of the small numbers of patients with events in the low-likelihood group. Such risk stratification may actually be more effective among women than men, but the strategy to be applied in the course of stratification is the same in both groups (19,32,103,103,131,318,335).

Hachamovitch et al. (19) analyzed 2592 patients who came to diagnostic evaluation with MPS for possible CAD. All underwent scintigraphy and were otherwise treated based on clinical findings. Image findings correlated well with anatomy. Patient management was clearly and appropriately influenced by MPS findings. Both women and men with interpretable stress ECG and intermediate or high post(stress)-test likelihood of CAD, as well as all those with an uninterpretable stress ECG, demonstrated a significant risk stratification benefit from scintigraphic study. Scintigraphic prognosis was much better defined and prognostic subgroups better separated in females. In another study (*32*), quantitative MPS was able to substratify risk well among risk groups already stratified by the Duke Treadmill Score among 2203 consecutive patients (Fig. 3).

MPS is broadly applicable to risk stratification and prognosis in CAD (*9,49,124–128,222–225,318,332–336*). When the relationship of clinical variables and the findings on stress testing and perfusion imaging were carefully related to the occurrence of coronary events, a rational approach to image application evolved (*49,222*). In populations without known CAD and an intermediate or high pre(stress)-test likelihood of disease, stress MPS demonstrated prognostic value exceeding all other variables (*48,128*). In these populations, stress MPS is appropriately applied to risk stratification (*47,48*). The application of the combined exercise and scintigraphic data in those with an intermediate and high likelihood of disease also appears cost effective for the identification of patients at high coronary risk (*126*). These SPECT scintigraphic findings appear similarly accurate in female patients (*10,11,47,48,126,128,337*).

Given the appropriate clinical setting and/or after initial stress testing, patients with a low-risk post-test likelihood of subsequent cardiac events should be treated conservatively, whereas those with a high risk of subsequent cardiac events should be treated aggressively. After integration of all available clinical data and test results, those who present an intermediate risk would benefit from noninvasive risk stratification. The greatest value and most important application of MPS is risk stratification of this large group with intermediate risk of death or infarction (*20,31,128,291,333–337*).

The Abnormal Scan. The greater event rates associated with abnormal scans have largely been established with ^{201}Tl and ^{99m}Tc sestamibi but appear independent of the imaging agent, protocol, stress or acquisition method. In addition, the added and independent prognostic power of MPS, beyond all other historic and clinical variables, has been demonstrated in both males and females (*10,11,32,51,52,126–128,335*) and is independent of patient age, coronary history and previous infarction. Reversible stress perfusion defects are strong predictors of outcome (*285,308,309*), but the extent of the stress image defect, related to the amount of ischemic and infarcted myocardium, is often the best powerful predictor (*10,32,285,320*). This has been confirmed regardless of the nature of the patient population or findings on stress testing (Figs. 33–36).

Prognosis is often predicted independently by both perfusion defect severity, a correlate of stenosis magnitude, and defect extent, a correlate of the amount of myocardium supplied by the involved stenotic vessels (*10,11*). In some studies, these variables are related exponentially to event rate (*8,10,11*) and are further modified by the associated provocative double product. Such quantitation is well within the realm of the method and adds greatly to its ability to risk stratify.

The prognostic value of perfusion image findings was shown by Ladenheim et al. (*10,11*) to be closely related to the associated level of stress or workload applied and the achieved "double product," an indirect and rough measure of the coronary flow demand, during dynamic exercise in a large medically managed population. Although prognosis and event rate were related almost exponentially to the size and severity of related induced image defect, this relationship was magnified and the related event rate augmented greatly, in association with a similar defect when found in patients who failed to achieve 85% of predicted rate for age (*10,11*) (Figs. 41,42).

More than 50% of MPS studies are currently performed with ^{99m}Tc-based agents, most commonly sestamibi. Iskander et al. (*338*) analyzed all 14 published reports in English, including more than 12,000 patients studied by

SPECT perfusion imaging with ^{99m}Tc-labeled perfusion tracers in their laboratory, and found that the group with normal scans had a rate of death or infarction of 0.6%/yr, whereas those with abnormal scans had a hard event rate of 7.4%.

Other image indices, such as lung uptake of ^{201}Tl on stress images (310) and transient dilatation of the left ventricle during exercise or with pharmacologic stress (8,339), have been found to be powerful predictors of outcome. Recent preliminary data demonstrates that LVEF acquired by the first-pass and gated methods performed with myocardial perfusion SPECT adds incremental prognostic information over that present in clinical, exercise and perfusion-related data combined (80,202,204,206) (Figs. 46,47). A normal peak-exercise ejection fraction measured using first-pass technique or with gated poststress acquisition identifies lower risk subgroups, whereas a depressed LVEF with stress or immediately after stress, identifies higher risk groups among patients with both normal and abnormal perfusion studies. Further, combined perfusion and function data provide the information needed to assess the relative likelihood of death or infarction among high-risk subjects. This profile will help guide therapy in high-risk patients. However, acquisition of accurate first-pass data, especially during exercise, requires special equipment and expertise that may not be widely available or even possible in some patients.

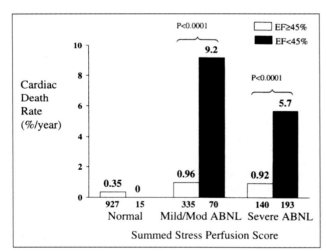

Figure 46 Cardiac death rate (%/yr) as a function of perfusion abnormality and poststress left ventricular ejection fraction (LVEF). The number of patients within each category is indicated below each column. As should be expected, the likelihood of cardiac death is far greater when associated with a poststress LVEF < 45%. Subsequent research suggests that cardiac death relates to LVEF modified by perfusion defect size, and subsequent infarction is more related to the presence and size of defects. The LVEF is not measured on stress echocardiography. ABNL = abnormality; Mod = moderate. (Reprinted, with permission, from Sharir T, Germano G, Kavanagh PB, et al. Incremental prognostic value of post-stress left ventricular ejection fraction and volume by gated myocardial perfusion single photon emission computed tomography. *Circulation* 1999;100:1035–1042.)

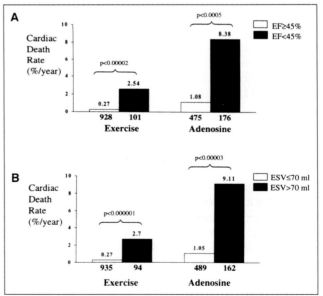

Figure 47 Prognostic value of poststress left ventricular ejection fraction (LVEF) and LV end-systolic volume (ESV). The rates of cardiac death per year are shown in patients undergoing exercise and adenosine stress as a function of (A) LVEF and (B) LVESV. Both LVEF and LVESV measured on MPS were important predictors of subsequent events. Neither is measured on stress echocardiography (Reprinted, with permission, from Sharir T, Germano G, Kavanagh PB, et al. Incremental prognostic value of post-stress left ventricular ejection fraction and volume by gated myocardial perfusion single photon emission computed tomography. *Circulation* 1999;100:1035–1042.)

The prognostic value of stress MPS was demonstrated by Brown (7), Staniloff and Ladenheim in 2 papers (9–11). In patients with normal rest ECGs, incremental prognostic value of MPS was demonstrated in patients with stress-induced ST depression and intermediate pretest CAD likelihood and in patients with a high CAD likelihood and discordant stress test results. The very low event rate in patients with normal stress SPECT MPS and the significantly higher rate in those with abnormal MPS has been confirmed now in studies involving >20,000 patients! A review noted previously, evaluating >12,000 patients and demonstrating an event rate of 0.6%/yr in those with normal studies and a 7.4%/yr event rate among those with abnormal scans (338), was true in both sexes, all age groups and for the gamut of presenting symptoms (5,9,11,32,80,338, 340–342).

More detailed risk stratification was demonstrated by Hachamovitch et al. (21). The incremental statistical and clinical prognostic abilities of MPS in patients without known CAD have been well documented with both exercise and pharmacologic stress for ^{201}Tl and ^{99m}Tc sestamibi (333) but are yet being formulated for tetrofosmin. In many studies and in different patient subgroups, the negative prognostic value of a normal MPS is much higher than that of a normal stress echocardiogram (338,343,344).

Risk stratification of stress MPS in patients with stable angina has been confirmed in 6 studies comprising about 350 patients with an event rate of 1%/yr in those with normal MPS (12,147,318,338,343,344). Studies by Iskandrian et al. (215) and Parisi et al. (303) demonstrated the prognostic value of MPS in patients with known CAD. Iskandrian et al. found a graduated CAD risk related to the MPS findings among 316 patients with proven CAD. Perfusion defect size was the single best predictor of prognosis, exceeding coronary anatomy, with a defect of 15% of the left ventricle related to a much poorer prognosis than a smaller defect. Parisi et al. demonstrated that a reversible MPS defect in patients with 1- or 2-vessel disease related to an 18% mortality during 5 yr, compared with an 8% mortality with a normal scan. A relationship between defect size and mortality rate was not evident for the stress ECG.

The Normal Scan. The event rate associated with a normal perfusion scan has been shown by numerous investigators to be <1% per year of follow-up (12,303,336,343–345). The finding has been further supported by prospective studies demonstrating the role of MPS in patient management and referral to angiography (16,215,303,345,346). This rate has been found in many studies to be independent of the radiopharmaceutical used, the stress or imaging method or acquisition protocol (planar or SPECT) applied. The rate appears to be maintained in the presence of CAD (215,223,341) and is uninfluenced by pre- or poststress–test likelihood of CAD, presenting symptoms or patient sex (128,308,309,347). However, the nature and vigor of the stress applied must be considered. Although some studies demonstrated the superior diagnostic ability of MPS, even at suboptimal heart rates (1,43), a normal MPS performed in association with a suboptimal exercise test may also be suboptimal (348). On the other hand, an abnormal MPS was shown by Cox proportional hazards regression analysis to be an excellent predictor of cardiac events in patients with high exercise tolerance, an overall low-risk subgroup (349). This uniformly low event rate is of critical value to CAD risk stratification and cannot be equaled by the predictive value of a negative stress echocardiogram (14,350–353). Here, any patient with a normal scan is at low risk and, in a prognosis-based approach to management, these patients would appropriately be managed conservatively without coronary angiography.

This high predictive value of a negative test can be expressed as:

$$\text{Predictive value of a negative test} = \frac{\text{True negatives}}{\text{True negatives} + \text{false negatives}},$$

and represents the ability of the test to identify patients without future cardiac events (over a subsequent 1-yr period). Identification of a patient in this population with an otherwise ambiguous presentation permits generally safe and conservative management, even in the presence of known CAD (*223*). It is a strong and clinically important feature of scintigraphic risk stratification, equaled by no other method.

Incremental Prognostic Value of Exercise Myocardial Perfusion Scintigraphy in Patients with Suspected But Without Known Coronary Artery Disease

Although the prognostic value of MPS is now well established (Table 15), support for its current position was initiated when Brown et al. (*7*) first described its incremental prognostic value over the clinical history and exercise test. Here, among 100 consecutive patients without prior MI, who were studied by exercise MPS and followed for a mean period of 3.7 yr, the number of reversible ^{201}Tl defects was the only significant predictor of cardiac events and was more predictive than the number of diseased coronary arteries at angiography. The prognostic power of MPS during 1-yr follow-up in patients without MI was also assessed by Staniloff et al. (*9*) in a group of 819 patients. Normal or equivocal studies were associated with a low event rate of <1%. The low event rate associated with a normal ^{201}Tl study has been further confirmed by Pamelia et al. (*346*). In the study by Staniloff et al. (*9*), the presence of 1 or more myocardial segments with a ^{201}Tl defect of moderate or severe intensity was associated with a 17% cardiac event rate.

In the subsequent study by Ladenheim et al. (*11*), the number of reversible ^{201}Tl defects and defect severity provided independent prognostic information that was further influenced by the achieved exercise heart rate among 1689 patients without MI or known CAD, followed for up to 1 yr. The cardiac event rate increased exponentially with increasing severity and extent of the perfusion defects, which added significant prognostic information to the clinical and exercise test data and introduced the concept of the incremental prognostic value of the perfusion scintigraphic method. Image findings were related to a much increased event rate when associated with a low achieved heart rate. Based on these 3 variables, patients could be classified into those with a low cardiac event rate of <1%, patients with a normal exercise ^{201}Tl study and a high achieved heart rate, and those with an event rate approaching 80%, when severe and extensive reversible defects occurred at a low achieved heart rate (Figs. 41,42). Nor were "high-risk" patients a homogeneous group; even here, substratification was possible. Interesting was the fact that the greatest discrimination of high- and low-event subgroups occurred in patients with a high pretest likelihood of CAD and equivocal or positive exercise ECG. A comparison of ROC curves demonstrated that the group with an abnormal baseline ECG and an abnormal stress ECG gained enhancement of risk stratification with MPS, as did those with a normal baseline ECG and an intermediate pretest disease likelihood, those with an equivocal stress ECG and those with a high pretest likelihood and a negative stress ECG. This also presented significant cost savings (*354*).

Kotler et al. (*311*) followed for 1 yr 268 patients with CAD on angiography but no intervention, among 4567 consecutive patients who had undergone perfusion scintigraphy. These investigators separated patients with suspected CAD into 9 groups, based on the pretest likelihood of disease and the results of exercise ECG. Within all 9 of the subsets, an abnormal perfusion study carried a worse prognosis than did a normal study. As in other studies, such risk stratification was far more discriminating than that simply derived from the extent of anatomic coronary involvement. A subgroup of patients with 3-vessel coronary disease with an average 1-yr event rate of 17% could be further classified prognostically into risk subgroups ranging from 4.5%–57.1%, based on the extent and severity of reversible and nonreversible ^{201}Tl defects. Overall, selective coronary angiography stratified the group based on coronary involvement from 7% with 1-vessel disease, 11.2% with 2-vessel disease and 16.8% with 3-vessel disease. Defect size and density permitted a broad range of risk stratification from 0%–44%, with 14 grades of intermediate risk (Table 12).

In another study, Kotler et al. (*310*) further demonstrated that, in a nonrandomized population, surgically treated patients had a coronary event rate similar to that of those who received medical therapy, if the number of reversible ^{201}Tl defects was no more than 1. Only in a subgroup of patients with 2 or more reversible segments was bypass surgery shown to be superior to medical therapy with respect to 1-yr event rate (11% versus 4%). The prognostic value of quantitative planar ^{201}Tl study was also assessed (*355*). The size of the myocardial perfusion defect on the stress study was quantitated as the area enclosed between the abnormal portion of the patient profile and the lower limit of the normal profile. The degree of defect reversibility was quantified by comparing the stress with 4-hr redistribution profiles. By multiple logistic regression analysis, a history of typical angina and the quantitative degree of defect reversibility were the most important predictors of coronary events. ROC curve analysis demonstrated that better accuracy for predicting coronary events could be achieved by combining the clinical variables with the scintigraphic variables.

Gill et al. (*312*) reported that increased ^{201}Tl pulmonary uptake on exercise planar images was the most significant predictor of coronary events in 467 patients with suspected CAD during a 5-yr follow-up period. The typically powerful predictors, in decreasing order of power, were history of typical angina, prior MI and exercise ST segment depression. The prognostic importance of pulmonary ^{201}Tl uptake has been further confirmed by Kaul et al. (*313*), who found that a quantitative index of pulmonary uptake of ^{201}Tl, the heart-to-lung ratio of ^{201}Tl, was the single most powerful variable for prognosis in symptomatic, ambulatory patients undergoing catheterization. In these planar ^{201}Tl studies, this variable was superior to clinical, exercise testing, angiographic and other quantitative imaging variables.

Machecourt et al. (*356*) demonstrated the relationship between the coronary mortality rate and the extent of perfusion defect using a 9-segment model in a large number of patients studied from 1987–1989. Here, a normal scan related to a mortality rate of 0.24%, whereas defects involving 1, 2 or 3 segments related to a subsequent mortality of 2%, 5% and 6%/yr, respectively, and involvement of 4 or more segments related to a mortality rate of 17%/yr!

Kaul et al. (*317*) also evaluated a population of 383 patients who were followed for a period of 4–8 yr. Multiple regression analysis of historical, clinical, exercise ECG, perfusion imaging variables and angiographic findings show that cardiac events were best predicted by the number of diseased vessels with ≥50% stenosis, followed by the number of ^{201}Tl segments with a reversible defect. The latter variable, however, was the best predictor of nonfatal MI. Furthermore, the combined prognostic power of catheterization and exercise ^{201}Tl variables, including the magnitude of change in heart rate between rest and exercise and the presence of ST segment depression, was found to be additive.

Berman et al. (*128*) demonstrated the prognostic value of stress MPS and its ability to risk stratify regardless of the pretest CAD likelihood or results of stress testing (Figs. 33–36). Hachamovitch et al. (*32*) examined 2203 consecutive patients who had no history of previous MI, coronary revascularization or coronary angiography before perfusion imaging (*32*). As in other patient subgroups, a normal perfusion scan predicted an excellent outcome, <1% event rate per yr of follow-up, irrespective of sex, the likelihood of CAD or presenting symptoms. Further, defect extent and severity added independent and incremental prognostic value to clinical and exercise variables, even in a patient population at low overall risk for adverse cardiovascular outcomes, with a 1.8% hard event rate.

These findings have been extended in a large consecutive series of patients (*19*) using the dual-isotope rest ^{201}Tl/stress ^{99m}Tc sestamibi SPECT protocol. Here, imaging yielded incremental prognostic value in 2592 patients with low, intermediate and high postexercise likelihood of CAD when compared with the quantitative Duke Stress Test Score. In all of these patient groups, a normal scan was associated with a low event rate. As in other studies (*357*), the most useful application of perfusion imaging related to patients with uninterpretable rest ECGs or intermediate Duke Treadmill Scores. In this large group of 1187 patients with an intermediate Duke score, the group with normal scans had a mortality of 0.4%, whereas a dense abnormality was associated with an 8.9% mortality (Fig. 3). The authors also found that exercise perfusion imaging added significant prognostic information based on ROC curve analysis. The stress scan also indicated better discrimination for identifying high-risk women than men. The odds ratio relating the image findings and the event rates of 1 group to those of another were much higher in women, again suggesting that coronary risk stratification was, in fact, better in women.

Miller et al. (*358*) used multivariate analysis to study the relationship between prognosis in CAD and a variety of stress test and stress ^{201}Tl imaging parameters in a large number of patients evaluated in a community population. The number of abnormal image segments, the number of redistributing segments and age were the only significant prognostic factors. Exercise time, the magnitude of ST-segment depression and stress-induced left ventricular dilatation were not significant predictors of outcome in this study.

Miller and Gersh (*359*) present an analysis of diagnostic and risk stratification strategies to identify patients with stable angina who are at lower risk for events but who would benefit greatly from aggressive medical management. Evidence presented makes a strong case for the cost-effective application of noninvasive stress perfusion imaging.

Incremental Prognostic Value of Pharmacologic Stress Myocardial Perfusion Scintigraphy

Many of the points discussed previously also apply to pharmacologic stress with a coronary dilator, such as dipyridamole or adenosine. Much of the research discussed includes patients studied pharmacologically or have parallels in studies performed with these direct dilators. These pharmacologic methods are gaining further support and are being applied in greater numbers for risk stratification after infarction and before high-risk noncardiac surgery (*360*) (Table 16). They also have been found to be cost effective in this setting (*361*). Dipyridamole is now available in an inexpensive generic form and is relatively simple to formulate and dispense in-house. These methods have distinct advantages over dobutamine stress in their consistent maximal effect, brevity of protocol, reproducibility and accuracy and possess all the advantages of the scintigraphic method. They are of great value in patients who are unable to exercise or unable to exercise satisfactorily. The subject has been thoroughly reviewed in *Self-Study Program III. Cardiology. Topic 2: Pharmacologic Stress.* In that volume, vasodilator-induced ST depression was noted to be a specific indicator of a tight coronary lesion, generally associated with a reversible image defect. However, infrequently, dipyridamole- or adenosine-induced ST depression may be seen with a normal MPS. Mathews et al. (*362*) have now reported 40 such cases with angiographic correlation and demonstrated that normal images relate to a low hard event rate even in association with vasodilator-induced ST changes.

Table 16
CONSIDERATIONS FOR PREOPERATIVE RISK ASSESSMENT FOR NONCARDIAC SURGERY

Assess risk related to individual surgery.

Recognize both the short- and long-term implications of preoperative myocardial perfusion scintigraphy.

Most patients with positive tests will have no events.

No test is perfect.

Image quantitation will help increase the predictive value of a positive test.

Decision to perform angiography is based on clinical factors, not simply because of elective surgery.

Perform angiography only in those who have high (moderate)-risk images and who would benefit from this study regardless of upcoming surgery.

The Frequency of Serial Study

The duration of the "warranty period" of a benign future and low event rate related to a normal or probably normal SPECT MPS has been evaluated (*342*). Here, the event rate was determined serially over a 3-yr period in a large number of patients undergoing MPS with normal or probably normal findings, with and without known CAD, to determine if there was a specific period after which the event rate escalated. Patients with CAD were noted to have a mild but significant bump in their event rate in their second year of follow-up, whereas those without known CAD were noted to have a mild bump in event rate after 2–3 yr. The latter, increasing from 0.9 in year 1 to 2.8 and 3.8 in the second and third follow-up years was well related to age, with those older than 65 yr demonstrating a 4% event rate in the second poststudy year and those younger than 65 continuing to demonstrate a low event rate. This also suggests the approximate, appropriate and necessary interval between MPS evaluations in patients thought to be at continued potential coronary risk: after 2 yr in those with CAD and after 3–4 yr in those without known disease. Others have also demonstrated the likelihood that the "warranty period" may vary, depending on the likelihood of disease (*342,363*).

Events, Prognosis and Lesion Severity: The Substrate of Subsequent Infarction

Seemingly incompatible with the relationship between CAD risk and defect severity are reports that coronary events, specifically acute infarction with acute coronary occlusion, occur in relation to coronary lesions that are not necessarily the most severe or even physiologically "significant" (*364–371*) (Fig. 48). Such studies are retrospective and evaluate selective populations in whom the infarct-related vessel was evaluated on a previous angiogram performed from months to >10 yr before the event in patients studied earlier for clinical reasons. The authors do not assess the state of the vessel hours or days before the event but generally exclude patients with prior revascularization and the most severe lesions, presenting a severe intrinsic bias. However, with their flaws, these studies

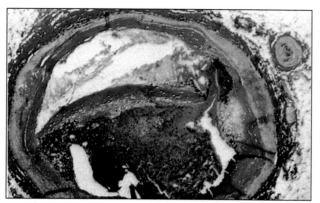

Figure 48 Acute coronary occlusion. A trichrome-stained pathologic example of a complete coronary occlusion with an atheromatous plaque rupture and intraplaque hemorrhage is shown. In which vessels does this occur? Can we predict this event?

demonstrate that infarcts, which generally relate to coronary occlusion, may not uncommonly involve vessels that are not necessarily the most stenotic when studied at variable times before occlusion and may not be significantly involved on angiography. That is, some condition other than the degree of stenosis determined subsequent coronary occlusion. However, perfusion scintigraphy has been shown to provide an excellent measure of percentage of lesion stenosis and of the CFR and bears an excellent relation to prognosis as well. Other parameters of ischemic risk, such as ST depression or wall motion, also are based on lesion severity and are prognostic in some studies. Thus, events and the coronary stenosis to which they often relate probably bear some relationship to CFR assessed by stress testing and perfusion scintigraphy and to the physiologic parameters determining stenosis significance. How can these apparently mutually exclusive observations be reconciled?

In fact, when analyzed quantitatively, on a vessel-by-vessel basis, and as a result of the inverse relationship between lesion severity and the percentage incidence of such vessels, the likelihood of an event precipitated by occlusion of a tightly stenotic vessel far exceeds that related to occlusion of any insignificantly stenotic vessel, even when most events occur in less stenotic vessels (365,367, 369,371,372) (Fig. 49). There does appear to be a relationship between the severity of coronary disease and the "ischemic burden," characterized by the full extent of more widespread and less severe disease (28,164,192,302,372) (Figs. 50,51).

Also, some studies do, in fact, relate lesion severity to specific regional ischemic risk (Fig. 52). A previous study looked at the location of infarcts as determined by the presence of fixed defects on scintigraphy in patients who presented with recent infarction in the presence of a prior exercise perfusion scintigram (373,374). The location of new infarction related well to the area of prior exercise-induced scintigraphic defect when infarction occurred spontaneously, and the area at risk accurately paralleled the area subsequently lost. In a study by Miller et al. (375), most infarctions occurred in regions with defects on prior imaging study and previously demonstrated MIR among 25 patients who had an acute infarction some time after perfusion scintigraphy. The incidence of infarction in regions with a reversible defect was 14/26 (54%), among those with fixed defects was 3/7 (43%) and among those without defect was 8/42 (19%). In this study, as in others, a substantial number of infarctions, 8/25 (32%) occurred in regions without related perfusion defect. Similarly, there was a strong correlation between regional ischemia and the site of subsequent infarction when MPS was performed in relatively close temporal relation to the subsequent event (376). An exception was infarcts occurring perioperatively after bypass surgery, in which the relationship was more variable, as might be expected when intraoperative events and surgical technique strongly influence natural pathophysiology (377,378).

Yet, the conclusion is unavoidable that coronary occlusion may occur in vessels with stenosis of varying degree. This may relate to factors regulating the stability of atheromata or those influencing the clotting system. However, the prognostic nature of methods based on lesion severity must still be explained.

Perhaps the relationship of ischemic parameters to prognosis and events is the result of the fact that severe ischemic disease identified by these methods also probably occurs in the presence of numerous lesser lesions, which occur in some proportion to lesion severity. All contribute to the "total ischemic burden" (366). Rather than any single lesion, this more global factor of coronary risk potential, possibly related to the extent of MIR (302), could be the factor linking events to lesion severity. Interesting is the fact that the degree of exercise-induced ST depression does not correlate well with the "ischemic burden" as identified and correlated with the stress perfusion scintigram (28,164,192,235,302,372).

It would appear, then, that cardiac risk is related directly or indirectly to the extent and pathophysiologic, if not anatomic, severity of coronary lesions, often viewed as a more physiologic index, the "ischemic burden" (368). The "ischemic burden" is generally well correlated with the CFR. The findings on stress perfusion imaging provide the best available correlation with the CFR and "ischemic burden" (379). Once the risk of cardiac events is established, aggressive or conservative management can be applied appropriately (16,379,380). This ability to prognosticate events based on induced ischemia and related or unrelated stenoses is imperfect. It remains impossible to predict timing, and specific localization of coronary occlusion in individual coronary patients may be tenuous. Yet, MPS can stratify low-, moderate- and very high-risk subgroups better than any other method (19,32). Neither the quantitative measure of coronary stenosis nor its effect on CFR permits the prediction of plaque rupture or other circumstance precipitating an acute coronary event (364–375). Perhaps some combined measure of the lipid profile, coagulation profile and factors yet undiscovered that relate to plaque stability will complement tests based on provoked ischemia and the CFR, and so provide another more refined method to substratify coronary-related risk.

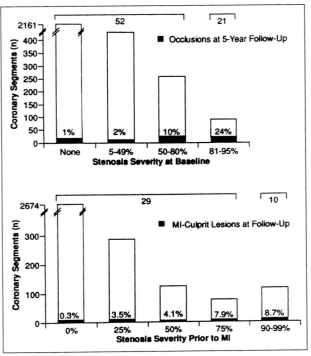

Figure 49 Frequency of coronary occlusion related to the percentage baseline stenosis. Analyzed quantitatively on a vessel-by-vessel basis, the likelihood of an event precipitated by occlusion of a tightly stenotic vessel far exceeds that related to occlusion of any insignificantly stenotic vessel, even when most events occur in less stenotic vessels. This is because there are many more coronary segments with less severe lesions than segments with severe lesions. Severe stenoses must be considered at greatest risk of subsequent occlusion. MI = myocardial infarction. (Adapted, with permission, from Alderman EL, Corley SD, Fisher LD, et al. Five-year angiographic follow-up of factors associated with progression of coronary artery disease in the Coronary Artery Surgery Study (CASS). *J Amer Coll Cardiol* 1993;22:1141–1154.).

Because many events relate to the rupture of an atherosclerotic plaque or occlusion of a vessel that did not earlier relate to a significant alteration in CFR, much of medical treatment and research is focused on altering plaque composition, increasing plaque stability or reducing thrombogenicity. Revascularization improves blood flow without influencing the factors that advance atherosclerosis or lead to coronary occlusion. Although revascularization protects myocardium that may be infarcted and reduces mortality in some subgroups, medical treatment alone may better address the factors that may stabilize atheromata or aid their regression, thus preventing infarction. On this basis, MPS is being applied increasingly to identify and monitor high-risk coronary patients and to assess the potential benefits of various treatments and their resultant implications for management decisions (381). It further

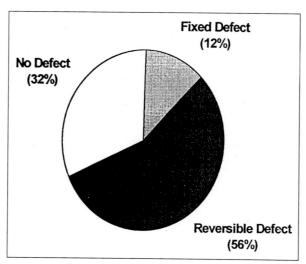

Figure 50   The substrate for subsequent infarction. The findings of prior SPECT images in the region of subsequent infarction are shown. Suprisingly (or not?) most infarcts occurred in regions previously shown to have fixed or reversible defects. (Reprinted, with permission, from Miller GL, Herman SD, Heller GV, et al. Relation between perfusion defects on stress technetium-99m sestamibi SPECT scintigraphy and the location of a subsequent myocardial infarction. *Am J Cardiol* 1996;78:26–30.)

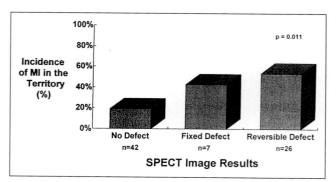

Figure 51   Subsequent infarction among segments. The incidence of subsequent myocardial infarction (MI) is shown in 75 regions among 25 patients studied based on appearance on SPECT. The likelihood of MI was greatest in those with reversible defects. (Reprinted, with permission, from Miller GL, Herman SD, Heller GV, et al. Relation between perfusion defects on stress technetium-99m sestamibi SPECT scintigraphy and the location of a subsequent myocardial infarction. *Am J Cardiol* 1996;78:26–30.)

presents the possibility of differentiating those at risk for death from those at risk for acute infarction and so presents a rational basis for management among high-risk coronary patients.

MYOCARDIAL PERFUSION SCINTIGRAPHY IN SPECIFIC CLINICAL SETTINGS

Patients with Known Coronary Artery Disease

The incremental value of exercise perfusion scintigraphy has been documented in patients with known CAD. Both positive and negative predictive values are well maintained in this population (*19,32,211,215,223,309,313,317,382,383*) (Tables 6A–E). Because of these findings, patients with persistent or recurrent and obviously ischemic symptoms indicating a failure of medical therapy should be referred for angiography to determine suitability for revascularization. Patients with controlled, stable or ambiguous symptoms or who are asymptomatic but in need of prognostic evaluation are candidates for perfusion imaging.

Use in Unstable Angina

For many years we have assumed that those with unstable angina have a dynamic syndrome requiring active and early intervention, angiography and revascularization. Similarly, those with non-Q wave infarction may have experienced a partial event with the worst yet to come. Although patients with unstable angina and non-Q infarctions often are managed aggressively, with frequent angiography and percutaneous transluminal coronary angioplasty (PTCA), these groups are heterogeneous in risk and many respond well to medical treatment, without serious events. Evidence has been accumulating that patients with

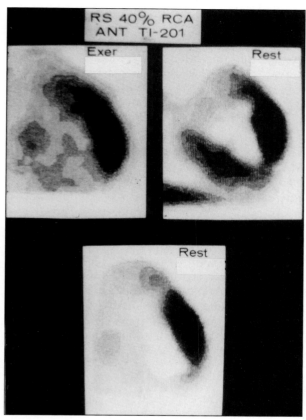

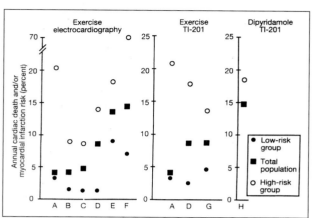

Figure 53 Noninvasive risk stratification in unstable angina. (Left to right) The risks related to the results of the exercise electrocardiogram and dynamic and pharmacologic perfusion scintigraphy, respectively, in high- and low-risk groups. Scintigraphy provides a superior risk-group discrimination. Results of stress echocardiography are not presented, because such studies had not yet been performed. Yet, scintigraphic and echocardiographic methods were recommended with equal weight! (Reprinted, with permission, from U.S. Department of Health and Human Services. *Unstable Angina: Diagnosis and Management.* Clinical Practice Guideline #10. Washington, DC: U.S. Department of Health and Human Services; 1994.)

Figure 52 Myocardium at ischemic risk. (Top) Stress (left) and rest (right) myocardial perfusion scintigrams from a patient with right coronary artery (RCA) stenosis estimated to be 40%. The scintigram clearly reveals evidence of reversible inferior ischemia. (Bottom) Subsequently, the patient had a spontaneous infarction of the same region, as shown on this rest image. This study illustrates the difference between angiographic anatomy and scintigraphic pathophysiology, and provides 1 form of evidence for the ability of scintigraphy to identify myocardium at ischemic risk (see references *379–390*). RS = right stenosis; ANT = anterior. (Reprinted, courtesy of Dr. M. Goris, Stanford University, Stanford, CA, and, with permission, from Botvinick E, Dae M, O'Connell JW, Ortendahl D, Hattner RS. The scintigraphic evaluation of the cardiovascular system. In: Parmley WW, Chatterjee K, eds. *Cardiology*. Philadelphia, PA: J.B. Lippincott; 1991.)

these syndromes represent a heterogeneous group with a spectrum of disease. Many respond well to conservative medical management. This variability relates to the nature of the pathophysiology, in which the condition is generally associated with a nonocclusive yet unstable atheromatous process or an occlusion, with collateral support or other ameliorating factor. Several clinical trials in patients with both unstable angina and non-Q wave infarction (*384–387*) and late follow-up study (*388*) have demonstrated the lack of significant differences in the rates of death or nonfatal infarction among those with unstable angina and non-Q infarction treated medically or with revascularization. Some studies that demonstrate improved survival among those with 3-vessel disease or reduced left ventricular function are open to question, because these studies were not randomized (*384–386*).

Randomized Trials. Both Veterans Affairs and National Institutes of Health randomized trials in unstable angina demonstrated no overall survival benefit of surgical compared with medical treatment. Convincing data demonstrate that medical therapy has a strong beneficial effect on unstable angina, with death and MI rates falling from 15%–40% to 3%–6% (*387,389*). In a study of 125 patients, Grambo and Topol (*390*) reported that the percentage of unstable angina patients refractory to medical therapy would fall from 55% to 9% with intensification of medical therapy (*390*). More recently, the Thrombolysis in Myocardial Infarction (TIMI) IIIB trial randomized 1473 patients with unstable angina or non-Q MI to: (1) conservative medical therapy with angiography only for refractory symptoms or evidence of ischemia on the stress ECG or MPS; or (2) an aggressive angiographic approach, with intervention, angiography and revascularization, when possible within 16–48 hr after admission. There was no difference in rate of death (2%) or MI (6%) between the two groups at 10 mo or 1 yr. Grambow and Topol (*390*) also demonstrated that more vigorous medical therapy after initial therapy could ameliorate symptoms in 54 of 65 continued symptomatic patients among the 125 patients treated. Because this and other studies suggested that most patients with unstable angina could be controlled symptomatically with medical therapy, an effective noninvasive method may permit reduced risk and cost of revascularization in all but those with refractory symptoms or who have evident high risk of future events in spite of symptomatic control.

Exercise Testing. Although exercise testing can be performed in unstable angina patients after they are stabilized with medical therapy, it provides little or no prognostic value. However, although exercise-induced ST depression related to an increased incidence of subsequent events (death, infarction or revascularization) in 2 studies, so too did the lack of ST changes with an event rate of 21%, and ST changes could not differentiate between high- and low-risk groups (*391,392*). In fact, in the study by Wilcox et al. (*391*) the exercise test performed at predischarge provided prognostic information that was independent from clinical and ECG data in medically treated patients with unstable angina. Yet, the stratification provided was not as great as that generally associated with stress MPS. In another study of 13,500 patients, induced ST depression did identify a higher risk group. Yet even a "low risk" was substantial, and 26% of the patients studied had a prior non-Q infarction (*393*)!

Stress Testing and Stress Myocardial Perfusion Scintigraphy. The role of the stress ECG alone in risk stratifying those with unstable angina has been only lightly studied. Stress MPS and the extent of MIR have been employed to assess risk in several studies in patients with unstable angina (*394–397*). Among 52 patients with unstable angina studied with exercise MPS by Brown (*394*), the only significant predictor of hard events among all clinical and exercise variables was the presence of a reversible defect. The group with reversible defects had a hard event rate of 26%, whereas the group with none had a 3% rate over the 39 mo of the study (<1%/yr). Stratmann et al. (*395*) confirmed these results in 126 medically stabilized unstable angina patients. Here, 10 of 40 (25%) patients with reversible defects suffered hard events, as did only 1 of 86 (1%) without reversible defects (*P* < 0.001) (*234,241,243*). Among 158 unstable patients studied by Madsen et al. (*396*) with symptom-limited exercise MPS performed after admission for a noninfarction chest pain syndrome, reversible defects related to a 21% hard event rate, with 3% among those without reversible defects over a mean 14 mo follow-up period. Hillert et al. (*398*) found that 15 of 19 patients with reversible ^{201}Tl defects suffered infarction or recurrent unstable angina compared with 2 among 18 ($P < 0.001$) with no evidence of redistribution on 12-wk follow-up. Marmur et al. (*399*) evaluated the predictive value of a positive stress ECG, stress MPS, Holter and coronary angiogram in 54 patients who were studied with each method, and presented with unstable angina responsive to medical therapy. The authors found that the only significant multivariate predictors of outcomes were a history of prior MI and the extent of reversible defects. In none of these studies were fixed defects or stress ECG findings predictive of outcome, and all revealed a high negative predictive value of a normal stress MPS in unstable angina.

Several studies demonstrate the value of pharmacologic stress MPS in acute coronary syndromes and unstable angina (*400–403*). Dipyridamole sestamibi imaging was performed by Stratmann et al. (*400*) before discharge of 128 medically treated patients with unstable angina who were at intermediate pretest clinical risk. They were then followed for 16 ± 11 mo. Events, both "hard" and "soft," were noted in 10% with normal studies and 69% with defects ($P < 0.01$), and the scan findings were the only independent predictor of outcome. It appears that a noninvasive strategy of risk stratification based in stress perfusion imaging can well separate high- from low-risk subgroups and serve as a basis for selecting those to most likely benefit from aggressive management.

Unstable Angina Guidelines: Politically (Not Scientifically) Correct. Recent clinical practice guidelines developed under the sponsorship of the Agency for Health Care Policy and Research (AHCPR) have indicated a clear role for the use of nuclear testing in patients admitted with unstable angina (*31*) (Fig. 53). These guidelines suggest that a significant number of such patients may be medically treated after appropriate risk stratification. This strategy is, as previously discussed, widely supported by the published data and is applied daily in the many patients presenting to the stress testing laboratory for evaluation in the setting of atypical or rest pain (*401*) (Fig. 54). Here, although their symptoms are ambiguous at presentation, many of these patients evaluated with stress testing demonstrate scintigraphic evidence of ischemia. Given the nature of their presenting symptoms, the diagnosis of unstable angina is applied to their syndrome. Such patients were safely evaluated with the demonstration of a spectrum of MIR and related prognoses.

The perfusion scintigraphic method is particularly applicable in patients who have minimal risk factors or in patients with clear-cut unstable angina who respond quickly to medical therapy. In these medically stabilized patients, either exercise or pharmacologic stress testing with perfusion imaging can effectively stratify patients into low- and high-risk subsets (*394,395,404,405*). Madsen et al. (*405*) used planar thallium imaging in a group of patients who had been admitted with unstable angina and were then followed for a 15-mo period. In this cohort, the presence of a reversible defect identified a high-risk patient subset with a 20% event rate. Similar findings by Brown (*394*) were reviewed previously. An advantage of rest MPS is its long-documented ability to identify abnormalities in the setting of unstable angina (*395,401*), even hours after pain resolution (*402*) (Fig. 55).

According to current AHCPR guidelines, failure of medical treatment to control ischemia or the presence of hemodynamic instability would result in referral to catheterization. Hemodynamically stabilized patients with medically controlled ischemia would be candidates for a noninvasive management approach. Within this approach, those patients at low risk by clinical factors, patients who

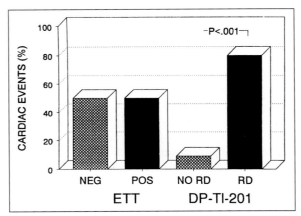

Figure 54 Myocardial perfusion scintigraphy (MPS) after acute infarction. The frequency of cardiac events is shown as a function of exercise electrocardiographic (ETT) and dipyridamole MPS (DP-TI-201). Although ETT had no significant prognostic value, the presence of thallium-201 (^{201}TI) redistribution was associated with a significantly increased risk of cardiac events. NEG = negative stress electrocardiogram; POS = positive stress electrocardiogram; RD = ^{201}TI redistribution. (Reprinted, with permission, from Leppo JA, O'Brien J, Rothendler JA, et al. Dipyridamole-thallium-201 scintigraphy in the prediction of future cardiac events after acute myocardial infarction. *N Engl J Med* 1984;310:1014–1018.)

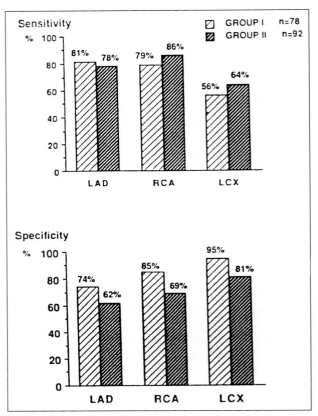

Figure 55 Dipyridamole coronary sensitivity. The sensitivity and specificity of diypridamole thallium-201 scintigraphy for individual coronary arteries are shown in patients with unstable angina. As with planar imaging in general, there was a reduced sensitivity for detection of left circumflex (LCX) stenoses. Group I was composed of patients with atypical or ambiguous chest pain. Group II included patients who proved to have unstable angina. LAD = left anterior descending; RCA = right coronary artery. (Reprinted, with permission, from Zhu YY, Chung WS, Botvinick EH, et al. Dipyridamole perfusion scintigraphy: the experiences with its application in one hundred seventy patients with known or suspected unstable angina. *Am Heart J* 1991;121:33.)

probably did not have unstable angina initially, can be managed as outpatients and referred to stress testing within 72 hr of initial admission. Patients at intermediate to high risk who have been stabilized and are free of recurrent angina or evidence of pump dysfunction or significant ventricular dysrhythmias are also candidates for this approach. The initial test in these patients would be exercise testing in those capable individuals with normal resting ECG who are not on digoxin. Presumably, patients with an abnormal rest ECG or who are on digoxin would undergo exercise stress MPS. Those unable to exercise satisfactorily would be evaluated with pharmacologic stress using a direct coronary dilator, such as dipyridamole or adenosine.

One figure (Fig. 53) included in the AHCPR guidelines demonstrates the far greater difference in event rate between normal and abnormal stress perfusion scintigrams than between normal and abnormal stress ECGs, attesting to the greater ability of the scintigraphic method to risk stratify these patients. Again, given the too frequent inaccuracy of the exercise ECG and the superior prognostic ability of the scintigraphic method, proceeding directly to stress MPS should be a commonly applied option. Stress echocardiography also may be performed in these patients in association with exercise or dobutamine stress. However, dobutamine stress would not appear to be well suited for patients with ongoing or recently symptomatic unstable angina. Further, data presented in the AHCPR guidelines demonstrates the lack of stress echocardiographic data in patients with unstable angina at that time. Nonetheless, these guidelines recommend that the decision to apply stress echocardiography or stress perfusion imaging should be determined on the basis of local availability and expertise. The experts who formulated these guidelines recommend a stress imaging method, stress echocardiography, with no support from the literature. This is the recommendation of a group of cardiologists who are strongly motivated politically and also, probably, by their vested interests. Beyond this, the AHCPR guidelines omit a variety of studies available at that time supporting the refined prognostic value of perfusion scintigraphy. Little has changed since this publication. There remain few published articles applying stress echocardiography to risk stratification and even fewer applying these methods to risk stratify patients with unstable angina. A recent article applied exercise echocardiography to >200 patients with unstable angina and found that the risk stratification ability of the method was no better than that of the stress ECG (*406*). All guidelines must be analyzed critically in this way. Methods applied should be based not only on the suggestions made but also should be influenced strongly by the whole literature and the observations and experience of the practitioner.

Patients Presenting with Acute Chest Pain and Possible Acute Myocardial Infarction

The Problem. Each year, >6 million people present to emergency departments (EDs) in the United States with chest pain or other symptoms or signs of an acute MI. More than half of these people are admitted to coronary care units (CCUs) or monitored hospital beds, with a diagnosis of "rule out MI" (ROMI). Yet, less than one-third of these patients are eventually shown to have had an acute coronary event. Although patients with noncardiac chest pain and a normal or nonspecifically abnormal ECG should be sent home and those with classic pain and acute ST elevation should be admitted and treated aggressively, patients with atypical pain and nonspecific ECG findings generally are admitted with a subsequently low event rate, in the range of only 10%–20%. This latter group is the largest patient group admitted! In spite of this, about 60,000 patients with acute coronary syndromes and 20,000 with acute myocardial infarction (AMI) are sent home without diagnosis.

The ED evaluation of chest pain is difficult and ambiguous. The evaluation, as currently performed, is inaccurate because of the low specificity and sensitivity of the resting ECG. However, discharge from the ED with an AMI has a poor outcome (*407*), and a missed AMI is the leading cause of medical malpractice litigation. For these reasons, most physicians treat presenting patients conservatively and admit too many patients to the hospital with what eventually proves to be noncardiac chest pain. Because of this practice, AMIs amount to <30% of CCU admissions. Although the group with a diagnosis of ROMI have excellent short-term prognoses, they absorb most of the costs.

The overall cost of such management, a current source of income to hospitals, is in the range of $3–5 billion annually! However, this adds to the health

Table 17
CHARACTERISTICS OF THE IDEAL EMERGENCY
DEPARTMENT CHEST PAIN TRIAGE METHOD

Analytic characteristics
    Simple assay
    Rapid turnaround
    High precision
    Quantitative

Biologic characteristics
    High myocardial "concentration"
    Not present in other tissues
    Not detected in normal individuals
    Released rapidly in response to injury
    Persists for a reasonable duration
    Released in proportion to injury
    Little-to-no population variation

Clinical characteristics
    Very sensitive and specific
    Optimal for diagnosis, prognosis
    Can influence therapy and outcomes

care budget, which already amounts to 14% of the gross national product. With continued reforms and the wider application of managed care, it will be the "providers" who will be paying this bill, as such funds will go into the category of expenses rather than profits. It is then important for all to develop a more efficient and cost-effective manner to triage patients presenting with a diagnosis of ROMI. In considering the options beyond acute cost savings, the contribution that the triage method will make to clinical management and long-term savings must be considered.

What Is Needed? In this age of cost containment, reduced frequency, duration and intensity of hospital stays are needed without sacrificing the quality of patient care. Although all that is actually needed is a method to accurately exclude AMI and an acute coronary syndrome, it would be important at the same time to identify risk and guide the management of those with such events. This represents the evident advantages of an exercise test or stress imaging study. Needed is a fast and inexpensive method (Table 17) to determine: the size, intensity and location of ongoing ischemia; the size, "density" and location of infarction; the extent and location of MIR; and to assess left (and right) ventricular function (Tables 18,19).

The underlying pathophysiology and eventual prognosis of unstable angina and AMI are similar, and both must be recognized in patients on ED presentation (Tables 18,19). Not only do we seek to identify patients with a low likelihood of AMI, but, optimally, we want to identify patients with a low risk of complicated AMI, patients with a low risk of coronary events, patients with unstable angina, patient prognosis, the extent of MIR, AMI (lesion) location, the culprit vessel and regional and global ventricular function. If we can characterize patients on presentation according to these, we will not only successfully triage patients but make an important contribution to the determination of the course and speed of patient management. Can a single method provide all of this information? Is there a method with a sufficiently high predictive value of a negative test to permit patient discharge? To which population should it be applied?

The Options. Alternatives to the CCU for patients with low-to-moderate likelihood (risk) are being developed and applied. Steps are being taken to develop coronary observation units (*408*) to reduce the length of stay and the intensity of nursing care after admission of patients with a low AMI likelihood. However, these units, too, are dependent on the rapid and accurate triage of patients and the generation of clinical patient profiles to guide treatment and

Table 18
WHERE DO WE DRAW THE DIAGNOSTIC LINE?*

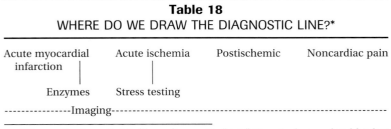

*The method applied is like a diagnostic "net." How inclusive should it be? Perfusion imaging is the only method that spans all groups.

speed management. We wish to determine the minimal time, services and tests to ROMI. The methods that can potentially be applied to the triage of ROMI patients and that present the opportunity to guide management are shown in Table 20.

Clinical Algorithms. Based on population studies relating the rest ECG and available clinical parameters to the likelihood of AMI, clinical algorithms offer the simplest approach to estimating the risk of AMI in patients presenting to the ED with possible acute infarction (*409*). Lee et al. (*410*) designed a multivariate algorithm to identify patients presenting to the ED with chest pain and a low risk of having an AMI. After application of this algorithm and stratification of likelihood among >2500 patients, 33 (3.5%) of 946 patients assigned to the low-risk group with normal or nondiagnostic ECG nonetheless had a final diagnosis of either AMI or unstable angina. Goldman et al. (*411*) have expanded on earlier work, applying a clinical patient profile algorithm to predict those needing intensive care among all who present to the ED with acute chest pain. Although, this and other algorithms separate patients into high- and very low-risk subgroups, there are major errors and omissions. Many with intermediate categorization are indeterminate in diagnosis, risk and management plan. Further, algorithms are targeted at infarct diagnosis and not unstable angina. We seek a method to make a diagnosis and, moreover, to determine risk and guide management. Algorithms alone are not enough.

Acute Testing to Telescope the Diagnosis and Evaluation: Serum Enzyme Analysis. Biochemical markers, enzymes that appear in the serum after myocardial cell death, have been considered the "gold standard" for the diagnosis of AMI. Such a method, if sensitive and timely enough, allows ruling out AMI if the results are negative. Myocardial-specific enzymes offer considerable promise for speeding the diagnosis of AMI and increasing its specificity (*412*). Sadly, but predictably, only about 30% of patients with the clinical diagnosis of unstable angina demonstrate elevated enzyme levels. The diagnostic accuracy of these enzymes depends on their individual kinetics and their temporal relationship to the course of chest pain. For all cardiac enzymes, however, the negative predictive value of the initial sample is generally not adequate to rule out AMI. Cardiac levels of troponin T and I seem to be highly sensitive and specific for myocardial necrosis and to increase quickly and remain elevated for prolonged periods. However, when Duca et al. (*413*) studied the appearance of image abnormalities and elevation of troponin I and T among

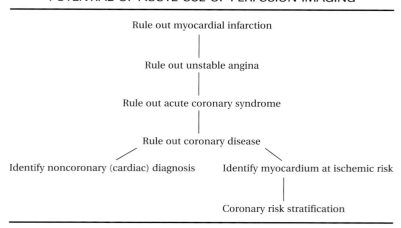

Table 19
POTENTIAL OF ACUTE USE OF PERFUSION IMAGING

Rule out myocardial infarction

Rule out unstable angina

Rule out acute coronary syndrome

Rule out coronary disease

Identify noncoronary (cardiac) diagnosis   Identify myocardium at ischemic risk

Coronary risk stratification

Table 20
POTENTIAL METHODS FOR THE TRIAGE OF EMERGENCY DEPARTMENT PATIENTS WITH CHEST PAIN

Apply clinical algorithms (to reduce hospital admissions to rule out myocardial infarction)

OR

Perform acute testing to telescope diagnosis/evaluation
Serum enzyme analysis
Exercise testing
Echocardiography
Perfusion scintigraphy

75 patients admitted to the ED with chest pain and a nondiagnostic ECG, acute rest sestamibi/tetrofosmin was more sensitive for AMI diagnosis than serum enzymes, with preserved specificity.

Patients presenting early with AMI, before enzyme elevation, or unstable angina without enzyme release, and a nondiagnostic ECG, must be identified and differentiated from those whose chest pain is of noncardiac origin. As a consequence, there is an urgent need to find yet another diagnostic strategy to accurately triage patients presenting to the ED with chest pain.

Stress Testing. The group to be targeted by this and other acute diagnostic approaches includes patients in whom the suspicion of CAD is high enough to consider admission to the hospital but low enough that the decision is questionable. Stress testing is finding an increasing role among low-likelihood patients able to exercise, with normal baseline ECGs. Exercise testing has been applied by Lewis et al. (414) for the identification of exercise-induced ischemia, to diagnose an acute coronary syndrome and so to triage ROMI patients. The exercise test identified most patients with events, as well as a low-risk subgroup who could be discharged or admitted. However, this study had no control subjects, and a select population was studied with a very low AMI rate. However, even a negative test did not, in many cases, influence management. Did the method truly reduce admissions?

The same researchers (415) conducted a prospective study of 212 heterogeneous low-risk ED patients with chest pain, as indicated by clinical and ECG criteria. Here, immediate exercise testing was performed before serum cardiac enzymes were measured! Positive tests revealed 13 with CAD, and negative tests were related to no events in follow-up. However, there were no AMIs in the population on follow-up. Stress testing was said to influence the early discharge of many with negative tests and was therefore highly cost effective as a triage measure in this population.

What is the value of acute exercise testing in such a low-likelihood population with not a single diagnosed AMI? In this low-likelihood group, the simple decision to exercise the patient acutely, without waiting for enzyme results, was probably enough to exclude AMI and permit an outpatient evaluation!

Stomel et al. (416) reported on the effects of the establishment of a chest pain center with the implementation of stress testing screening in patients presenting with chest pain syndromes with intermediate risk. Although hospital admissions fell 21%, referrals to the center increased by 1726%. Among 333 patients with an intermediate risk, there were no deaths and only one non-Q infarction. However, stress testing was normal in 11 patients with subsequently proven CAD and 4 with revascularization, and there were 9 false positives among 13 patients with positive stress tests!

Stress testing alone often has been found to be insufficient for risk stratification in unstable angina and after infarction and certainly suffers in comparison with stress MPS. Is it well applied as a triage method in patients presenting with chest pain? In some subgroups? When the problem is thoughtfully assessed, there will be an expanded role for dynamic and pharmacologic stress MPS to complement the standard stress test in this setting as in others.

Echocardiography.

Rest Echocardiography. The utility of echocardiography in identifying patients with unstable angina has been evaluated in a limited number of studies involving a small number of patients. Generally, rest echocardiography has been applied. Stein et al. (417) reported a sensitivity of 92% and a specificity of 69% for predicting major in-hospital complications in 63 patients.

Rest echocardiography has been applied to the evaluation of patients presenting with ROMI with somewhat varying criteria and limited success. Wall motion abnormalities have been found to resolve rapidly if imaged serially after chest pain presentation with ST abnormalities but no infarction. Such imaging must be performed during chest pain, or sensitivity falls to unacceptable levels (418).

Sabia et al. (419) applied 2-dimensional echocardiography in 180 high-risk patients presenting to the ED. Tailored criteria for CAD diagnosis brought a high sensitivity and predictive value of a positive test with a poor specificity and predictive value of a negative test.

Rest echocardiography was applied in acute coronary syndromes in a series of studies (420–422). It demonstrated a high sensitivity in patients with a Q-wave MI and a moderate sensitivity in 79 patients with a non-Q MI (420). However, overall there was difficulty recognizing wall motion abnormalities with small transmural or non-Q MI, and diffuse wall motion abnormalities were nonspecific for CAD. Kontos et al. (421) found a modest sensitivity and specificity in 140 patients evaluated with rest echocardiography with possible acute coronary syndromes. The method may be best applied in ambiguous cases with ongoing chest pain, abnormal ECG and prior known normal left ventricular function.

Stress Echocardiography. Stress echocardiography has not been applied widely to the evaluation of CAD in patients with unstable angina. Studies are generally subjective and qualitative, with few studies of risk stratification and outcomes. The latter generally relate to LVEF, which is not measured at stress echocardiography, either with exercise or pharmacologic stress.

Lin et al. (406) evaluated the "incremental prognostic value" of exercise echocardiography in 226 medically treated patients with unstable angina. The stress echocardiogram was not used for decision making, and 18% of patients who went to revascularization were never studied. A positive stress echocardiogram was related to a 9% event rate, but the event rate in those with a normal stress echocardiogram was still >3%/yr.

Trippi et al. (422) applied dobutamine stress echocardiography to triage patients presenting to the ED with chest pain (422). Studies were performed by the ED staff and the technician on call in chest pain patients with a low risk of infarction and CAD. The study was transmitted to the on-call cardiologist, who read the study on a lap-top computer. The discharge of 41 patients after normal dobutamine stress echocardiograms brought a decrease in costs without adverse events at 30 days. There were still many needless admissions. Is dobutamine the pharmacologic agent of choice in patients presenting with a possible acute coronary syndrome? Is the echocardiographic method reproducible and accurate enough to apply in such cases?

The echocardiographic method is ubiquitous, highly portable and readily available to cardiologists and ED physicians. Yet, the method is not widely advocated as a method to risk stratify patients with unstable angina or non-Q MIs nor as an ED triage method. This speaks more eloquently than the literature and serves to summarize the findings. The generalized clinical use of echocardiography to triage patients for AMI or unstable angina has demonstrated poor sensitivity and specificity and has not been recommended or implemented.

Rest Perfusion Imaging. For many years, rest perfusion imaging has been applied successfully with ^{201}Tl using planar imaging to accurately diagnose unstable angina and AMI in patients presenting with a diagnosis of ROMI (423–425). The method was successfully applied to evaluate the extent of MIR and to

Table 21

DISADVANTAGES OF PLANAR THALLIUM-201 IMAGING FOR TRIAGE OF PATIENTS PRESENTING TO THE EMERGENCY DEPARTMENT WITH CHEST PAIN

Low sensitivity—overcome with SPECT

Temporal factor—redistribution

Physical factor—attenuation reduces specificity

Availability—cyclotron-produced

determine prognoses in patients with unstable angina and also has been used to determine the cause of rest ECG abnormalities. It demonstrated a high sensitivity and specificity for acute ischemic events in patients presenting with chest pain and related well to outcome, even when performed early after the resolution of chest pain (*423–426*).

Although MPS provides an excellent estimate of infarct size, size is likely overestimated when measured early (12–48 hr) after the event. This relates to the probable inclusion in the defect of viable myocardium at risk. Also, wall motion abnormalities related to stunning may relate to perfusion defects produced by the partial volume effect. A resolution of the defect may be heralded as resolution of hibernating myocardium, when, in fact, it simply relates to improved function after resolution of stunning! Prior infarction remains a confounding variable in the evaluation of MPS in the acute setting.

In addition to its suboptimal imaging characteristics, ^{201}Tl is cyclotron produced and not readily available (Table 21). Further, it redistributes and must be imaged soon after administration in order to assess the distribution of perfusion at the time of injection. Technetium-99m agents have much improved imaging characteristics, are generator produced and are readily available. Their general lack of redistribution permits delayed imaging of the injected dose with determination of the perfusion distribution at the time of administration. Concern for recognition and, when possible, exclusion of artifacts must be part of perfusion image analysis in general. Here, in its application to the patient with acute chest pain, it must be obsessively applied.

Technetium-99m sestamibi has been applied widely in the acute setting to determine the cause of spontaneous chest pain (*427*) (Figs. 56,57) (Table 22), as well for the diagnostic and prognostic evaluation of patients with unstable angina (*428*), the implications and distribution of AMI and the effects of thrombolysis and acute PTCA.

Recent studies have demonstrated the promise of rest sestamibi (and tetrofosmin) imaging performed in the ED (*429–432*). The studies suggest that this is a cost-effective tool to triage patients and assess the likelihood of AMI or an acute coronary syndrome among those presenting with chest pain and an ambiguous ECG to ROMI. A number of these studies demonstrate a high diagnostic accuracy of the method, with resultant dramatic reductions in hospital stays and related costs.

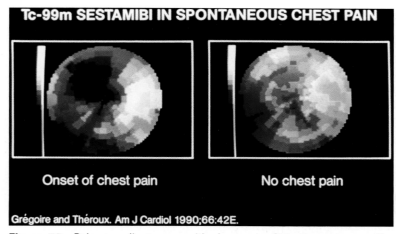

Figure 56 Polar coordinate map with chest pain. Objective polar coordinate maps from a SPECT perfusion image acquired in a patient during spontaneous chest pain (left) and after resolution (right). A similar principle, with administration of sestamibi at the time of presentation with acute chest pain, may aid early screening of patients for possible infarction and represent a cost-effective measure. (Reprinted, with permission, from Bilodeau L, Theroux P, Gregoire J, et al. Technetium-99m sestamibi tomography in patients with spontaneous chest pain: correlations with clinical, electrocardiographic and angiographic findings. *J Am Coll Cardiol* 1991;18:1684–1691.)

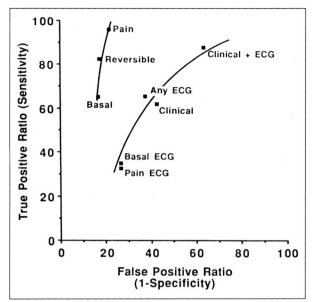

Figure 57 The diagnostic value of evaluation for myocardial infarction during spontaneous chest pain. When obtained during spontaneous chest pain (Pain), technetium-99m sestamibi SPECT studies were the most sensitive and specific of all clinical, electrocardiographic (ECG) and imaging criteria. A reversible sestamibi defect was a very sensitive indicator. SPECT myocardial perfusion scintigraphy acquired in the pain-free state (Basal) has a sensitivity in the range of 60%–65%, compared with that of basal ECG abnormalities with a sensitivity of 35%–40%. (Reprinted, with permission, from Bilodeau L, Theroux P, Gregoire J, et al. Technetium-99m sestamibi tomography in patients with spontaneous chest pain: correlations with clinical, electrocardiographic and angiographic findings. *J Am Coll Cardiol* 1991;18:1684–1691.)

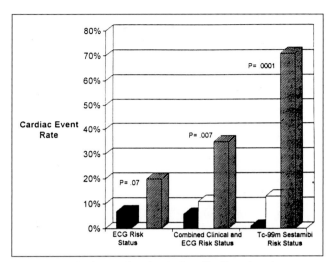

Figure 58 Risk stratification in low-likelihood patients presenting to the emergency department (ED) with chest pain. This bar graph relates the findings on electrocardiographic (ECG) analysis (left), combined clinical and ECG analysis (center) and sestamibi imaging (right) to the event rate among a population of 102 patients with relatively low CAD likelihood presenting to the ED with chest pain. Black bars = normal test result; white bars = equivocal test result; gray bars = positive test result. The superior risk stratification ability of the perfusion imaging method is clear. (Reprinted, with permission, from Hilton TC, Thompson RC, Williams HJ, et al. Technetium-99m sestamibi myocardial perfusion imaging in the emergency room for evaluation of chest pain. *J Am Coll Cardiol* 1994;23:1016–1022.)

Varetto et al. (*429*) used rest sestamibi to study 60 consecutive patients presenting to the ED for admission to ROMI with a nondiagnostic ECG. Patients with prior MI were excluded, and many of those imaged were pain free at the time of radionuclide administration. Among 30 with an abnormal sestamibi study, 27 (90%) had events. The method had a diagnostic sensitivity of 100%, a specificity of 92%, a predictive value of a positive test of 90% and a predictive value of a negative test of 100%. These workers also compared the accuracy of rest echocardiography with that of rest MPS for ED triage and found the echocardiographic method to have a much lower sensitivity.

The cost of a rest ^{99m}Tc sestamibi SPECT study should be in the range of $300–$500, comparable with that of other methods. This provides the potential for the advantages of reduced hospital (CCU) days, reduced costs and expeditious evaluation and management. Hilton et al. (*430*) studied 102 patients with typical angina and normal or nondiagnostic ECGs. Those with a history of MI were excluded. Patients were injected during pain. The radionuclide was available from 8:00 AM to 12:00 PM. Only 10% of eligible patients were not studied because the imaging agent was unavailable. Those with coronary events could not be separated from those without on the basis of age, sex, type of pain,

Table 22
TECHNETIUM-99M SESTAMIBI (TETROFOSMIN) PERFUSION
SCINTIGRAPHY FOR TRIAGE OF PATIENTS PRESENTING
TO THE EMERGENCY DEPARTMENT WITH CHEST PAIN

Advantages	Disadvantages
Perfusion + function	Cost? Single rest study
Perfusion more sensitive and specific than wall motion	Availability, logistics
Reproducibility	Differentiate acute and remote myocardial infarction
Defects persist long after clinical ischemia	Not real-time
Objectivity (normal data base)	"Radiation"
Quantitative relation to myocardial infarction, ischemia and prognosis, as continuous variables	
Choice of pharmacologic stress method; dilator stress sensitive	
Inadequate studies are rare	

coronary risk factors, physical exam or ECG results. However, none of 34 patients with normal sestamibi images had CAD on subsequent stress testing and/or coronary angiography and all were event free after 18 mo of follow-up. Overall, only 1 patient among 70 with a normal scan had an event (bypass surgery), with a predictive value of a negative test of 98%. Among 17 patients with a positive image, 12 had events, a positive predictive value of 71%. Two patients among 15 with equivocal tests had events. Multivariate regression analysis identified an abnormal sestamibi study as the only predictor of an adverse event ($P = 0.009$). An abnormal image had a sensitivity of 94% and specificity of 80% for all events, with sensitivity of 100% and specificity of 78% for AMI. The ED sestamibi study separated 85% of the population into low-risk (1%–2%) and high-risk (>70%) groups.

Further, the high specificity permitted reduction of admission based on image findings. With conventional triage, 50%–70% of those presenting to the ED are admitted, with an event rate of 20%. With the findings in this study by Hilton et al. (*430*), only 30% of patients were admitted, with an event rate >70% (Figs. 58–61). Figure 62 demonstrates the superiority of rest MPS with ^{99m}Tc sestamibi over rest echocardiography for the triage of patients presenting to the ED with chest pain.

In 3 studies (*430–432*), a normal rest ED sestamibi study had a benign long-term outcome, with no events in 166 patients followed for 3–18 mo. In another study, Wackers et al. (*445*) demonstrated the benefits of a normal rest SPECT perfusion image performed with tetrofosmin in patients presenting to the ED with chest pain and normal or nondiagnostic ECG.

Tatum et al. (*434*) used rest SPECT sestamibi imaging to study 135 patients presenting to the ED with chest pain. Of these patients, 27 had abnormal images, including 18 among 19 (95%) with CAD and AMI or unstable angina. Among 88 with normal images, CAD was documented in only 1, an overall specificity of 88% (87/96), with positive and negative predictive values of 67% and 98%, respectively. There were wall motion abnormalities in 8 patients without CAD.

The same group (*435*) studied the potential cost effectiveness of initial myocardial perfusion imaging for the triage of patients presenting to the ED with chest pain. In the "scan strategy," those with abnormal images were admitted, whereas those with normal scans were sent home. The "no scan strategy" employed clinical and ECG variables to triage patients. Those with ≥3 risk factors or abnormalities were admitted, whereas all others were sent home. The costs were greatest among those patients who were admitted and who had adverse events: $21,375/patient. The costs were lowest among patients discharged from the ED: $715/patient. Overall, the "scan strategy" cost $5,019/patient, whereas the "no scan strategy" cost $6,051/patient.

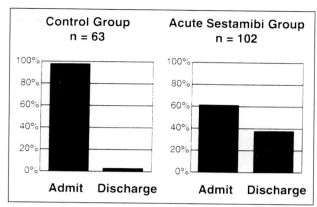

Figure 59 Effects of altered practice patterns. These bar graphs show the percentage of low-likelihood patients presenting to the emergency department with chest pain that are admitted or discharged, in a control group (left) and a group of 102 patients after screening with the addition of rest sestamibi imaging (see Fig. 61). (Reprinted, with permission, from Hilton TC, Thompson RC, Williams HJ, et al. Technetium-99m sestamibi myocardial perfusion imaging in the emergency room for evaluation of chest pain. *J Am Coll Cardiol* 1994;23:1016–1022.)

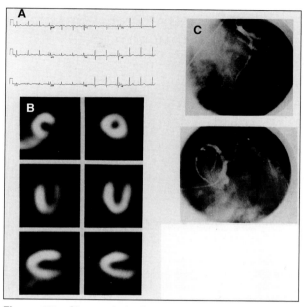

Figure 60 Chest pain in the emergency department (ED). Case example: (A) Normal electrocardiogram in a patient presenting to the ED with chest pain and a grossly abnormal rest technetium-99m sestamibi SPECT scan. (B, left panel) Coronary angiography demonstrated a left circumflex coronary occlusion, (C, upper panel) which was opened (C, lower panel) with subsequent normalization of the repeated perfusion scan (B, right panel). (Reprinted, with permission, from Hilton TC, Thompson RC, Williams HJ, et al. Technetium-99m sestamibi myocardial perfusion imaging in the emergency room for evaluation of chest pain. *J Am Coll Cardiol* 1994;23:1016–1022.)

In their largest report, Tatum et al. (*436*) applied rest sestamibi images to risk stratify 1187 consecutive patients with acute chest pain. The image sensitivity for AMI diagnosis was 100%, and specificity was 78%. Here, 32% with abnormal scans, but only 3% with normal scans, had revascularization. Over 1-yr follow-up, there was not a single death or nonfatal infarction in any patient with a normal scan. A 19% "hard event" rate was reported among those with abnormal scans.

Kontos et. al (*437*) reported the diagnostic value of gated rest SPECT sestamibi images and serial myocardial specific enzymes sampled over 8 hr in a group of 620 patients presenting to the ED with a low-to-intermediate likelihood for an acute coronary syndrome. There were 59 (9%) patients with acute MI, 81 others (13%) had CAD and 58 of the latter had revascularization. Sensitivity for detecting AMI was similar for imaging and serial troponin levels (92% and 90%, respectively). However, although rest gated MPS had an 82% sensitivity for the detection of AMI and all CAD, serial troponin had a 53% sensitivity and the initial troponin had only a 10% sensitivity. Rest MPS had a 76% specificity for AMI and all CAD, compared with 97% for serial troponin. The study concluded that the 2 methods provide complementary information for the identification of patients with acute coronary syndromes.

Kontos et al. (*438*) also compared the use of rest sestamibi to screen low-risk patients presenting to the ED with a similar prior group presenting in the same way but not so evaluated. Those evaluated by MPS had a lower rate of referral to catheterization but a greater proportion of significant disease and no greater risk.

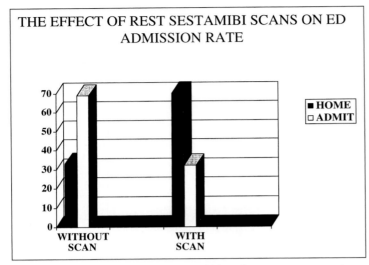

Figure 61   The effect of rest sestamibi imaging on emergency department admission rate. Shown graphically is the reduction in hospital admissions achieved in the study by Hilton et al. when coronary risk was considered and a control group was not employed. Here, 69 of the 102 study patients were initially classified as intermediate or high coronary risk. After study with rest technetium-99m sestamibi, only 32 patients had abnormal or equivocal scans that would bring admission. With an additional effort, the equivocal group could be significantly reduced and the advantage of the method enhanced yet further. However, in practice, many more low-likelihood patients are admitted (see Fig. 59). (Reprinted, with permission, from Hilton TC, Thompson RC, Williams HJ, et al. Technetium-99m sestamibi myocardial perfusion imaging in the emergency room for evaluation of chest pain. *J Am Coll Cardiol* 1994;23:1016–1022.)

The sum of other studies presented at the American Heart Association (AHA) meeting in 1999 indicated that 240,000 unnecessary admissions could be avoided and $85 million saved if rest ^{99m}Tc sestamibi studies were applied to triage ambiguous and relatively-low likelihood patients presenting to the ED with chest pain.

A large prospective randomized trial was conducted at 7 clinical centers in the northeast United States. Here, 2456 patients (50% women, 50% men) with low AMI likelihood presenting to the ED to ruleout AMI, with ambiguous symptoms and nondiagnostic ECGs, were assigned randomly to conventional care or conventional care with rest SPECT sestamibi study (*439*). In the scan group, there were no instructions as to how the ED team was to use the findings. Nevertheless, overall there was a 20% reduction in hospital admissions without loss of sensitivity for AMI or unstable angina diagnosis. If applied nationwide, the results indicate a reduction of 240,000 admissions and a savings of many millions of dollars.

The ability of the rest MPS method to identify those benefiting from acute revascularization in the absence of diagnostic ECG changes was well documented by Christian et al. (*400*) in a small population presenting with classic symptoms of AMI but with nonspecific ECG findings prohibiting acute thrombolysis. This early and specific diagnosis, relating image defects to a coronary occlusion in 12 of 14 patients studied, permitted early intervention and revascularization. These were just the "tip of the iceberg," because most patients with AMI and occlusion cannot be recognized by ECG changes. The method may not only benefit rapid diagnosis but aid and speed delivery of needed treatment or aggressive management. Here, diagnostic specificity and sensitivity are required. This study suggests that the method may permit not only economies of management but also present new insight into pathophysiology and prognosis. The method has demonstrated its ability to identify the extent of MIR in AMI (*440*) but is thought to be at some disadvantage in the presence of a prior infarction (image defect). This can be turned to advantage and impressive comparisons made with this reproducible, quantifiable method in the presence of a readily accessible prior study.

In a small study by Sciammarella et al. (*441*) of 30 patients admitted with ambiguous presentations to ROMI, 7 had image abnormalities, each with an acute coronary syndrome. Only 1 of the remainder was seen to have ischemia on subsequent stress imaging. Most of the other 22 patients subsequently demonstrated a noncardiac cause of symptoms. Some patients were evaluated by stress imaging, which showed larger defects compared with the ED rest study, whereas others demonstrated rest ED sestamibi defects comparable with those previously or subsequently demonstrated on stress imaging. Many patients

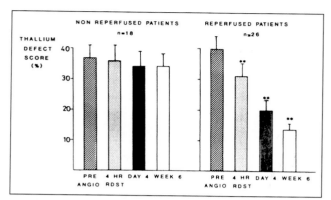

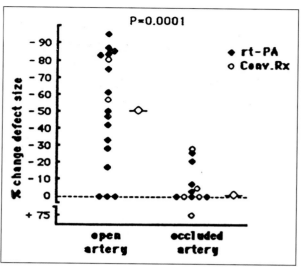

Figure 73 The effects of thrombolysis on defect size. Shown is the mean value of thallium-201 (^{201}Tl) defect scores in patients presenting with an acute infarction before (preangio) and 4 hr after streptokinase (4-hr redistribution; RDST), as well as 4 days and 6 wk later in nonreperfused (left) and reperfused patients (right). Serial improvement in ^{201}Tl defect score does not occur precipitously but is evident over the entire period. (Reprinted, with permission, from DeCoster PM, Melin JA, Detry JM, et al. Coronary artery reperfusion in acute myocardial infarction: effect of intravenous followed by intracoronary streptokinase application on estimates of infarct size. *Am J Cardiol* 1985;58:889–895.)

Figure 74 Defect size after thrombolysis. The status of the infarct-related artery in patients receiving technetium-99m sestamibi before and after thrombolytic therapy (rt-PA) or after conventional treatment (conv Rx) was the single most important factor, unrelated to anatomic location of the effected vessel, which determined the change in perfusion defect size. (Reprinted, with permission, from Wackers FJTh, Gibbons RJ, Verani MS, et al. Serial quantitative planar technetium-99m isonitrile imaging in acute myocardial infarction: efficacy for noninvasive assessment of thrombolytic therapy. *J Am Coll Cardiol* 1989;14:861–873.)

Such studies demonstrated the feasibility of the scintigraphic method as a substitute for clinical events as an end point in the evaluation of interventions in AMI. Animal experiments were performed to measure the extent of MIR. These determined that the region of risk was modulated by the extent of collateral flow, the duration of occlusion and the severity of myocardial oxygen demands (*502*). This method can better distinguish the effects of therapy than LVEF, for example, where the latter may be preserved in the presence of a small risk region unaffected by therapy or with a large risk region salvaged with prompt restoration of local arterial patency. A population of 40,000 was included in the GUSTO Trial to demonstrate the mortality benefit of thrombolytic therapy (*290*). However, Gibbons et al. (*468*) used the perfusion imaging method in only 50 patients to demonstrate, with a high level of statistical dependability, the similar effectiveness of direct PTCA and thrombolytic therapy.

After instrumentation, of course, the possibility of altered lesion stability plays a large role, along with lesion severity, in the likelihood of subsequent occlusion or restenosis (*503*). Yet, as in the uninstrumented patient, such noninvasive image evaluation can aid selection of patients for subsequent intervention. MPS has been shown in several blinded studies (*273,504*) to be of great value for the assessment of the benefit of thrombolysis. It has been the noninvasive research method employed, with comparison of pre- and postintervention perfusion studies (*280–284,504*), to determine the value of thrombolysis and other pharmacologic methods of revascularization (*283,505*). Its utility was established with assessment of relatively small patient numbers, in whom perfusion defect size was used as a surrogate end point for death or MI (*275–277*). In this way, the

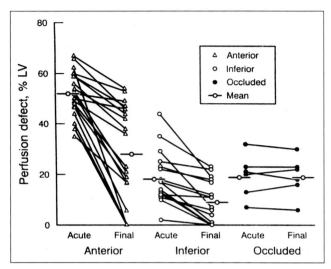

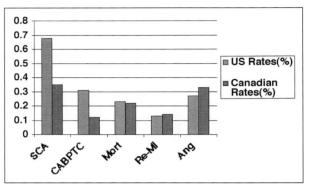

Figure 75 Determinants of defect size after thrombolysis. Shown is the perfusion defect size determined before reperfusion therapy (Acute) and at discharge (Final) with technetium-99m isonitrile SPECT imaging, related to the infarct location and restoration of arterial patency. Although anterior infarcts were larger because of the extent of the perfusion zone of the effected vessel and demonstrated a greater reduction in defect size after revascularization, both anterior and inferior infarcts showed a significant reduction in defect size after reperfusion therapy ($P < 0.001$ for both). (Reprinted, with permission, from Christian TF, Gibbons RJ, Gersh BJ, et al. Effect of infarct location on myocardial salvage assessed by technetium-99m isonitrile. *J Am Coll Cardiol* 1991;17:1303–1308.)

Figure 76 Patient management after myocardial infarction (MI) and associated clinical outcomes. Shown are rates of selective coronary angiography (SCA), revascularization (CABPTC), mortality (Mort), "reinfarction" (Re-MI) and angina (Ang) in the United States and Canada. After infarction, patients are studied invasively and revascularized at a much higher rate in the United States, without obvious improvement in outcomes, subsequent infarction or death, but with a somewhat lower frequency of angina. Perfusion scintigraphy is employed sparingly and selectively, but with a greater influence on management decisions in Canada, where it is concentrated in major centers that offer invasive evaluation and treatment. Do we do perform too many coronary angiograms in the United States? Do we perform too many perfusion scintigrams—or too few? (Reprinted with permission from Rouleau JL, Moye' LA, Pfeffer MA, et al. A comparison of management patterns after acute myocardial infarction in Canada and the United States. *N Engl J Med* 1993;328:779–784.)

benefits of thrombolysis and other interventions, such as acute angioplasty or stents, can be determined in hours. With the administration on presentation of ^{99m}Tc sestamibi or other ^{99m}Tc-based perfusion agent and subsequent imaging after intervention, image evidence of the presenting perfusion defect, the results of intervention and the extent of myocardium salvaged can be documented.

The perfusion scintigraphic method has become the noninvasive method of choice for the evaluation of "complex and difficult" patients. This saves costs and directs appropriate patient management based on pathophysiologic findings, compared with the invasive approach, in which decision making is based solely on the anatomy, which is too often ambiguous. In fact, lesser rates of angiography, with greater weight in decision making applied to the clinical and noninvasive findings, has demonstrated no worsening of the clinical outcome at a considerable cost saving, such as has been implemented in the Canadian health care system (*506–509*). In Canada, noninvasive imaging is currently widely used as a guide to the performance of more selective invasive studies and appears to be a reasonable way to guide invasive evaluation (*16*) (Fig. 76).

Gating. A recent study indicates that acute infarct size is most accurately measured on nongated images (*510*). Recent studies have confirmed previous impressions demonstrating that quantitative sestamibi MI size, measured without gating at the time of admission and including infarcted and ischemic myocardium, predicts subsequent mortality (*217*). Therefore, gating can be used to assess systolic function. The rest data file can then be "collapsed" to yield the ungated set, with greatest prognostic perfusion value. Subsequent stress MPS can be applied to assess the amount of MIR and prognosis.

The Strategy for Postinfarction Risk Stratification. Prognosis and risk stratification, rather than diagnosis, are always the indications for stress testing post-MI in patients with a high pretest likelihood and significant CAD risk (Table 25). MPS is the leading prognostic method in CAD, with clear advantages over simple stress testing and other imaging methods based in function evaluation and is superior in many studies to coronary angiography (*511,512*). MPS is indicated wherever coronary risk is the variable to be assessed in patient groups with intermediate-to-high pretest likelihood. Excluding those who are at known high risk based on clinical presentation or course and those with known unambiguous native or postrevascularization anatomy, all post-MI patient groups are potentially suited for such evaluation.

Postinfarct patients who are stable after several days can be risk stratified well with stress testing then or just before discharge. However, the recommendations of published guidelines lag behind current data and are strongly influenced by economic and political considerations. Although studies have demonstrated the value of stress perfusion imaging for prognosis in patients with an intermediate or high CAD likelihood, specifically post-MI, the ACC/ American Heart Association (AHA) Task Force *Report on Acute Myocardial Infarction* (*513*) recommends exercise testing alone as a submaximal test for prognosis and functional evaluation, performed 4–6 days after the event, or as a symptom-limited test given early after discharge, at 14–21 days. However, the recommended delay in testing leaves patients vulnerable to unseen events in the interim and unnecessarily delays appropriate management. Furthermore, exercise testing alone appears to be unsatisfactory for risk stratification after infarction, with a 25% sensitivity to events among 10 studies reviewed by Brown, in which ST changes were themselves nonpredictive of events (*357*). Exercise perfusion imaging or echocardiography are also recommended by the guidelines as most appropriately indicated (class I) but only when the stress ECG is uninterpretable (as a result of LBBB, digoxin, LVH, etc.). Vasodilator stress perfusion imaging or dobutamine stress imaging were both recommended less enthusiastically with the same Class IIa classification, to be applied only in those who cannot exercise satisfactorily. In spite of this equal standing, vasodilator stress with MPS is widely applied, whereas dobutamine and exercise echocardiography have been lightly applied in this setting and dobutamine could be problematic in the setting of acute ischemia. Although the TIMI II Trial (*514*) and others demonstrated high coronary risk among those unable to exercise and relatively low risk among those who can exercise to stage II of the Bruce Protocol or >6 METS, these patients represent a heterogeneous group, well and safely substratified by pharmacologic stress imaging with a coronary dilator. Although several studies demonstrate safe and effective risk stratification with a coronary dilator (dipyridamole or adenosine) stress test performed within 1–4 days of the event (*479–486*) and this is in common practice among many patient

---

Table 25

WHEN IS PERFUSION IMAGING COST EFFECTIVE FOR CORONARY ARTERY DISEASE (CAD) DIAGNOSIS OR PROGNOSIS?

With an interpretable rest electrocardiograph:
    For diagnosis—in selected patients with intermediate pretest likelihood of CAD
    For prognosis—in those with intermediate or high pretest likelihood of CAD

When the rest electrocardiograph is uninterpretable or with vasodilator pharmacologic stress testing:
    In all groups

---

subgroups, these are designated as class III (contra)indications. As with the Unstable Angina Guidelines (*31*), there is no effort made to distinguish between documented advantages of the different methods and modalities, although the amount of data available demonstrating the prognostic value of stress echocardiography is sparse. Yet, in a review of 10 studies of exercise testing after MI, Brown (*36*) demonstrated the disappointing sensitivity (27%) of exercise testing for prediction of events and showed that the presence of ST changes was as predictive of a subsequent event as their absence! The TIMI II Trial (*2,278,514*) demonstrated that those who can exercise were a relatively low-risk group, whereas those who could not were a heterogeneous group harboring many high-risk patients. These facts indicate the appropriate class I indication of pharmacologic stress MPS for all stable patients who cannot exercise adequately.

Currently, many researchers advocate the routine catheterization of all patients with AMI, despite the limited recommendation of this intervention in current guidelines. Based upon published data (*16,506–509*), an alternate strategy may be applied to stable post-MI patients without clear indication for revascularization (*510*). Here, catheterization is avoided or delayed until clinical indications present themselves or the patient is noted to be at high risk by stress test indicators primarily based in MPS. Post-MI patients with recurring angina, evidence of left ventricular dysfunction, heart failure or significant arrhythmias would be considered high-risk patients who should be referred to angiography directly, without need for initial noninvasive evaluation. However, post-MI patients who are clinically stable and asymptomatic or with nonspecific symptoms may be referred to stress MPS. Patients demonstrating high-risk scintigrams, whether performed using pharmacologic or exercise stress, should be treated aggressively and generally are referred to angiography because of related risk, even in the absence of ongoing symptoms (Tables 11,12,14).

After Interventions

Evaluation of Patients at Coronary Angiography. Reproducibility and Relationship of Visual Stenosis Assessment to Flow Reserve. Superiority of Myocardial Perfusion Scintigraphy. Numerous studies have demonstrated the poor reproducibility and frequent inadequacy of visually interpreted coronary angiograms in determining the hemodynamic significance of coronary artery lesions (*513–519*). Doppler evaluation has confirmed this insensitivity of angiographic coronary anatomic evaluation (*520*) with the demonstration of abnormal flow reserve in patients with abnormal perfusion images and normal coronary arteries (*521*). Miller et al. (*522*) studied a cohort of patients with coronary stenoses of indeterminate significance, comparing the results of quantitative coronary angiography, sestamibi SPECT imaging and coronary reserve measured with an intracoronary Doppler flow probe. They demonstrated the best correlation to be between flow reserve measurements and sestamibi uptake (89% agreement; $\kappa = 0.78$) (Figs. 77,78). These studies suggest that among those patients with equivocal angiographic findings, MPS can identify those lesions that are physiologically significant and thus those patients who are at greater risk. Subsequently, in such cases, decisions about revascularization, particularly with PTCA, can be based on both physiological and anatomical data. The same authors (*523*) measured basal and hyperemic proximal and distal coronary flow velocities in the instrumented vessels with intracoronary Doppler and performed rest–stress sestamibi SPECT MPS in 34 consecutive patients within 3 mo of successful PTCA. In spite of significant angiographic improvement after

revascularization. If positive, stress MPS may be considered or the patient taken directly to angiography.

Based on AHA–ACC guidelines, the goal early after revascularization is to assess the result of the intervention and the likelihood of restenosis after PTCA. Stress MPS has an excellent ability to assess perfusion after revascularization and predict subsequent stenosis. Late after PTCA, the goal is to recognize worsening CAD and nonrevascularized segments. Although MPS may be of value in symptomatic patients or incompletely revascularized patients after PTCA, it is not recommended (a class III indication) as a routine study in asymptomatic patients after PTCA. The periodic evaluation of high-risk asymptomatic patients after PTCA is a class IIB indication.

A recommended approach to the post-PTCA patient justified by the proven ability of the method and the clinical need is outlined later in this book in the section on Summary Strategy. If the purpose of the procedure is to relieve symptoms and to improve the quality of life, there is no basis for performing follow-up testing in the asymptomatic patient. However, the recurrence of symptoms or functional limitation comparable with those before the intervention are indications for either stress MPS or repeat catheterization, depending on the gravity or clarity of symptoms. The implications of symptoms different from or less severe than those of the initial presentation are grounds for noninvasive assessment to determine the presence, extent and severity of perfusion abnormalities and MIR. If PTCA was performed to modify outcome after infarction, the intermediate likelihood of restenosis resulting in significant recurrent risk presents adequate justification for stress MPS, even in the absence of recurrent symptoms. In patients who have positive exercise tests or exercise-induced symptoms before PTCA, an exercise test as the initial study rather than stress imaging may be appropriate. Those with intermediate-to-high postexercise test likelihood of ischemia would then be referred for MPS or angiography, depending on the findings on stress testing. Those patients who had no ischemic symptoms or ECG changes before PTCA (silent ischemia), those patients with an uninterpretable stress ECG, diabetics with an increased incidence of restenosis or patients considered to be at high risk because of coronary anatomy or ventricular dysfunction would be referred to stress MPS 3–6 mo after PTCA. From a technical perspective, SPECT imaging, as opposed to planar perfusion imaging or other imaging methods, is particularly suitable for this application because of its unique ability to provide a clear "roadmap" of coronary involvement, with delineation of regional ischemia or ischemic potential and its relationship to a specific vascular territory.

Evaluation of Patients After Coronary Artery Bypass Graft Surgery. Neither the workload achieved nor the stress ECG were able to risk stratify patients after CABG. Stress-induced ST abnormalities, even deep ST depressions, often persist in spite of adequate revascularization and symptomatic relief after CABG (195). In a group of 873 symptom-free patients studied with exercise perfusion scintigraphy after CABG, ^{201}Tl defects and exercise capacity were strong and independent predictors of subsequent death and nonfatal infarction (550). An exercise capacity <6 METS was the best predictor of hard events in some studies (22,515), but workload is an entirely nonspecific finding. Desideri et al. (551) demonstrated a greater predictive value and a significantly higher χ^2 for stress MPS than for the clinical history, symptoms or results of exercise testing. Age, time after CABG and quantitative defect score were 3 independent predictors of hard events after revascularization surgery (552,553).

As noted previously, the routine image evaluation of asymptomatic patients after revascularization is inappropriate (554). Published ACC/AHA guidelines

(*161,531*) support stress testing or stress imaging evaluation when post-CABG patients present renewed symptoms or in selected asymptomatic patients with ECG changes or an ischemic stress ECG response. Further, the study is appropriate to quantitate left ventricular function and may be applied in the setting of incomplete revascularization, baseline multivessel disease, after a perioperative infarction, with new or worsening heart failure, in those who cannot exercise, with ventricular arrhythmias and in diabetics, a high-risk subgroup prone to distal disease and progressive atherosclerosis. Similar to its application after angioplasty, MPS is applied well in patients with prerevascularization silent ischemia, those with uninterpretable ECGs and with mild or ambiguous symptoms. The pattern of perfusion should be correlated with the known angiographic anatomy to determine the vascular state of the region.

Four recent studies (*346,554–556*) demonstrated the strong predictive value of reversible or multiple perfusion defects as the strongest independent predictor of events 2–10 yr after CABG. Miller et al. (*556*) studied patients 2 yr after CABG and found the extent of stress-induced defect to be an important prognostic indicator. Here, small defects represented incomplete revascularization and were not prognostically important. The prognostic importance of induced defect size after CABG has been proven important by Palmas et al. (*555*) and others (*346,550,557*). Most with revascularization procedures are well revascularized and do not necessarily need a stress MPS study. It is recommended that asymptomatic patients need no study after CABG until at least 5 yr, when graft attrition begins to reach significance. One group possibly needing earlier evaluation is diabetics, who were shown to have significantly worse outcomes (*558*).

Applied early to the assessment of myocardial perfusion after bypass surgery, MPS is generally used to assess postrevascularization symptoms or to determine the significance of apparent angiographic progression. It became clear early on that even successful surgery not uncommonly results in much improved but incomplete revascularization. Modest abnormalities are common and acceptable after the procedure, because CABG may make the patient better but not normal. For that reason, ascribing symptoms to limited image defects seen after CABG is risky, because these are likely much improved compared with the preoperative study. It is a great advantage to have a preoperative study when evaluating symptoms after surgery (*559,560*). Without such a baseline, even if performed early after CABG, subsequent evaluation is difficult to interpret securely in a clinical context, except when grossly abnormal. It is known that scan defects may precede post-CABG ischemic symptoms. Preserved scan perfusion essentially excludes graft stenosis.

An approach developed by Hachamovitch et al. (*556*) to apply in patients who have undergone CABG is outlined later in the Summary Strategy. Although exercise perfusion imaging performed within 2 yr of CABG could stratify patients into low- and high-risk subgroups, the literature suggests that risk increases significantly 5 yr after saphenous vein grafts are placed (*556*). After that time, 15%–40% of patent grafts show abnormalities, ranging from luminal irregularities to significant stenoses, and an additional 20%–28% of grafts will be occluded, overall presenting an intermediate likelihood of significant ischemia at this time point (*561*).

Exercise myocardial perfusion SPECT was an independent and incremental predictor of outcome in patients >5 yr after CABG. Palmas et al. (*555*) demonstrated that the cardiac event rate >5 yr after CABG increased with the image ischemia score and with time after revascularization. After evaluation of treadmill exercise data, ^{201}Tl myocardial perfusion SPECT provided incremental prognostic information in such patients studied late after CABG (*555*), with results similar to those found in a general population using planar thallium imaging (*562*).

Here, the excellent prognostic value of stress perfusion imaging performed late (>5 yr) after CABG was demonstrated. However, after 10–15 yr, there was a somewhat increased event rate, even in those with normal stress images. Nallamothu et al. (346) demonstrated that the predictive value of MPS is greater than that of the angiographic anatomy in patients >5 yr after CABG. Here, image defects were seen with nongrafted vessels, entrapped grafts, disease beyond grafts and diseased grafts. These specific scenarios can be predicted by relating image defects to vascular anatomy and can be related at angiography to the patient-specific anatomy. Individuals in this cohort had an excellent prognosis in the setting of a normal scan, but those patients with severe and/or extensive abnormalities had poor prognoses and more frequent referral to revascularization late after testing. The use of clinical risk factors in combination with MPS appears to be a cost-effective approach in this population. In light of these findings, it seems prudent to consider stress MPS for patients >5 yr after CABG and in those who are symptomatic at any point after surgery. Referral to cardiac catheterization should follow imaging in those patients in whom moderate to severe ischemia is present. In >2000 patients evaluated after CABG, prognosis again appeared directly related to the extent of reversible defect size (346,550,555,556).

Gating has been applied to the evaluation of the results of CABG (195,554). Abnormal perfusion images were not uncommonly detected in the presence of normal left ventricular function and LVEF. The combination of perfusion and function, here as elsewhere, promises augmented clinical value. In a study of 489 patients evaluated after PTCA or CABG by both radionuclide angiography and stress perfusion scintigraphy, perfusion image findings were found to add to those of left ventricular function as a predictor of cardiac death or nonfatal infarction (198).

Risk Stratification Before Noncardiac Surgery

Exercise MPS certainly may be performed to risk stratify high-risk patients before major noncardiac surgery. However, because many of these patients cannot perform the intense exercise often needed to gain a high negative predictive value, pharmacologic stress with maximal coronary dilatation and test of the CFR is generally applied. This is discussed in depth in *Self-Study Program III. Cardiology. Topic 2: Pharmacologic Stress.*

Application of Stress Myocardial Perfusion Scintigraphy in Women

The application of MPS in women has been made an issue of even higher importance by detractors misrepresenting the method (Tables 27,28). Often quoting old or selected literature, some reviewers suggest that MPS is at a major disadvantage compared with

Table 27
METHODS THAT AID IMAGE EVALUATION IN WOMEN (AND MEN!) AND THAT AID IDENTIFICATION OF ATTENUATION ARTIFACT

With planar imaging
  Analysis of defect distribution (modest anterior defect, sparing apex and septum; limited lateral defect)*
  Correlation of findings with body habitus*
  Acquisition of image with breast retracted or in right lateral decubitus position*
  Use of technetium-99m–based imaging agents*
  Consultation with circumferential profiles

With SPECT imaging

SPECT imaging itself

Consultation with projection images

Consultation with polar maps

Prone imaging (reduced patient motion, diaphragmatic and breast attenuation)

Gating

Attenuation correction

Evidence of differential attenuation

*Applies to both planar and SPECT imaging

Table 28

ADVANTAGES OF STRESS PERFUSION IMAGING IN WOMEN

Increased diagnostic accuracy

Increased prognostic value

With vasodilator coronary stress

Lowest risk with a normal study

Cost-effective risk stratification to guide patient management

stress echocardiography for the diagnosis and risk stratification of CAD in women. They do not consider the current data as here presented and reviewed more thoroughly elsewhere. The issue is compounded further by concern regarding a sex bias in the application of diagnostic and therapeutic methods in CAD. Yet, the high diagnostic accuracy of the method and its unbiased application in women is presented in the reviews of Miller (*563*) and Travin and Johnson (*564*).

Stress Testing. Given the problems of the stress ECG in women, the advantages of MPS are potentially increased. Here, a reliable MPS may prevent needless angiography or counter a disabling fear in women with atypical chest pain. However, as with all methods, MPS is not immune to the problem of false-positive tests. Inevitably, as disease incidence falls, both test specificity and the predictive value of a positive test suffer! MPS must have a relatively high specificity to reduce the problem, but this will not eliminate it in the evaluation of low-likelihood patients. When the female population evaluated is appropriate for study they will benefit, as do men, from both the diagnostic and prognostic advantages of the scintigraphic method (*5*) (Figs. 80,81).

Image Artifacts. Because of the failure to understand and then to recognize soft tissue attenuation artifact, planar and early SPECT studies demonstrated reduced diagnostic specificity in women and large patients of both sexes, a group that presents a special diagnostic challenge. The trained practitioner now can accurately apply the method clinically in patients of both sexes of all sizes and dimensions.

The cause and effects of attenuation now are well understood, and their recognition is at an advanced stage. Attenuation defect size and density have been significantly reduced by the use of SPECT imaging, with the application of ^{99m}Tc-based perfusion agents and by the utilization of associated planar projection, prone and gated images and polar maps, which help to interpret the findings (*149*) (Table 27) (Figs. 82–84). The application of these methods and tools has reduced the effects of breast attenuation and associated false-positive studies without reducing the high prognostic value of negative tests in women. In addition to anterior breast attenuation, the relatively smaller size of the female heart and end-systolic volume <20 cc have been reported to represent particular problems reducing test sensitivity (*307*) (Fig. 40).

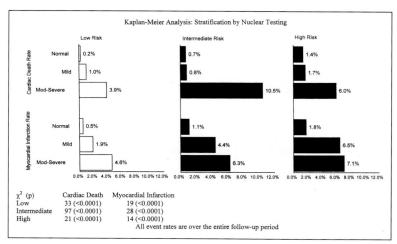

Figure 80 Differential risk. Shown is the higher rate of cardiac death (top panels) and myocardial infarction (MI) (bottom panels) among patients with moderate-to-severe scan defects, whereas mild defects related only to increased MI rates in 5183 consecutive patients undergoing stress myocardial perfusion scintigraphy. The relationships were most dramatic among those with intermediate (middle panels) or high (right panels) coronary risk. (Reprinted, with permission, from Hachamovitch R, Berman DS, Shaw LJ, et al. Incremental prognostic value of myocardial perfusion single photon emission computed tomography for the prediction of cardiac death: differential stratification for risk of cardiac death and myocardial infarction. *Circulation* 1998;97:535–543.)

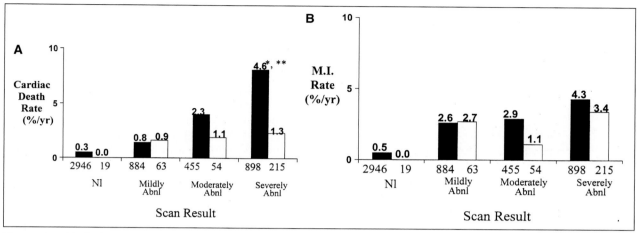

Figure 81 Perfusion scintigraphy guides therapy. Shown are rates of cardiac death (top) and myocardial infarction (MI) (bottom) per year as a function of scan result in a group of 5183 consecutive patients undergoing adenosine and exercise stress. Solid bars represent patients undergoing initial medical therapy after nuclear testing, and open bars represent patients undergoing revascularization early after nuclear testing. Surgical revascularization appeared to reduce death rate especially in those with severely abnormal scans but was not different from medical therapy in the prevention of infarction. *P < 0.01 versus patients undergoing revascularization early after nuclear testing. **P < 0.001 within patients treated with medical therapy after nuclear testing. NI =normal; Abnl = abnormal; Mod = moderately; Sev = severe. (Reprinted, with permission, from Hachamovitch R, Berman DS, Shaw LJ, et al. Incremental prognostic value of myocardial perfusion single photon emission computed tomography for the prediction of cardiac death: differential stratification for risk of cardiac death and myocardial infarction. *Circulation* 1998;97:535–543.)

Breast attenuation is influenced by breast size and density. Although reducing attenuation by only 14% compared with the 73 keV photon of ^{201}Tl, ^{99m}Tc-based agents also present less Compton scatter, better image resolution and optimized gating. Even reversible defects may relate to technical causes, such as varying position of attenuating structures, variable patient motion or other factors. Gating permits the identification of normal wall motion and thickening in fixed defects that result from attenuation but not those that result from extensive infarction (*207*). Nonetheless, limited infarction and reversible ischemia may relate to normal systolic function.

Some studies demonstrate improved accuracy with a variety of attenuation correction methods, generally improving specificity if not sensitivity, with increased homogeneity in attenuation-corrected normal studies (*291,292,565*). However, in practice, sensitivity may suffer as well, and the methods are not ready for general application.

Diagnostic Sensitivity. Many studies demonstrate the diagnostic value of MPS in women and its advantage compared with other methods (*566*). In a multicenter study, Van Train et al. (*567*) demonstrated similar sensitivity, specificity and normalcy in men and women. Iskandrian et al. (*568*) also found a similar sensitivity and normalcy in men and women. Although sensitivity was high in patients of both sexes with multivessel disease (82% in women; 93% in men), it was lower in women (52%) with single-vessel disease than in men (87%) with single-vessel disease. This was thought to be the result of a low achieved double product in the women. Specificity was somewhat reduced in women, probably as a result of the confusion of breast attenuation with perfusion defects in this relatively early SPECT study. Later, the same researchers (*44*) demonstrated that the results of exercise perfusion imaging predicted well the presence of extensive CAD, as opposed to those with exercise-induced ST depression or any other clinical factors, in 834 patients including 217 women. They found that the presence of a multivessel

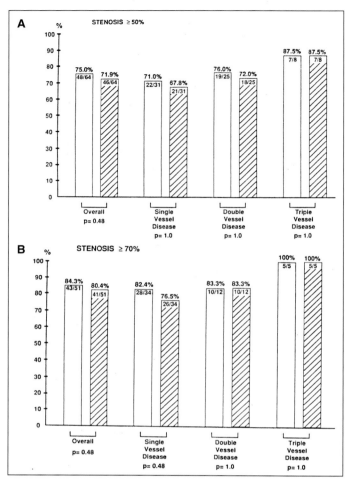

Figure 82 Myocardial perfusion sensitivity: disease involvement. Shown is the sensitivity of thallium-201 (open bars) and technetium-99m sestamibi (striped bars) perfusion studies for the detection of single-, double- and triple-vessel coronary arterry disease in patients with ≥50% (top) and ≥70% (bottom) coronary stenoses. The differences between this and the values with 50% or greater stenoses relate to the variability in lesion hemodynamic severity, the presence and contribution of collaterals, the degree of linearity of tracer distribution with flow and many other factors. (Reprinted, with permission, from, Taillefer R, DePuey EG, Udelson JE, et al. Comparative diagnostic accuracy of Tl-201 and Tc-99m sestamibi SPECT imaging: perfusion and ECG-gated SPECT in detecting coronary disease in women. *J Am Coll Cardiol* 1997;29:69–77.)

defect was a far better predictor of ischemia and CAD ($\chi^2 = 107$) than the exercise heart rate achieved ($\chi^2 = 27$) or ST depression ($\chi^2 = 8$). Image data were far more powerful predictors than clinical or exercise data.

In a group of 243 women evaluated for CAD, multivariate analysis identified the exercise heart rate and the number of reversible perfusion defects as the 2 predictors of high-risk, multivessel disease (*569*). In another study (*218*), data from 1 center were used to develop incremental logic algorithms that were then applied to 865 patients studied with stress MPS and coronary angiography at 4 other centers. There was a significant increment in accuracy related to stress MPS for both the presence and extent of CAD, which were similar in both men and women.

Amanullah et al. (*570*) found adenosine ^{99m}Tc sestamibi SPECT to be an accurate and effective protocol for the detection of CAD in women and was equally sensitive in women presenting with nonanginal symptoms. The overall sensitivity (93%), specificity (78%) and predictive accuracy (88%) in 203 patients were no different than those among the 103 patients without prior infarction (91%, 78% and 86%, respectively). The normalcy rate was 93%. The sensitivity was 93% and specificity 69% in women with nonanginal symptoms and 92% and 82% in those with angina. Sensitivity was maintained and similar in those with high, intermediate or low likelihood of CAD. The authors also found a sensitivity of 91% and specificity of 70% for the specific diagnosis of severe or extensive CAD (*571*).

When ^{201}Tl and ^{99m}Tc sestamibi were compared (*139,118*), there was a diagnostic concordance of 94% between 4622 planar image segments studied with the 2 agents in many patients of both sexes. Although planar imaging with both ^{99m}Tc sestamibi and ^{201}Tl demonstrated an incremental sensitivity for coronary diagnosis in the presence of 3-vessel disease (92% and 95%, respectively) compared with single-vessel disease (73% and 77%, respectively), SPECT image analysis demonstrated similar sensitivities for each agent in the presence of both single- (90% and 90%, respectively) and 3-vessel (98% and 96%, respectively) disease. A prospective study (*149*) was conducted in 85 consecutive female patients and 30 female volunteers who had low likelihood of CAD (Figs. 82–84). The sensitivities for the diagnosis of stenoses >50% and >70% with stress imaging performed in the same patients with each radionuclide were high: 75% and 84%, respectively, for ^{201}Tl and 72% and 81%, respectively, for ^{99m}Tc sestamibi. In this study, sensitivity did not differ between agents and was not

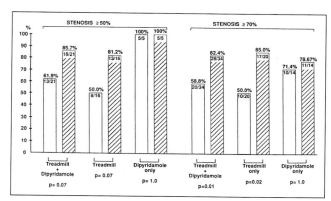

Figure 83 Myocardial perfusion specificity: treadmill/dipyridamole. Shown is the specificity of thallium-201 (open bars) and technetium-99m (^{99m}Tc) sestamibi (striped bars) studies for the detection of coronary artery disease in female patients undergoing either treadmill or dipyridamole stress testing, or both. Specificity appeared to be generally augmented by appliction of ^{99m}Tc sestamibi. (Reprinted, with permission from, Taillefer R, DePuey EG, Udelson JE, et al. Comparative diagnostic accuracy of Tl-201 and Tc-99m sestamibi SPECT imaging: perfusion and ECG-gated SPECT in detecting coronary disease in women. *J Am Coll Cardiol* 1997;29:69–77.)

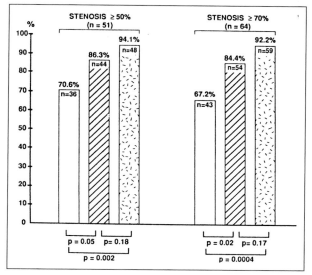

Figure 84 Myocardial perfusion specificity: nongated/gated. Shown is the specificity of thallium-201 (open bars), technetium-99m (^{99m}Tc) sestamibi (striped bars) and gated ^{99m}Tc sestamibi perfusion SPECT (speckled bars) studies for women patients without coronary artery disease and a group of normal volunteers. Data from gated studies adds to test specificity. (Reprinted, with permission from, Taillefer R, DePuey EG, Udelson JE, et al. Comparative diagnostic accuracy of Tl-201 and Tc-99m sestamibi SPECT imaging: perfusion and ECG-gated SPECT in detecting coronary disease in women. *J Am Coll Cardiol* 1997;29:69–77.)

influenced by gating. However, specificity for stenoses >50% was 62% for ^{201}Tl and 86% for ^{99m}Tc sestamibi ($P < 0.03$), whereas specificity for stenoses >70% was 59% for ^{201}Tl and 83% for ^{99m}Tc sestamibi ($P < 0.02$). When gated wall motion and thickening were added, the specificity of ^{99m}Tc sestamibi images was >92%.

Most recently, in a large multicenter analysis, Marwich et al. (*572*) examined the prognostic value of stress MPS among 5009 men and 3402 women with symptomatic or suspected CAD undergoing exercise (7486 patients) or pharmacologic (925 patients) stress MPS. A pretest clinical risk index was calculated for all subjects, who were followed for events during a mean of 2.4 yr. After adjustment for exercise variables, the number of abnormal territories was the strongest correlate of mortality in women undergoing exercise MPS.

Santana-Boada et al. (*335*) studied 702 consecutive patients without prior MI who underwent stress ^{99m}Tc sestamibi SPECT, 68% with exercise and 32% with dipyridamole (when exercise was insufficient). The "select minority" included 163 patients with coronary angiography performed for clinical reasons within 3 mo of stress imaging, and the "silent majority" included 539 patients without coronary angiography. The mean age was 58 ± 10 yr. Sensitivity and specificity were calculated for the select minority based on angiographic findings, and, for the silent majority, based on the method of Diamond (*49*). Here, a correction was formulated for the positive and negative predictive values in this population without the "gold standard" correlation. Here, sensitivity and specificity are constant and the demonstrated variability of positive and negative predictive values relate to the application of the same test in populations with varying disease prevalence. The prevalence could be formulated from the analysis of Diamond and Forrester (*102*) and the sensitivity and specificity applied, as in the angiography group, to determine the negative and positive predictive values based on disease prevalence. The authors found a lower disease prevalence in women (32%) than in men (80%) ($P = 0.0001$). The probability of a positive test was also lower in women (34%) than in men (65%). In the catheterization group, the sensitivity for women (85%) was slightly lower than that for men (93%) ($P = 0.01$). There was no difference in specificity (91% versus 89%) and, with correction for prevalence, there was no difference in either sensitivity (87% versus 88%) or specificity (91% versus 96%) between women and men. In the population overall, the sensitivity and specificity was similar in both men and women!

In an editorial written to accompany the Sanatana-Boada article (*335*) and based on its findings, Hachamovitch and Cacciabando (*573*) presented 2 approaches to the evaluation of CAD in women and men: an anatomic approach, based on the gold standard anatomical diagnosis of CAD, and a physiologic, prognostic approach, based on scintigraphic findings employed to assess related risk and the need, if demonstrating moderate-to-severe defects, for coronary angiography (Fig. 85). This approach is similar to that presented in the Summary Strategy section of this book. In such an approach, diagnostic evaluation requires that those with low CAD

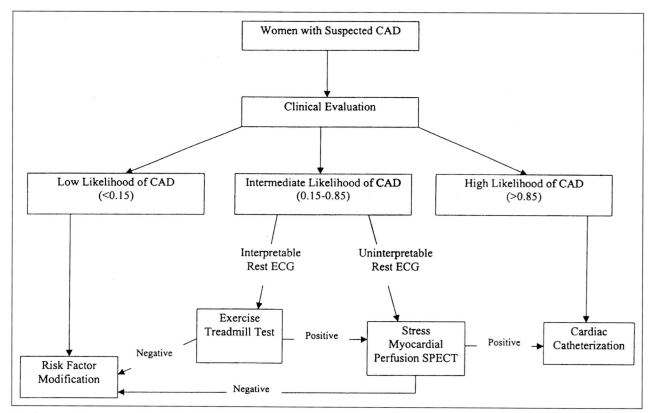

Figure 85   Myocardial perfusion scintigraphy: prognostic evaluation in women. Shown is an appropriate clinical algorithm for the prognostic evaluation of women with suspected coronary artery disease (CAD) using a risk-based approach to testing, in which the value of test results relates to patients based on the pretest likelihood of CAD. The algorithm is well applied in men. ECG = electrocardiogram; ETT = exercise treadmill testing; LV = left ventricular. (Reprinted, with permission, from Hachamovitch R, Cacciabando JM. Stress myocardial perfusion SPECT in women: is it the cornerstone of the noninvasive evaluation [abstract]? *J Nucl Med* 1998;39:756–759.)

likelihood, regardless of the nature of their rest ECG, simply have risk factor modification, whereas those with intermediate likelihood and a normal ECG get stress testing without imaging and go on to MPS only if the stress test is abnormal. These patients are then considered for angiography if imaging is abnormal. Those with an intermediate likelihood and an abnormal rest ECG would go for stress imaging and, with a normal or mildly abnormal image, have risk factor modification or, if imaging is moderately or severely abnormal, be considered for angiography. Those with a high likelihood of disease would go directly to angiography. However, although for prognostic evaluation those with low likelihood are treated similarly, those with high pretest likelihood of CAD are grouped with those of intermediate likelihood and sent to stress imaging and to angiography only with moderately or severely abnormal images. Those with normal or mildly abnormal images will have risk factor modification (Fig. 86).

The physiologic approach to patient evaluation appears well justified. Shaw et al. (653) demonstrated the cost-effective application of stress MPS in a large population of women with stable angina. In this study, the method was an appropriate and efficient "gatekeeper" for angiography.

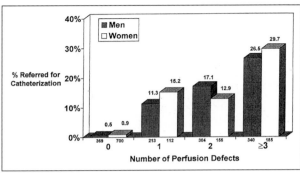

Figure 86 Relationship of perfusion defects to catheterization rate in men and women. Shown is the rate of catheterization in relation to the number of technetium-99m sestamibi defects in the same 2378 consecutive patients without history of coronary disease, prior infarction, catheterization or revascularization. Overall, 19.4% of men and 20.4% (P = NS) of women with abnormal images were referred for catheterization. Numbers below columns are the numbers of patients in each group, and numbers above columns represent the catheterization rates over the follow-up period. (Reprinted, with permission, from Travin MI, Duca MD, Kline GM, et al. Relation of gender to physician use of test results and to the prognostic value of stress technetium-99m sestamibi myocardial single photon emission tomography scintigraphy. *Am Heart J* 1997;134:73–82.)

The Case for Sex-Related Diagnosis, Referral and Management Bias. When asked which illness presented their greatest mortality threat, women identified cancer, specifically breast cancer (574). However, cardiovascular disease, most prominently CAD, is the leading cause of death among women, exceeding by a factor of 2 the likelihood of death from cancer (575) and responsible for the loss of 500,000 women each year and one-third of all deaths in women (576).

Symptoms generally occur 10 and infarction 20 yr later in women than in men. Anginal symptoms developed earlier in women and were more benign, but there was a higher infarct-related fatality rate when events eventually did occur in older women (577). Similarly, women have higher perioperative morbidity and mortality at CABG, probably as a result of their average greater age at the procedure, concomitant illnesses and possibly the more advanced state of CAD at the time of surgery. There is much evidence, however, that MPS brings CAD diagnosis and prognosis in women and men to near equality at a high level of success.

The diagnosis and treatment of CAD in women may be delayed because of the mistaken underestimation of CAD risk, the often erroneous ideas that women of any age are less likely to have CAD, that angina always has a better prognosis in women, that treatment is less successful and more dangerous in women or that noninvasive diagnosis with stress testing and MPS is useless in women. The early identification of CAD in women is clearly important to avoid a prophecy based on misconception and expedite treatment before CAD and other illness progress to make intervention more dangerous and less beneficial. Yet, some early studies suggested that the less frequent, later diagnosis and less aggressive treatment of CAD in women than in men is the result of a sex-related referral bias, with the more frequent testing and subsequent cardiac catheterization of men compared with women with apparent similar clinical and risk profiles (*578*). Thereafter, a flood of literature has evaluated sex-related differences in test utility and post-test angiography, as well as relative mortalities after cardiac events (*579–584*).

Mark et al. (*585*) reported the lower referral rate of women to coronary angiography compared with men. Although some investigators who view the findings superficially consider them illustrative of a sex-related bias in the diagnosis and management of CAD, a deeper analysis of this and several other studies has found that such sex-related differences are appropriate when corrected for baseline group differences and the results of MPS. Shaw et al. (*584*) evaluated the prognostic value of exercise or dipyridamole planar perfusion imaging in 840 patients (340 women, 500 men) without history of prior MI. Fewer women than men with positive tests underwent angiography. Yet, cardiac death and infarction were greater in women (6.9%) than in men (2.4%). They found that when all related variables were accounted for, men in similar clinical subgroups were referred for angiography more often than women. However, catheterization and revascularization rates appeared related to defect size and intensity and suggested no clear evidence of sex bias.

Lauer et al. (*586*) prospectively evaluated the pattern and logic behind referral to angiography in both men and women. This prospective study analyzed consecutive patients (2351 men and 1318 women) evaluated by exercise ^{201}Tl MPS who had never undergone coronary angiography. Women had a lower incidence of induced ischemia, CAD, angiography, mortality and overall end points than men. Again, sex-related differences in referral for coronary angiography after exercise perfusion imaging could be explained by the higher rate of abnormal tests in men.

The potential sex differences in the use and prognostic value of stress sestamibi imaging were studied over a period of 15 ± 8 mo in 1226 men and 1151 women (*587*) (Figs. 86,87). Here, the referral for catheterization and CABG increased in both sexes with the extent and severity of defects. There was no difference in catheterization referral rates between sexes, normalized for defect size. Image defect size was an independent predictor of events. For both men and women, image findings were strongly correlated with prognosis, and event rates associated with abnormal images were similar in men and women, 19.6% and 18.2%, respectively. Conversely, normal images were related to low event rates in both men (1.7%) and women (0.8%). In a larger study, Hachamovitch et al. (*19*) demonstrated a strong and appropriate relationship between findings on stress MPS and subsequent management in women.

Hachamovitch et al. (*318*) performed an extensive prospective study evaluating events and rates of referral to coronary angiography after stress MPS, consecutively performed in 1074 women and 2137 men. The overall event rates for women (3.4%) and men (2.9%) were not significantly different. Although more men were referred for catheterization than women (10.6% versus 7.1%; $P < 0.001$), when corrected for the amount of underperfused myocardium, there were no sex-related differences in the rate of referral or in rates of revascularization after risk stratification. Although women underwent scintigraphy less often than men, women were sent to angiography in the setting of severe scintigraphic ischemia more often than men (Table 29). This seems appropriate, because women with severely abnormal images had a higher event rate than men (17.5% versus 6.3%, $P < 0.0001$). In fact, given the higher event rate with the same defect size among women compared with men, it would have seemed appropriate to refer women to angiography at an even higher rate. Potential differences in catheterization referral rates between

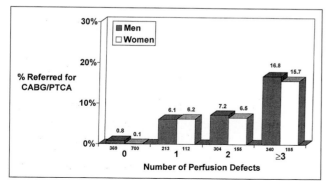

Figure 87 Relationship of perfusion defects to revascularization. Shown according to the same format as Figure 86 is the referral rate for revascularization (percutaneous transluminal coronary angioplasty [PTCA] or coronary artery bypass graf [CABG]) in relation to the number of technetium-99m sestamibi defects. Overall, 10.7% of men and 10.2% ($P =$ NS) of women with abnormal images were referred for revascularization. (Reprinted, with permission, from Travin MI, Duca MD, Kline GM, et al. Relation of gender to physician use of test results and to the prognostic value of stress technetium-99m sestamibi myocardial single photon emission tomography scintigraphy. *Am Heart J* 1997;134:73–82.)

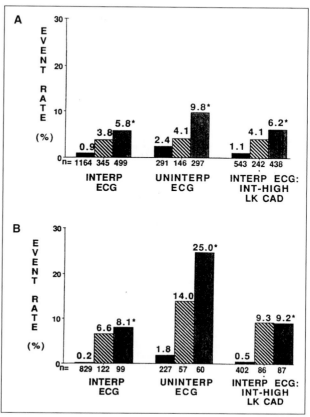

Figure 88 Event rates in men (A) and women (B) according to the findings on the rest electrocardiogram (ECG) and myocardial perfusion scintigraphy. Data was analyzed for interpretable ECGs (INTERP ECG), uninterpretable ECGs (UNINTERP ECG) and interpretable ECGs, excluding patients with a low (<0.15) likelihood of coronary artery disease (INTERP ECG:INT-HIGH LK CAD). Within each of these subgroups, a significant difference was found in the hard event rate as a function of defect score in both men and women. Among those with INTERP ECG:INT-HIGH LK CAD there was no difference in risk stratification compared with those with INTERP ECG, suggesting that the excluded low-likelihood group contributes little and may be initially well tested without imaging (Reprinted, with permission, from Hachamovitch R, Berman DS, Kiat H, et al. Comparison of incremental prognostic value, risk stratification and cost effectiveness of rest/exercise Tl-201/Tc-99m sestamibi SPECT in women and men. *J Am Coll Cardiol* 1996;28:34–44.)

men and women may be explained by the underlying differences in prevalence of abnormal scans, reflecting the underlying differences in CAD prevalence and severity in the population referred for SPECT.

The sex-related bias in referral to angiography may favor women or men, not based on sex but on the presence of known CAD and on the degree to which the physician involved is concerned about the diagnosis and dynamic nature of the disease process (*588*). The likelihood of referral is also influenced by the confidence of the physician in the test result. This may reduce the test specificity of MPS

Table 29
RELATIONSHIP OF PERFUSION DEFECTS TO EVENTS
IN MEN AND WOMEN

Scan subgroup	Events (%)	
	Men	Women
Normal	1.0	0.8
Mildly to moderately abnormal	2.8	5.6
Severely abnormal	6.3*	17.5*

*$P < 0.01$.

These figures represent the annual percentage of cardiac events (death and infarction) in relation to defect size and sex among 2203 consecutive patients without history of coronary disease, prior infarction, catheterization or revascularization, studied by Hachamovitch et al. (*318*) with perfusion imaging and followed prospectively. Results demonstrate a progressive increase in the incidence of cardiac events with increasing defect size. In fact, a large defect bore a worse prognosis in women. The related angiographic rate was proportional to the event rate, except in women with severely abnormal scans who were studied less often than might be advised given their extremely high event rate.

more than that of other methods, if it is the recipient of greater trust compared with other stress imaging methods.

Chowdhry et al. (*589*) evaluated the contribution of quantitative stress perfusion image findings to the referral to angiography in 11,063 consecutive men (7006) and women (4057), compared with the influence of other clinical and stress test findings. Severity and extent of image ischemia was, by far, the leading predictor of angiography, with a lower threshold for referral in men among all scan categories. However, rather than being indicative of an antifeminine bias, the outcome data suggested that women were studied at an appropriate rate, whereas men were studied too often, especially when scan findings were normal or mildly abnormal, and at a rate not justified by the outcome (*589*).

Roeters van Leenep et al. (*590*) demonstrated that, after correction for the presence and severity of stress MPS defects, both men and women were referred to coronary angiography at similar and proportional rates. There was no association between sex and the likelihood of referral to angiography but a strong relationship in both sexes between defect size and referral to angiography. These findings demonstrate the lack of a sex bias in referral to angiography.

Prognostic Value of Perfusion Scintigraphy in Men and Women

Miller et al. (*591*) presented the results of a multicenter study evaluating the prognostic value of stress perfusion imaging in 314 women and 1262 men. Both men and women had low event rates in the presence of a normal scan (1.4% and 0.6%, respectively). However, although the risk related to an abnormal scan was high in both groups, it was higher in women (10.9%) than men (6.9%), presenting women with an 11-fold risk ratio compared with a negative test and a risk ratio of 6 for men.

Pancholy et al. (*307*) found that MPS was predictive of outcomes in women and added incremental prognostic information over clinical and exercise variables in a catheterized population. The study evaluated the independent and added prognostic value of SPECT ^{201}Tl MPS in 212 women undergoing coronary angiography. Multivariate survival analysis demonstrated that a large perfusion abnormality and age were the only independent predictors of events and, reminiscent of the findings of other researchers (*318,354,430,446,447*), that women with large perfusion abnormalities (>15% of the left ventricular myocardium) had significantly worse event-free survival rates than women with no or small defects (15%; $P = 0.0001$). They did not compare their prognosis with a male group.

Hachamovitch et al. (*592*) demonstrated that hard coronary events in women could be predicted by the findings on stress perfusion SPECT modulated by the pretest likelihood of disease. Here, the 1-yr rate of death or infarction was 1% in association with normal scans and 4% with abnormal scans in a low-likelihood group, but 1% and 12% when normal and abnormal scans were evident in women with a high pretest likelihood of coronary disease.

This was again confirmed by Boyne et al. (593), who studied the value of exercise ^{99m}Tc sestamibi SPECT to predict events in a total of 229 patients with a "comparable" population of 114 men and 115 women. Again, the event rate related to a normal scan was 0.8%/yr, but that related to an abnormal scan was 5.4%/yr ($P < 0.005$). In addition, when used in a strategy incorporating clinical and exercise variables toward a prognostic end point, perfusion imaging cost less per patient in women than in men (594).

In a larger cohort of patients representing consecutive referrals and coming to diagnostic evaluation for possible CAD with dual-isotope myocardial perfusion SPECT (2742 men, 1394 women), Hachamovitch et al. (19) again found MPS to add incremental prognostic value to clinical and exercise variables in both men and women (Figs. 88–91). Both women and men with an interpretable stress ECG and an intermediate or high postexercise test likelihood of CAD, as well as all those with an uninterpretable stress ECG, demonstrated a significant risk stratification benefit from scintigraphic study. Normal images related to a very low event rate in both sexes. MPS appears to be well utilized to identify patients at greatest risk, with excellent correlation to subsequent anatomy. Hard events, cardiac death, infarction and remote revascularization during the 2 mo after scintigraphy were well predicted in these groups on the basis of image findings. Scintigraphic prognosis was much better defined and prognostic subgroups better separated in women, in whom scintigraphic abnormalities related to a worse prognosis and a higher event rate. Here, the odds ratio, comparing events with an abnormal to those with a normal scan, was far greater in women, again suggesting that coronary risk stratification was better in women. Patient management was strongly influenced by scintigraphic findings, in which the larger the reversible defect, the more likely was

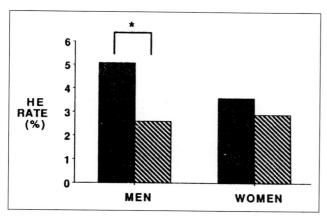

Figure 89 Hard event (HE) rates in men and women according to presenting symptoms. This study analyzed 2592 patients of both sexes, who came to diagnostic evaluation for possible coronary artery disease (CAD). The event rate in men with anginal symptoms (solid bars) was significantly higher (*) than in men with nonanginal symptoms (hatched bars). Symptoms were not as prognostic in women. ECG = electrocardiogram. (Reprinted, with permission, from Hachamovitch R, Berman DS, Kiat H, et al. Comparison of incremental prognostic value, risk stratification and cost effectiveness of rest/exercise Tl-201/Tc-99m sestamibi SPECT in women and men. *J Am Coll Cardiol* 1996;28:34–44.)

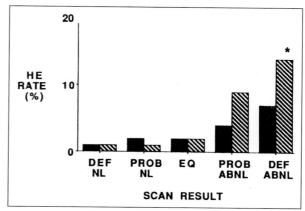

Figure 90 Hard event (HE) rates in men and women according to scan result. The hard event rate in women (hatched bars) with definitely abnormal (DEF ABNL) scan results was significantly higher (*) than in men (solid bars) ($P < 0.001$). DEF NL = definitely normal; EQ = equivocal; PROB ABNL = probably abnormal; PROB NL = probably normal. (Reprinted, with permission, from Hachamovitch R, Berman DS, Kiat H, et al. Comparison of incremental prognostic value, risk stratification and cost effectiveness of rest/exercise Tl-201/Tc-99m sestamibi SPECT in women and men. *J Am Coll Cardiol* 1996;28:34–44.)

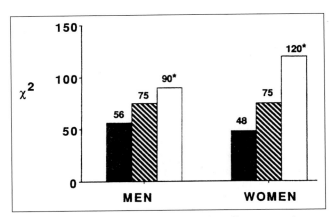

Figure 91 Incremental prognostic value. Shown are the results of the determination by Cox proportional hazards model of the evaluation of the incremental prognostic value (χ^2) of clinical variables (solid bars), clinical + exercise variables (hatched bars) and clinical + exercise + perfusion image data (open bars). The χ^2 of the model including perfusion scintigraphy was significantly greater than the others. (Reprinted, with permission, from Hachamovitch R, Berman DS, Kiat H, et al. Comparison of incremental prognostic value, risk stratification and cost effectiveness of rest/exercise Tl-201/Tc-99m sestamibi SPECT in women and men. *J Am Coll Cardiol* 1996;28:34–44.)

angiography. Therefore, contrary to popular belief but similar to other reports (*19,32,318,591,594–597*), in a variety of clinical settings, MPS stratified coronary risk better and appropriately affected management in females, in whom the same scintigraphic abnormality appeared to relate to a worse prognosis than in males (*598*). This had no relation to the selection process, in which the likelihood of coronary angiography was related to the same defect size and related provocation in both sexes. The prognostic value of the exercise test alone was far less than the SPECT study and similar in men and women.

Hachamovitch et al. (*32*) performed another extensive prospective study of the incremental prognostic value, role in risk stratification and impact on patient management of SPECT MPS in 2203 consecutive patients without history of CAD, prior infarction, catheterization or revascularization, who were followed for 566 days. Multiple logistic regression analysis and calculation of the global χ^2 revealed that scan data contributed 95% of the information (global $\chi^2 = 169$) that brought patients to angiography and that 5% was contributed by historic and stress test findings (global $\chi^2 = 31$)! The scan results substratified risk well among all groups based on their pretest CAD likelihood, in which normal scans were low risk in all groups and risk increased with worsening scan findings. Referring physicians used this test to determine management, and early postscan referral rates to angiography and revascularization paralleled the hard event rates in each category, which directly related to each category of scan result. Here, there were very low referral rates when the scan was normal or probably normal, with increasing rates in relation to worsening scan findings, with scan findings paralleling event rates in all scan categories. Nor did the findings on exercise variables, such as the Duke Treadmill Score (Fig. 3), pretest CAD likelihood, symptoms, sex or age eliminate the incremental prognostic value of MPS. Scintigraphic findings brought additional risk stratification, even after consideration of presenting symptoms, age, sex, disease likelihood and the Duke Treadmill Score. Both the hard event rate and the catheterization rate were well stratified on the basis of scintigraphic findings within patient groups, demonstrating low, intermediate and high Duke Treadmill Scores. It was the image defect score, rather than the ECG and stress test parameters, that related to event rate and determined management! The hard event rate was 0.4% among those with an intermediate-risk Duke classification but a normal scan. Scintigraphic risk stratification was beneficial among those with interpretable stress ECGs and intermediate-to-high postexercise test likelihood of CAD or in those with an uninterpretable rest ECG, regardless of pretest likelihood. When subdivided into groups based on sex, image findings stratified event rates well among both men and women. However, the risk related to a severe image defect in women far exceeded the risk of such an image defect in men. Although the catheterization rate increased with the severity of scan findings, the catheterization rate in women was similar to that in men for

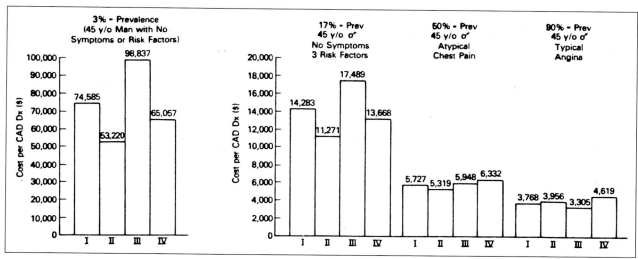

Figure 92 Prevalence versus cost effectiveness. Presented are the costs per coronary artery disease diagnosis (Cost per CAD Dx($)) in 4 representative patients with increasing CAD likelihoods of 3%, 17%, 50% and 90%, from left to right, with the application of 4 diagnostic strategies (I = stress electrocardiography [ECG] with angiography if abnormal; II = stress myocardial perfusion scintigraphy [MPS] first and angiography if abnormal; III = angiography first; IV = stress ECG with stress MPS if abnormal and angiography if MPS is abnormal). Generally, approach II, based on stress MPS, is most cost effective, except at highest likelihood. The diagnostic costs, however, appear exorbitant in the very low-likelihood group, and the stress MPS method is often valuable for prognosis in those with highest likelihood. The costs, overall values and management principles have evolved with time and methodologic improvements. However, the basic principles remain suprisingly constant, although with variations based on specific clinical and ECG characteristics and test indications. (Reprinted, with permission, from Patterson et al. [633].)

as one of multiple factors related to coronary risk (see *Self-Study Program III. Cardiology. Topic 2: Pharmacologic Stress*). Recent studies have demonstrated the ability of MPS to stratify coronary risk, even in a low-likelihood population, but with a relatively low cost effectiveness (*19,32,129*). Elliott et al. (*636*) have demonstrated the utility of the method to provide long-term risk stratification among asymptomatic candidates for renal or pancreas transplants.

Mammograms are recommended in women older than 50, but debate still rages over the application in younger women, with a relatively reduced specificity and lower incidence of disease. A chest radiograph is accepted practice in screening for tuberculosis. These are appropriate because of the importance of the related diagnosis, the sensitivity of the method applied, its relative specificity and the low risk and cost of subsequent confirmatory procedures. The stress evaluation of asymptomatic individuals with CAD risk factors is often performed before joining an exercise program, to qualify for life insurance, for patient reassurance or for other considerations. Stress testing in such patients should generally involve a simple dynamic exercise study, and MPS should be reserved to clarify abnormal findings on stress testing. In those rare cases in which both studies are abnormal, evidence suggests a significant proportion of true positives. However, great will power and restraint must be applied on the part of the managing physician in the setting of such positive results, because, even in the setting of CAD, in asymptomatic patients there is no controlled study or any good evidence of benefit from any intervention other than risk factor modification.

Asymptomatic patients with risk factors should be evaluated and treated medically with vigorous risk-factor reduction. Some clinicians would perform ultrafast CT scanning for the identification of coronary calcification. However, these tests appear too often abnormal in the setting of normal stress tests, stress

MPS and in asymptomatic patients, and, regardless of the CT findings, the best management is often conservative and medical.

The evaluation of asymptomatic patients may be worthwhile to uncover occult disease and implement risk-factor modification. Bayesan analysis suggests that symptomatic patients with an intermediate-to-high likelihood of CAD are best suited for evaluation (637). This has been well documented in studies in which MPS results suffer impressively when applied to aymptomatic low-likelihood patients (638,639). For this reason, routine screening of asymptomatic patients is not recommended. Rather, the application of MPS to selected high-risk groups is potentially beneficial. Those with more modest risk but who are embarking on an exercise program or hold responsible jobs, such as airline pilots or train engineers, in which sudden incapacitation may risk the lives of others, may be suitable subjects.

PATIENT OUTCOMES AFTER STRESS PERFUSION IMAGING

Evidence-Based Approach/Outcomes-Based Approach to Management

The extensive evidence of the physiologic and prognostic value of stress MPS is widely documented here. This evidence can be applied in individual cases to risk stratify patients to a high degree of accuracy. Once established, the nature and likelihood of related outcomes may be determined. The derived coronary-related risk becomes an important consideration in patient management.

The Influence of Myocardial Perfusion Scintigraphy on Patient Management

An anatomic approach to study efficacy evaluates method sensitivity, specificity and negative and positive predictive values. More recently, a prognostic or risk-based indication for study has been developed, based on the objective of cost effectiveness. This is supported by the demonstration of the prognostic value of MPS and its statistically significant ability to risk stratify in CAD, to demonstrate an incremental prognostic ability and to present a more refined risk stratification based on the response to treatment. The latter ability has developed a closer link between the MPS method and patient management decisions (630,631).

In addition to its diagnostic and prognostic value, the impact of MPS on subsequent patient management and outcome also has been assessed. This has been done by measuring the rate of referral to coronary angiography and revascularization after testing as a function of scan result, compared with clinical and exercise test information in many studies (16,17,19,20,32,128,129,305,306, 335,589). On the basis of such results and the findings of others who document the value of the scintigraphic method in identifying coronary patients at greatest risk (305,640,641), a number of publications indicate the important role of stress scintigraphic study in the evaluation and management of patients with known or suspected CAD.

In an early study of a population of 61 patients assessed with dipyridamole MPS, Schechtmann et al. (642) evaluated the influence of test findings on clinical management. Pretest disease probability was calculated, and test influence on patient management was determined by set criteria. Patients included those with a low pretest probability and reversible image abnormalities who went on to catheterization or aggressive medical management, patients with a high pretest probability and a benign image who were discharged or managed conservatively, patients with an intermediate pretest probability or those with known but ambiguous CAD who were sent to image evaluation and demonstrated image findings consistent with subsequent management. Dipyridamole scintigraphy influenced management in almost 80% of this initial group of patients with known or suspected coronary disease and who could not undergo dynamic stress testing. Further, because scintigraphic and angiographic findings were generally consistent, such influence was apparently appropriate (4,643). When compared with other methods, this level of test influence is extremely high and, in addition to the accuracy of test results, relates to the diagnostic difficulty presented by these patients, the lack of acceptable diagnostic alternatives and the need and willingness, moreso in these patients, to let image results guide management decisions. This was not the case with stress echocardiography (251,603,605,644), which demonstrated a modest influence on patient management. Mereles et al. (644) demonstrated that management was affected in <15%, and negative findings in patients with intermediate-to-high likelihood of CAD did not necessarily keep patients from angiography, nor, in those with low-to-intermediate likelihood, did abnormal findings generally propel them to angiography. When tests are ordered but not vigorously acted upon, it exposes a lack of confidence in their findings and an alternate motivation for their performance. It also suggests a lower level of post-test referral bias, which may lead to a higher apparent specificity. Many studies have been published to support the utilization of the MPS method for management decision making.

In the studies by Hlatky et al. (4,643), the percentage of patients whose physicians recommended coronary angiography fell dramatically among all groups of pretest disease probability with the negative results of ^{201}Tl planar perfusion scintigraphy. This resulted in a reduction in the number of negative angiograms performed and resulted in significant savings. The effect was greatest among those with the highest pretest likelihood. Not only do negative images reduce the incidence of angiography, but, judging from current prognostic data, they do so safely (251). New methods promise to enhance this ability (645). Similar effects of a normal MPS on resource utilization were demonstrated by Miller et al. (646). Berman et al. (647) demonstrated the full "gatekeeper" function of the method in a large population. Among a large number of patients with chest pain syndromes, Amanullah et al. (648) demonstrated the most powerful predictor of revascularization to be the presence of reversibility on stress SPECT MPS.

Nallamothu et al. (346) presented extensive data regarding the current role and value of MPS in patient management. The authors studied the influence of diagnostic exercise ^{201}Tl SPECT MPS, performed in 2700 patients, on subsequent angiography, revascularization and outcomes. Only 3% of the patients with normal images went to angiography within 6 mo of SPECT study. Among those 673 with abnormal SPECT studies, 36% went to angiography ($P < 0.001$). Among those with defects, the defects in patients undergoing angiography were larger than the defects of those who did not have angiography. Multivessel disease was present in 13% of those with angiography and normal images and in 55% of those with angiography and abnormal images ($P < 0.001$). Revascularization was performed in 2% of those with normal images and in 30% of those with abnormal images ($P = 0.0001$). There were no events among those with normal images who were treated medically, but 10% of those with image abnormalities who were treated medically had events ($P = 0.02$). Those with events had significantly larger defects than those with none. Perfusion imaging had a great influence on patient management.

Kang et al. (223) sought to determine the angiographic rate and eventual out-come among patients found to have normal sestamibi MPS. Only 132 patients, ~3% of >4000 patients with normal dual-isotope ^{201}Tl rest/^{99m}Tc sestamibi stress SPECT perfusion images, underwent coronary angiography 6 mo before or after imaging and were followed for 22.5 ± 6.4 mo. The normal group as a whole had an event rate <0.5%. Among those studied invasively, 59 (45%) had abnormal angiograms, 31 with single-vessel disease, 17 with 2-vessel disease and 11 with left main or 3-vessel disease. Among these, hard events were evi-dent in only 3 patients, each with 2-vessel disease—a hard event rate of only 1.2%/yr. In patients undergoing angiography, a normal SPECT sestamibi perfu-sion scan was associated with a good prognosis and complemented the angio-graphic assessment of risk. The study at once confirms the imperfection of the method and yet also affirms the overall benign prognosis of a normal image and supports further the application of scintigraphic findings to patient manage-ment. Amanullah et al. (649) reported the outcome of patients treated medically with left main and 3-vessel disease after adenosine MPS evaluation and found that scintigraphy was a strong predictor of outcome, even in this high-risk group (649). The identification of advanced anatomic CAD, as occurs occasionally in the presence of a normal stress MPS study, was aided by an assessment of left ventricular volumes and LVEF from gated studies (650).

Referral to catheterization after SPECT appears to be driven by several fac-tors. As demonstrated by Kang et al. (223) in patients who have undergone ex-ercise stress, the extent and severity of ischemia present is the single most im-portant variable. Although the presence of anginal symptoms also appears to influence the rate of referral, stress-induced pain is a diagnostic finding and does not relate to prognosis. Additionally, many such patients are sent for scintigraphy to assess the cause or prognostic importance of pain symptoms or their equivalent, so management is based on image findings and not the pres-ence of angina. In patients without previously documented CAD, the rates of re-ferral to catheterization increased significantly as a function of scan abnormal-ity. However, for any given scan result, the referral rate was greater in patients with a higher likelihood of CAD (16,32,319,651,652).

Referral rates to catheterization after MPS were explained by the underlying differences in prevalence of abnormal scans reflecting the underlying differ-ences in the prevalence and severity of CAD in the large population studied by Hachamovitch et al. (318) (Fig. 93).

On the other hand, it appears that patients referred for SPECT who undergo pharmacologic stress are referred to catheterization less frequently than those patients who undergo exercise stress, despite the greater overall coronary risk of these patients (318,319,651,652). In addition, clinical variables that clearly in-fluence the decision to refer to catheterization after exercise MPS do not influ-ence the decision to refer to catheterization after pharmacologic stress. The un-derlying clinical reasoning behind this finding is unclear but may relate to the fact that the population undergoing pharmacologic stress is sicker and, because of greater interventional risks, requires greater image abnormalities to balance disease risks with potential benefits.

Shaw et al. (653) compiled and analyzed outcomes data from 4638 women with stable chest pain studied at 7 centers, either with early coronary angiogra-phy (3375) or with stress MPS and angiography only if at least 1 reversible seg-mental perfusion defect was evident (1263) (Figs. 94–96). Perfusion defects and referral to angiography increased in women in parallel with increasing pretest CAD likelihood. Cardiac death rates ranged from 0.5% to 2.2%/yr without

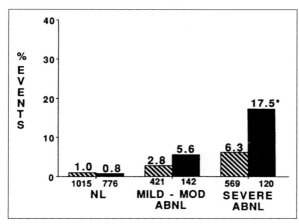

Figure 93 Event rate and defect score. This extensive prospective study evaluated events and rates of referral to coronary angiography after stress perfusion scintigraphy, consecutively performed in 1074 women and 2137 men. Here, the incremental risk related to increasing defect severity, quantitated based both on extent and density, is well shown. Women (solid bars) were more likely to have a normal scan, whereas men (hatched bars) were more likely to have abnormal scan results. Women also had a higher event rate than men with a similar severe image score. MILD − MOD ABNL = mild-to-moderate scan abnormalities; NL = normal scan; SEVERE ABNL = severe scan abnormality. (Reprinted, with permission, from Hachamovitch R, Berman DS, Kiat H, et al. Gender-related differences in clinical management after exercise nuclear testing. *J Am Coll Cardiol* 1995;26:1457–1464.)

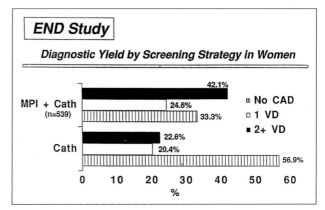

Figure 94 Diagnostic yield by screening strategy in women with chest pain. Shown are the findings on coronary angiography in stress myocardial perfusion scintigraphy (MPI + Cath) and catheterization-first (Cath) groups. There was twice the incidence of normal angiograms among the Cath groups. The 33% incidence of normal angiograms among those studied invasively in the MPI + Cath group likely relates to patient selection and the image criteria applied. CAD = coronary artery disease; VD = vessel disease. (Reproduced, with permission, from Shaw LJ, Heller GV, Travin MI, et al. Cost analysis of diagnostic testing for coronary artery disease in women with stable chest pain. *J Nucl Cardiol* 1999;6:559–569.)

difference between management groups. However, the revascularization rate and cost per patient were higher among the angiography-first group, ranging from $2490 for low-likelihood to $3687 for high-likelihood angiography-first subjects versus $1587–$2585 for the same subsets among MPS-first subjects. There was a far higher rate of women catheterized with normal coronary arteries among those who went first to angiography.

Anatomic Versus Risk-Based Management Strategy. The management of patients with a high pretest likelihood of CAD raises an interesting dilemma. In an algorithm based on an anatomic end point, these patients would all be referred to catheterization rather than MPS. In a prognosis- or risk-based testing strategy, these patients, if clinically stable, would be referred to stress MPS. In a benefit-oriented algorithm, only those patients with symptoms or compromised quality of life would be referred to such testing. This referral would be based on the principle that a significant proportion of these patients would have low-risk scans and thus would not require further testing. If, in a particular population, an excess of patients do not have low-risk scans, then direct referral to catheterization in that group would be appropriate. This potential risk-related strategy is supported by a report investigating the prognostic application of perfusion imaging and its use in the risk stratification of patients with a high likelihood of CAD or with previous MI (*319*).

Bateman et al. (*16*) performed a large retrospective study of rates of coronary angiography in 4162 patients who were evaluated with MPS in a clinical group

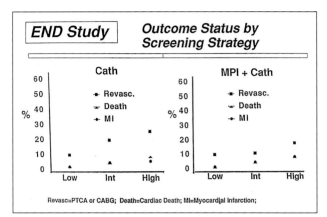

Figure 95 Outcome status by screening strategy in women with stable angina. Total and risk-stratified event rates did not differ significantly between catheterization-first (Cath) and myocardial perfusion scintigraphy-first (MPI + Cath) groups. Low = low pretest coronary artery disease (CAD) likelihood; Int = intermediate pretest CAD likelihood; High = high pretest CAD likelihood; MI = myocardial revascularization; Revasc = revascularization. (Reproduced, with permission, from Shaw LJ, Heller GV, Travin MI, et al. Cost analysis of diagnostic testing for coronary artery disease in women with stable chest pain. *J Nucl Cardiol* 1999;6:559–569.)

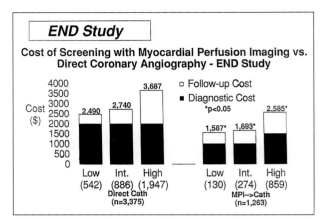

Figure 96 Cost of screening with myocardial perfusion imaging versus direct coronary angiography in women with Stable angina. Economics of Noninvasive Diagnosis Study. On average, there was a 30% greater cost incurred per woman with chest pain when approached with angiography first (Direct Cath) than when studied angiographically after an abnormal myocardial perfusion scintigraphy (MPI–Cath). Significant cost differences were seen in each pretest coronary artery disease (CAD) probability subset. Low = low pretest CAD likelihood; Int = intermediate pretest CAD likelihood; MI = myocardial revascularization; High = high pretest CAD likelihood; Revasc = revascularization; Cath = cardiac catheterization; MPI = myocardial perfusion imaging. (Reproduced, with permission, from Shaw LJ, Heller GV, Travin MI, et al. Cost analysis of diagnostic testing for coronary artery disease in women with stable chest pain. *J Nucl Cardiol* 1999;6:559–569.)

practice and followed for a 26-mo period. Most patients had known CAD, 35% with prior MI, and ~705 with prior PTCA. Sixty percent of those studied had reversible defects. Forty-two percent of those with reversible defects, as opposed to only 3.5% of those with normal scans (n = 1663), went to angiography within 3 mo of study. Among those with "high-risk" patterns of reversibility (LAD or multivessel disease and/or abnormal lung uptake) (n = 1141), 60% went to angiography, compared with only 9% in those with mild to moderate defects (n = 1358). Reversibility and "high-risk" image reversibility were the strongest predictors of angiography. The data in these images were utilized to a high degree. Further, after 3 yr, the hard event rate among those with normal scans or those with mild defects was 3%, cumulatively, so these patients should be treated medically. Even here, when studies were self referred, consulting cardiologists based their decision on the image findings and specifically on those that indicated extensive MIR in patients who might benefit from revascularization. In all, 1189 of these patients, or 61% of the overall cohort, could be reclassified as low risk for cardiac death on the basis of MPS and, thus, probably not in need of catheterization unless refractory symptoms occur.

The findings suggest that patients are essentially managed in this manner, with only those with moderate or severe defects going on to angiography. Further, revascularization, performed frequently among those undergoing angiography and with a high incidence of moderate-to-severe defects, was more beneficial than medical treatment in those with such defects, whereas there was no difference between medical and revascularization treatment among those with mild image defects. Among those with moderate or severe defects, roughly 50%

now come to angiography, a number likely needing expansion. However, to apply this method successfully, quantitative definitions of mild, moderate and severe defects must be firmly established. In an anatomy-based strategy, however, the patients in this study (16) would have been referred to catheterization and possibly revascularization for treatment of their coronary anatomy, despite the absence of risk for an adverse outcome. Thus, a risk-based strategy can successfully identify low-risk patients from within a high-risk population and spare invasive evaluation. Studies have compared anatomic with risk-based management approaches and found no increase, or a reduced rate of interventions and events, with risk-based management (130,131,277,388,508,509,654–656). Medical treatment was related to fewer hard events than revascularization among patients with image findings of single-vessel disease, regardless of the vessel involved (657). These results parallel those determined previously, in which vascular involvement was established angiographically.

An analysis of management patterns and their relationship to image findings has been performed among 14,831 patients undergoing stress ^{99m}Tc sestamibi MPS (1991–1996) at 3 large referral centers where quantitative scoring by the 20-segment method was practiced (658). The study demonstrated an increasing and appropriate reliance on scintigraphic findings for management decisions. This occurred while there was no change in the event rates related to any scan score and the catheterization and intervention rates related to normal scans remained unchanged at levels of ~2% and 0.5%, respectively.

Decision-making algorithms based on studies with large patient numbers have been well developed for patients with symptoms and a low pretest likelihood of CAD and for patients with suspected (intermediate pretest likelihood) or known (high pretest likelihood) CAD. Noninvasive strategies are both appropriate and cost effective for risk stratification in CAD. Variables on MPS provide supplementary prognostic information to clinical and ECG stress test variables. Although these and other studies demonstrate a strong relationship between scintigraphic findings, the performance of angiography and revascularization, each such application of scintigraphy is not made in a vacuum but taken in association with symptomatology, coronary risk factors and left ventricular function (659).

MPS clearly serves as the "gatekeeper" for these next-most-expensive and dangerous diagnostic steps in patients with angina pectoris generally (647) and in other specific coronary subgroups, such as those evaluated after CABG (660), and in women (653). MPS has been shown to decrease costs without harm when used as the "gatekeeper" to angiography in women with chest pain syndromes (653). The data supports such an application of scintigraphy but does not support a similar use for any other noninvasive method. To apply stress echocardiography in this way would burden the patient with an unacceptably high event rate in the absence of a firm data base documenting the prognostic value of the method (14). Beyond this, a new chapter has begun, in which MPS findings appear potentially able to determine the specific nature of the risk and so aid determination of the appropriate treatment. Further, serial studies may not only be able to determine treatment success or failure but also assess the ability of such treatment to modify (improve) outcome. With such evaluation, MPS would serve as a guide for the need for alterations in therapy.

Prediction of Specific Risk: Cardiac Death Versus Myocardial Infarction

Until recently, the prognostic evaluation of MPS has been limited to the identification of combined "hard" end points: cardiac death and MI. Several recent reports, however, have shown that the method yields incremental prognostic value with respect to cardiac death as an isolated end point and is well able to separate patients with such a likelihood from those more likely to suffer a nonfatal infarction (*343,344,354,661*). The Economics of Noninvasive Diagnosis study reported a risk-adjusted SPECT model predicting cardiac death in 8411 patients (*334*).

The most thorough of such studies analyzed the incremental value of exercise SPECT MPS for the prediction of individual hard end points and its implications for risk stratification in a group of 5183 consecutive patients, followed for 642 ± 226 days after SPECT MPS, 119 with cardiac death and 158 with AMI (*21*) (Figs. 80,81). The event rate related to a normal scan was 0.5%. The frequency of both cardiac death and nonfatal infarction increased with worsening scan defects. Mild scan abnormalities were related to low rates of cardiac death but higher rates of nonfatal infarction (0.7% versus 2.6%; $P < 0.05$). Risk stratification was based on scan findings within groups determined by their prescan CAD likelihood. Those one-third of patients with a low pretest likelihood of CAD had a very low event rate, with cardiac death or nonfatal infarction <1%. They do not require image evaluation for prognosis, unless quality-of-life issues are considered. Those with mild scan abnormalities with an intermediate-to-high pretest CAD likelihood had a 4.4%–6.5% chance of developing a nonfatal MI in the next year and a 0.8%–1.7% chance of cardiac death. Moderate-to-severe induced scan defects related to a high incidence of both cardiac death (6%–10.5%) and nonfatal infarction (6.3%–7.1%). This analysis identified a patient cohort with mildly abnormal scans, who are severely threatened by infarction but not by cardiac death. Such patients would probably not benefit from revascularization, which is not proven to prevent infarction, unless refractory symptoms were present. Instead, they could perhaps be treated medically with a noninvasive strategy and aggressive risk-factor (lipids, smoking, weight, etc.) reduction and might not require coronary angiography (*662–664*). Those with moderate-to-severely abnormal scans could be treated aggressively with angiography and appropriate revascularization. These findings were consistent for patients having either pharmacologic or exercise stress MPS and were confirmed by the subsequent retrospective analysis of patients at the same institution. Here, a review of events demonstrated a similar relationship to scan findings and the prescan likelihood among a large number of patients. Further, when these patients were retrospectively analyzed according to therapy delivered, revascularization only reduced the incidence of death among those with moderate-to-severe scan defects and there was no difference in outcomes, whether treated medically or with revascularization, among those with mildly abnormal scans. These findings have significant implications for the use of MPS in the guidance of post-test patient management and the decision to refer to catheterization or treat medically (*217*). This could result in significant cost savings without change in outcomes. Of note is the fact that the incremental MI rate paralleled defect size and density and, so, indirectly supported the relationship between the severity of coronary stenosis and the occurrence of subsequent infarction.

Angiographic evidence of modest CAD or a scintigraphic pattern consistent with a low-to-intermediate risk of CAD (summed stress imaging score 4–8) related to a cardiac death rate of 0.85 and a nonfatal infarction rate of 2.7% and should also be approached with medical management and risk-factor modification that may actually modify the coronary pathophysiology. Here, the risk of events may be significantly reduced with lipid-lowering therapy (*662–664*). Aspirin, antioxidants such as as vitamin E or certain dihydropridine calcium channel blockers may also benefit outcome by modification of the disease process (*665*). In the absence of a high-risk perfusion scintigraphic pattern, defined as multivessel or LAD involvement or increased lung uptake, most patients will do well with medical therapy, with a <1%/yr risk of death or nonfatal infarction and a revascularization rate of <3%/yr (*16*).

Another View of the Proper Role of Stress Myocardial Perfusion Scintigraphy in Patient Management: Acute Infarction

The evaluation and management of patients with AMI is in evolution. Those with evidence of a dynamic or unstable state with recurrent symptoms, ECG changes, heart failure, reduced left ventricular function or hemodynamic instability comprise roughly 15% of post-MI patients and require angiography and revascularization as available. However, the remaining 85% of post-MI patients are stable and often will harbor only small amounts of scarred myocardium and MIR. Evidence suggests that such patients could benefit from the noninvasive evaluation of their ischemic potential and left ventricular function (*217,279*). Patients with little residual ischemia post-MI have a benign follow-up with a low event rate, regardless of whether they are treated medically or with revascularization. Its high predictive value when negative makes MPS a valuable method in the risk stratification of this population. Currently, 70%–80% of these patients undergo coronary angiography and often revascularization (*666*). However, the results of 2 large post-thrombolytic trials demonstrate no significant advantage of revascularization, with an equally beneficial outcome among patients treated in Canada and the United States, although U.S. patients were revascularized at a 3-fold higher rate (*506–508,667*) (Fig. 76). Do these figures indicate that procedures are often performed in patients at relatively low risk, who do not need or benefit from them or that aggressive medical treatment was as effective as revascularization? Studies noted previously suggest that this high number can be significantly reduced if angiography were to be reserved for patients with moderate-to-severe ischemia or ischemic potential. As data increases relating the extent of abnormality on MPS to outcomes, some suggest that the idea that revascularization is necessary to improve outcome and is superior to medical treatment in all post-MI patients with a moderate amount of induced ischemia may itself increase, beyond need, the number of patients undergoing angiography and revascularization (*210,316*).

Extensive previous medical–surgical comparison treatment studies (*210*) have demonstrated a general advantage of surgical compared with medical treatment in patients with advanced CAD and extensive ischemia, especially when these are combined with reduced left ventricular function. However, recent studies comparing the outcomes benefits of medical and revascularization therapy are few (*303,658,669*). Those that specifically apply the results of MPS to determine the advantages of those treatment options are relatively rare (*16,21,301,348,444,670–674*). This is especially important given the demonstrated advantages of current medical therapy of the post-MI patient (*131,301,510,665–667,670,674*). Several investigators have applied serial SPECT MPS before and after intensive medical therapy (*287,288,301*) or revascularization. These were performed in order to determine the value of the intervention to reduce ischemia or ischemic potential. For this purpose, reproducibility of the method must be high (*135*).

A Special Case: Gauging Risk Based on the Response to Therapy

It has been well determined that both exercise and pharmacologic stress MPS will satisfactorily risk stratify post-MI patients. Those with minimal ischemia or ischemic potential are at low risk for death or recurrent MI. Aggressive intervention and management is generally reserved for the patient with an apparent increased risk related to scans revealing "moderate and severe ischemic potential." Adenosine MPS has been shown to be performed safely within 2–3 days after the event and has been shown to stratify post-MI patients well into low-, intermediate- and high-risk subgroups on the basis of measures of total infarct image defect size (*217*). Here, those with total defect size <20% of the left ventricular mass had a 1-yr mortality of 0% and risk of recurrent MI <5%/yr (*216,301*).

One of the strong points of the pharmacologic method using direct coronary dilators, well supported in the literature (see *Self-Study Program III. Cardiology. Topic 2: Pharmacologic Stress*), is that it can be done while the patient is on anti-ischemic therapy, without loss of sensitivity or ability to risk stratify! This seems to relate to the fact that these dilators act on the coronary flow supply rather than on demands, whereas beta blockers affect demands. However, beta blockers reduce resting myocardial blood flow (*672*). With the subsequent administration of coronary dilators, there is an increase in the CFR in areas supplied by stenotic vessels. Although a similar effect must occur in the bed of normal vessels, this could potentially result in a relative reduction in the differential flow augmentation between stenotic and normal beds. This, in turn, could result in an apparent reduction of the related induced defect with a potential underestimation of related disease and risk (*302*).

As if taking advantage of this effect, the randomized study by Dakik et al. (*313*) applied adenosine MPS early after uncomplicated infarction in patients off anti-ischemic therapy to determine the risk and optimize the outcomes that occur with aggressive medical therapy and revascularization. They selected those patients with large defects on this initial adenosine stress evaluation, as defined in their earlier study (*217,316,464*), and then repeated pharmacologic stress MPS 6–8 wk later, while the patient was on maximal anti-ischemic therapy or after revascularization with angioplasty or stent. Those patients who had a small or reduced defect size on the late study compared with the initial study were found to have excellent prognoses and were treated conservatively with maximal medical therapy. However, if the defect size remained the same or increased, the prognosis was poor, with an ~35% event rate, recommending re-examination of the therapeutic regimen. If not maximal, medical therapy could be augmented and testing repeated. If therapy was maximal, then revascularization was recommended. This study, as others noted, demonstrated the ability of MPS to stratify the post-MI patient. However, it also suggests that not even all patients with evidence of moderate-to-large defects early after infarction need revascularization therapy and that serial MPS can determine optimal treatment on an individual basis.

These data suggest that the full diagnostic (and prognostic) value of the adenosine (and dipyridamole) method may be obtained only with the patient off beta blockers and antianginal drugs at the time of study! However, if subsequent prognosis after treatment relates to stress image findings on therapy, the patient must then be studied after revascularization and while on maximal medical therapy.

But why does the defect size in the Dakik study (*301*) decrease late after MI? Is this the result of the effects of beta blockers and other anti-ischemic medications on the response to the dilator? Even so, why should this provide prognostic information any more than reduced ischemia, induced in association with an exercise test performed with a blunted double product after beta blockade? Although such a response to stress testing may parallel a good therapeutic and symptomatic response, MIR (which in some way appears to relate to prognosis) could still be elicited if the appropriate stress were applied. If this is the cause of the findings, why then do we need to wait 6–8 wk to perform the second study? Although unlikely, is the finding the result of an actual pathophysiologic effect of treatment on the percentage of coronary stenosis or an alteration in regional vasoreactivity with improvement in the CFR? The study findings beg the question, "Is prognosis related to the pathophysiologic significance of the lesion or simply to the amount of ischemia elicited in relation to any given lesion?" Most would say the former. The latter also might be true but would be strongly influenced by the stress applied. This was suggested in the study by Ladenheim et al. (*10*), in which defect size and the stress (double product) that induced it were related. Neither hypothesis is in accord with studies that suggest that the risk of "hard events" is unrelated to lesion severity or associated ischemia. There are many publications that demonstrate the relationship between the severity of induced ischemia, measured by a number of parameters, and prognosis (*10,21,210*). Other studies demonstrate the relationship between prognosis and the frequency of induced ischemia (*303,346,669*), as well as the prognostic value of the response of stress MPS to therapy (*303*). However, this relationship is again generally thought to relate indirectly to lesion severity and the relative ease of ischemia induction. Although many studies and clinical experience demonstrate the ability of medical therapy to reduce symptoms, there are also some studies that indicate that the suppression of ischemia may itself reduce coronary risk and improve long-term outcome (*346,668,669*). Only this study by Dakik et al. (*301*) and the article by Sharir et al. (*302*) demonstrate that the findings on vasodilator MPS are significantly affected by anti-ischemic therapy. Only the study by Dakik et al. (*301*) suggests that the method can be accurately applied to determine the anti-ischemic effect of medical therapy and its influence on outcome. This methodology must be tested.

When To Apply Scintigraphy?

Dynamic stress (exercise) testing of all kinds remains the primary noninvasive method for the diagnosis and evaluation of CAD and its related risk. Studies noted earlier have shown that, in the presence of a low CAD likelihood determined from epidemiologic and clinical variables and an interpretable ECG, MPS adds little to the risk stratification of a patient who can exercise adequately. Exercise testing with symptomatic, hemodynamic and ECG monitoring may be all that is required in patients with low pretest likelihood of CAD and a normal resting baseline ECG, who can perform to a level sufficient to address the clinical question (*9*). However, pathophysiologic data related to MPS is generally more reliable. It has been shown to augment diagnostic accuracy beyond the ability of the stress test alone, in both sexes and at all ages, and is especially useful in those with an intermediate pretest CAD likelihood. Stress scintigraphy has been recommended to gain added information in those cases in which the results of the stress ECG and related findings do not answer the clinical question, such as in the presence of an uninterpretable stress ECG. In such cases, scintigraphic findings may swiftly guide appropriate management and actually reduce costs by permitting the rapid selection and implementation of appropriate methods and therapies. The method already has been shown in many cases, especially those with an intermediate-to-high pretest or post-test likelihood of CAD, to have an added prognostic benefit beyond even quantitative stress test analysis (Fig. 3). Studies cited previously demonstrate the strong relationship with outcome (*1,9,10,16,19–21,318,334,341,342,349*) and the strong and appropriate impact on management (*2,9,10,46–48,106–108,128–130,576–578*).

In those who cannot exercise satisfactorily to address the clinical question, pharmacologic stress MPS with a coronary dilator remains the method of choice. Other conditions and patient groups benefiting from pharmacologic stress MPS are enumerated in Table 4 of *Self-Study Program III. Cardiology. Topic 2: Pharmacologic Stress.* Here, those sent to angiography or treated conservatively and followed with an abnormal scan had a high incidence of CAD and related events. In those with benign images and who were not studied invasively, there was an event rate of ~1%/yr, equal to that of an asymptomatic population in the coronary age group (*11*). This relationship between a benign prognosis and a normal scintigram was true even in the presence of a high likelihood of or even with known CAD (*1,9,16,48,126–128*), based on clinical and demographic factors (*14,342*), and remains one of several important clinical features of the method.

From another vantage point, Hachamovitch et al. (*673*) make the following points and related suggestions designed to extract the most from the perfusion study:

- Angina is a clinical diagnosis. There may be anginal equivalents, most commonly a variant of classic exertion-related chest pain or shortness of breath with exertion. This latter is sometimes classified as a "functional" symptom needing wall motion (echocardiography) analysis for its best assessment. However, if coronary related, it is most likely the result of diastolic dysfunction with elevated pulmonary venous pressure, and its primary perfusion-related etiology makes MPS best suited for its diagnosis and risk stratification. Such ischemic symptoms often relate to the most severe ischemic abnormalities.
- In those able to exercise to a level satisfactory to answer the clinical question, dynamic exercise testing is the method of choice, providing valuable symptomatic, hemodynamic and ECG data.
- Patients with a high-risk (≥4% hard event rate/yr) clinical or stress-test profile of CAD should go directly to angiography (*31*).
- Patients with a low risk (<1% hard event rate/yr) clinical or stress test profile of CAD should be treated medically and with risk-factor stratification.
- Patients with an intermediate risk (>1% and <4% hard event rate/yr) clinical or stress test profile of CAD should be studied with stress MPS and so directed to conservative medical or aggressive angiographic management.
- Those with nonanginal chest pain should be evaluated for other systemic pathology and evaluated for coronary risk factors,
- Asymptomatic patients with risk factors should be evaluated and treated medically with vigorous risk-factor reduction. Some researchers would perform ultrafast CT scanning for identification of coronary calcification. However, the position of this modality in clinical evaluation is not yet established. There are no controlled studies demonstrating the value of revascularization specifically in asymptomatic subjects with CAD.

Shaw et al. (*674*) analyzed stress test, MPS and clinical data among 3620 medically treated patients (42% female, 58% male) with an intermediate poststress test risk, to develop a hierarchical approach to coronary risk stratification after exercise. The results demonstrated that symptomatic patients with an intermediate event likelihood after quantitative exercise testing will benefit from further evaluation with an exercise MPS (Fig. 97).

MYOCARDIAL ISCHEMIA AND NONCORONARY HEART DISEASE

General Considerations

MPS is based on a test of the CFR, which is itself a test of coronary vasoreactivity. The latter may be compromised early in the course of atherosclerosis and may be abnormal in the setting of limited atherosclerotic narrowing. This may produce false-positive tests for coronary narrowing but true positives in relation to vasoregulation abnormalities. MPS has demonstrated regional abnormalities in relation to several conditions that cause myocardial ischemia in the absence of typical epicardial CAD. This also may be the case in those with longstanding hypertension and ventricular hypertrophy, noncoronary cardiomyopathies and other conditions. Narula et al. (*675*) found that both LVH and MPS defect size were independent predictors of outcome in hypertensive individuals.

Coronary Spasm

Coronary spasm most often occurs in the setting of atherosclerotic disease. It may, of course, present as a relatively isolated abnormality of vasoreactivity. Coronary spasm is not generally precipitated by stress testing. However, when present, the radionuclide distribution will parallel induced flow abnormalities. Because spasm often relates to severe, transmural ischemia, image defects in this condition may be among the most severe. Induction of spasm with ergonovine or other agent may be risky but was done as a diagnostic test in the controlled environment of the catheterization laboratory. Some researchers have demonstrated it to be safe to apply MPS for the indirect diagnosis of spasm during its provocation in selected patients without CAD (*676*).

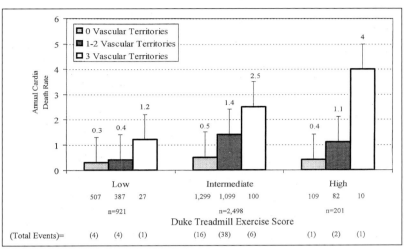

Figure 97 Added prognostic value of myocardial perfusion scintigraphy beyond the Duke Score. (Top) The annual death and infarction (event) rates related to low, intermediate and high Duke Exercise Treadmill Test Scores and exercise SPECT myocardial perfusion imaging results among 3620 study patients. The ability of the scintigram to risk stratify within Duke Score categories, here based on the extent of involvement of vascular regions, is apparent. The catheterization rate was also related to Duke Score and image findings. This latter relationship parallels that for events and supports the fact that image data is acted upon clinically in rough proportion to its clinical implications. (Reprinted, with permission, from Shaw LJ, Hachamovitch R, Peterson ED, et al. Using an outcomes based approach to identify candidates for risk stratification after exercise treadmill testing. *J Gen Intern Med* 1999;14:1–9.)

Arteritis and Cardiomyopathy

Coronary arteritis or embolization, ischemia related to a myocardial bridge or intramyocardial coronary vessels, coronary fistula (*677*) or a congenital anomalous coronary origin, may produce regional fixed or reversibly ischemic defects for obvious reasons. More global conditions, documented to produce ischemia and even life-threatening ischemia, are sometimes evident on MPS. These include LVH of any cause (*678*) and dilated and hypertrophic cardiomyopathy (*679*). Commonly, a perfusion study is requested to determine the cause of a dilated cardiomyopathy. Although a homogeneous pattern of uptake generally relates to a noncoronary etiology, the specificity of such evaluation suffers somewhat from the relationship of dilated cardiomyopathies to regional scar and even to regional, noncoronary-related ischemia. Although unusual, reversible defects may be seen here, as with hypertension or any cause of myocardial ischemia. Although defects in the myocardium of noncoronary cardiomyopathies often present spotty, widespread and limited fixed defects and a segmental defect distribution helps secure the diagnosis of CAD, this latter may also be seen, but less often, in noncoronary cardiomyopathies, as also may occasional reversible defects. Further, cavitary dilatation and wall motion abnormalities may themselves relate to image defects on the basis of a partial volume effect and not based in specific perfusion abnormalities. Right ventricular dilatation suggests a noncoronary cause but again is not wholly specific.

Among patients with cardiomyopathy, an ischemic cause was itself an independent predictor of mortality. Not noted specifically in this population is the prognostic value of the extent of MIR. However, studies related to the value of reperfusion in patients with dysfunctional but viable ischemic myocardium provide strong evidence related to the prognostic importance of scintigraphic findings (680).

Danilos et al. (681) demonstrated that the distribution of defects, their severity and reversibility all contribute to the likelihood of CAD in the presence of a congestive cardiomyopathy. Yao et al. (682) suggested that defect intensity alone could differentiate ischemic from nonischemic dysfunction. Gated SPECT also can help to differentiate an ischemic from a nonischemic cardiomyopathy by the finding of dysfunctional but perfused myocardium (683).

When approaching such patients, it is best to relate their global systolic function to noted perfusion defects. That is, rather than diagnose CAD based on the simple presence of perfusion defects or even reversible defects, ask the question, "Can these defects, fixed or reversible, explain the level of systolic dysfunction?" If the answer is "No," then the condition is probably noncoronary. Alternatively, the patient may have limited coronary disease that may not be the cause of widespread dysfunction. For example, a dilated and dysfunctional but relatively well-perfused ventricle in a patient studied before renal transplantation could have a hypertensive rather than a coronary cardiomyopathy. If the study is requested to determine not the diagnosis but the prognosis of the coronary patient with a severe dilated cardiomyopathy or to help guide the management of such patients, then the question is, at least in part, one of viability and should be answered in that context.

Cardiac Transplantation

Studies have not demonstrated a compelling advantage to any noninvasive imaging method for the early identification of transplant rejection. As in other settings, MPS has demonstrated value in the identification of recurrent obstructive coronary disease, whether of an atherosclerotic or immunologic cause. However, early recognition of the process has been unsuccessful. Recent work suggests that the serial evaluation of myocardial perfusion with ^{201}Tl imaging may well identify the early stages of allograft vasculopathy, the most common cause of death after the first year of transplantation (684). To this date, no method appears to replace the endomyocardial biopsy for the evaluation of rejection after heart transplantation. Serial study is often needed to recognize the decremental pattern of rejection (685). Perhaps the combined perfusion–function information of MPS will prove superior in this setting.

Collagen Vascular Diseases

A more unusual condition, also related to perfusion defects, is scleroderma heart disease (686). Although clinical correlation is always required to aid identification of the cause of ischemia and to differentiate among causes in such cases, the method generally maintains its specificity for CAD.

Valvular Disease

Not infrequently, patients with valvular heart disease may present symptoms or ECG changes suggesting associated CAD. There are surely many causes of potential ischemia in the setting of aortic stenosis, especially with concomitant LVH. Sometimes it is of value to differentiate among these and identify CAD in the presence of aortic stenosis or other valvular disease. Pharmacologic stress MPS has been demonstrated to be safe and accurate for the diagnosis of ischemia with associated CAD in the setting of aortic stenosis (*687*). Sometimes rest MPS is all that is needed to reassure that left ventricular dysfunction is most likely related to the hemodynamic effect of the obstructive lesion rather than the presence of (ischemic) scar.

Left Bundle Branch Block

Several studies have indicated the lack of specificity of exercise MPS for disease diagnosis in the setting of LBBB (*150–154*). Dipyridamole perfusion scintigraphy was demonstrated to be an excellent prognostic as well as diagnostic tool in a study evaluating 96 patients with LBBB (*688*). This appears to relate most prominently to scintigraphic defects, often reversible, in the interventricular septum. However, in high-risk, high-likelihood populations, the great number of normal and benign exercise scintigrams in LBBB relate to a benign prognosis, and most scintigraphic abnormalities in this setting relate to true CAD, with a similar sensitivity to that observed in the absence of LBBB. Realizing the deficiencies, the study is certainly of utility in the setting of LBBB, and exercise imaging may be performed when the evaluation of perfusion during exercise is needed. The findings of reduced specificity probably relate, in part, to a selection bias. The findings also relate to the difficult population with LBBB, with a high incidence of patients with reduced ventricular function and noncoronary cardiomyopathy (*154*). However, there is a pathophysiologic explanation for exercise-induced septal perfusion abnormalities in LBBB, in which regional septal myocardial oxygen demands may be relatively reduced as a result of the conduction-related contraction delay compared with other areas (*689,690*). The increased heart rate of exercise reduces further the already reduced diastolic flow in the late-contracting septum, whereas other regions augment perfusion in relation to demands, increasing the difference in relative regional perfusion. A number of studies indicate a maintained diagnostic specificity for CAD in relation to pharmacologic stress in the presence of LBBB, with agents such as dipyridamole or adenosine that primarily test the CFR and do not greatly augment heart rate or the double product (*155,156,295,691*). When highest perfusion-related specificity is required, dynamic exercise should be omitted in favor of direct coronary dilation as the method of choice to test the CFR in the presence of LBBB.

ASSESSMENT OF MYOCARDIAL VIABILITY

Overview

Dysfunctional myocardium in the setting of CAD may yet be viable. Identification of such dysfunctional but viable myocardium is a critical duty that often shapes treatment (see *Self-Study Program III. Cardiology. Topic 3: Cardiac PET Imaging* and *Self-Study Program III. Cardiology. Topic 5: Myocardial Perfusion Scintigraphy. Technical Aspects*) (Tables 30,31). Perfusion imaging appears to differentiate viable but dysfunctional "hibernating" myocardium

---

Table 30

EVIDENCE OF MYOCARDIAL VIABILITY AND FUNCTION REVERSIBILITY BASED ON SINGLE-PHOTON PERFUSION IMAGING

---

1. Extensive reversible perfusion abnormalities in regions with abnormal wall motion
2. Regional delayed redistribution of thallium-201 in regions with abnormal wall motion
3. Relatively modest fixed defect in regions with abnormal wall motion
4. Normal wall motion in the presence of fixed perfusion defects
5. Abnormal wall motion in the presence of normal or modestly reduced rest regional perfusion

---

from scar. In the presence of severe and/or extensive CAD, such patients with significantly reduced left ventricular function would more likely benefit from revascularization than from heart transplantation (692), with a good possibility of gaining improved function, improvement in New York Heart Association heart failure classification and prolonged survival (693). CAD must be sought in all with heart failure. Each of 2 recent series (694,695) demonstrated a significant ($\geq$4%) improvement in LVEF in roughly 30% of patients undergoing revascularization. Approximately 20% of these had an increase in LVEF >8%. The evaluation of myocardial viability and the likelihood of functional improvement after revascularization should be aspects of the evaluation of every patient with CAD and congestive heart failure.

Radionuclide Methods

Thallium-201: Uptake, Redistribution and Reinjection. The transmembrane passage of ^{201}Tl is an energy-requiring process. The intracellular localization of the radionuclide at once testifies to cell viability. The initial distribution of ^{201}Tl is primarily related to regional myocardial blood flow. However, several hours after administration, ^{201}Tl redistributes in the myocardium according to regional potassium space, marking cellular volume and indicating a more complete assessment of regional myocardial viability. Association of a reversible ^{201}Tl defect with regional myocardial viability was first demonstrated by Pohost et al. (696). This classic article first presented the concept and clinical implications of delayed defect reversibility on ^{201}Tl perfusion imaging. The authors studied this property with the injection of ^{201}Tl at rest during transient coronary occlusion and subsequently monitored serial radionuclide distribution after reperfusion in animals. Clinically, the question of regional myocardial viability is frequently raised in patients with CAD who have regional or global myocardial asynergy (304).

It is difficult to predict viability of myocardial regions with asynergy by the degree of regional wall motion abnormality, the status of coronary stenosis or the presence or absence of Q waves on the resting ECG (697,698).

However, Bodenheimer et al. (699) and Foster et al. (700) showed that reversible ^{201}Tl defects are associated with less severe myocardial asynergy. The contractility of these areas appeared to improve with nitroglycerin in >90% of cases (701). Rozanski et al. (702) evaluated the results of redistribution ^{201}Tl

---

Table 31

THE SPECTRUM OF MYOCARDIAL PATHOPHYSIOLOGY AND VIABILITY*

Myocardial state	Rest wall motion	Rest/stress perfusion	Metabolism
Normal	Normal	Normal	Normal
Scar	Abnormal	Abnormal–fixed	Absent
Ischemia	Normal	Reversible–defect	Normal
"Stunned"	Abnormal	Normal	Normal
Hibernating	Abnormal	Reversible or fixed defects	Preserved

*The expected relationships between the pathophysiologic state and related function, perfusion and metabolism.

scintigraphy for identifying myocardial viability in 25 patients who underwent radionuclide ventriculography before and after CABG. The presence of ^{201}Tl activity on the 4-hr redistribution study was associated with partial or complete improvement of wall motion in 81% (35/43) of segments after surgery. However, among the 29 asynergic segments with little corresponding ^{201}Tl activity on the redistribution study, only 4 (14%) showed postoperative improvement of resting wall motion abnormalities. Overall, redistribution on preoperative exercise ^{201}Tl images was highly predictive in identifying those 38 (54%) of 72 asynergic myocardial segments that would show subsequent improvement after CABG, irrespective of the severity of asynergy noted preoperatively. Similarly, Brundage et al. (703) demonstrated extensive focal improvement of asynergic segments related to preserved resting ^{201}Tl uptake or redistributing defects but a general lack of response in the absence of significant ^{201}Tl uptake or redistribution after subsequent CABG.

Late Reversibility. Several studies have confirmed that reversible ^{201}Tl defects are associated with myocardial viability but have emphasized that ^{201}Tl defects persisting on 4-hr redistribution imaging did not reliably predict infarcted myocardium (704). These nonreversible ^{201}Tl defects sometimes showed an improved or normal ^{201}Tl pattern after PTCA or CABG (705). Some defects that were apparently fixed after 4 hr, normalized 18–24 hr after ^{201}Tl injection (706) and demonstrated a high likelihood of functional improvement with revascularization. This late reversibility and viability was often, but not always, shown to be associated with less severe wall motion abnormalities and less frequent Q waves (698–701). The process of ^{201}Tl defect reversibility after exercise may take more than the conventional 4 hr.

In a subsequent study (707), the value of 4-hr versus 18–72-hr (late) ^{201}Tl redistribution tomographic imaging was compared in 21 patients who were imaged both before and after CABG (n = 15) or PTCA (n = 6). In a total of 201 tomographic myocardial segments with ^{201}Tl defects in which the related coronary arteries were subsequently successfully reperfused, the 4-hr redistribution images did not predict the postintervention scintigraphic improvement. Although 85% of 4-hr reversible segments improved after intervention, 72% of nonreversible segments also improved after intervention. In the same patient population, the late (24-hr) redistribution pattern was an effective predictor of postintervention scintigraphic improvement, with 95% of the late reversible segments improved after intervention and only 37% of the late nonreversible segments improved ($P < .0001$).

The frequency of ^{201}Tl late reversibility was prospectively assessed in 118 patients who underwent stress–redistribution ^{201}Tl SPECT (708). Late reversibility of at least 1 segment was present in 53% of the patients and in 22% of 762 segments with 4-hr nonreversible defects. Assessment of late-reversing segments appears critical for full viability assessment. Several factors may be responsible for the delay in ^{201}Tl redistribution after exercise injection of the agent. Rapid blood clearance of ^{201}Tl and subsequent low blood levels have been shown to be associated with a high frequency of nonreversible defects in viable myocardial regions. Poststress glucose loading with eating also results in decreased blood ^{201}Tl concentration in the initial 2 hr after ^{201}Tl injection, thus resulting in a high frequency of nonreversible defects in regions that have demonstrated reversibility at 4 hr when ^{201}Tl imaging was performed without glucose loading. Another potential mechanism for a delay in image reversibility is low regional myocardial blood flow. This is partly supported by the findings of a statistically significant inverse relation between the degree of coronary stenosis and the rate of ^{201}Tl defect reversibility. Here, the frequency of severe coronary stenosis (>90%) was 65% in association with 4-hr reversible defects and 85% in association with late reversible defects (707). Several studies support the fact that the likelihood of functional improvement after myocardial revascularization of dysynergic segments varies directly with the number of viable segments (692,709).

Rest–Redistribution. A similar logic also applies to the localization of radionuclide after rest injection. Here, again the initial, postinjection distribution parallels myocardial perfusion. In the presence of "rest ischemia" or "hibernating" myocardium, the defect seen immediately after rest injection can be misleading. Several studies document regional defect reversibility and viability related to improved image findings with delayed postrest imaging (692,710,711). A rest–4-hr delay redistribution protocol may be required to maximize viability assessment in some cases. The lack of significant ^{99m}Tc sestamibi redistribution may put it at a disadvantage for viability evaluation. Here, the relative intensity of fixed perfusion defects must also be considered, because viability has been better related to the amount of regional perfusion than to the presence of redistribution (712–714).

Reinjection. The administration of an additional 1-mCi dose of ^{201}Tl before delayed imaging, the reinjection method, has been shown to further maximize defect reversibility (713,714).

Imaging metabolism with flourine-18 (^{18}F) fluorodeoxyglucose (FDG) has long been the standard for myocardial viability, based on evidence of active glucose metabolism. The agent is a positron emitter, and positron emission tomography (PET) imaging is not always available. Bonow et al. (714) have demonstrated that the level of relative regional perfusion is itself evidence of viability and correlates strongly with active myocardial metabolism and FDG uptake. Here, relative perfusion ≥50% of maximal appears viable, even in apparently "fixed" defects. In addition, evidence of "redistribution," especially when applying the reinjection technique to dense defects <50% of peak radioactivity, aids viability assessment (714). The mechanism of improved relative uptake in viable myocardium is unclear and may relate to either a preferential uptake of radionuclide in the deficient region or, more likely, a generalized augmentation of activity in all regions. Both will relate to the visual impression of "redistribution." Similar findings have been confirmed more recently. Studies with quantitative PET indicate some overlap in relative and absolute regional perfusion between viable and nonviable segments, suggesting some difficulty in using perfusion measurements alone as viability markers (715). However, even in this quantitative PET perfusion study, overall higher perfusion related to a greater likelihood of viability. Thus, although an imperfect measure, there is significant support for the use of regional perfusion and uptake of a perfusion-related tracer in the assessment of regional myocardial viability. These agents all pass actively or passively through a viable cell membrane and bind to a cellular component in a living cell. Although perfusion brings the agent to the myocyte, localization within indicates viability. The relationship between ^{201}Tl uptake and regional viability, as evidenced by improved regional function after revascularization, has been demonstrated (250). Here, rather than a sharp cut-off at the 50% level of relative perfusion between viable myocardium and scar, there was an almost continuous relationship between the amount of radionuclide uptake and the likelihood of functional restoration after revascularization. Important here, as in other studies, was the higher negative predictive value of the perfusion scintigraphic method. This value is important if we are to offer revascularization to all who might benefit, rather than withhold it, on the basis of a falsely negative study, from those who could potentially benefit from revascularization. Yet, demonstrated as well, and also similar to other articles, was an overall greater specificity of low-dose dobutamine echocardiography for the determination of functional recovery compared with the scintigraphic method. Although the methods agreed in their findings among 82% of hypokinetic segments, the concordance was only 43% among 155 akinetic segments, where MPS identified many more viable segments.

Udelson et al. (446) demonstrated a similar relationship between the extent of radionuclide uptake and functional improvement in relation to ^{99m}Tc sestamibi imaging, with a positive predictive value of 75%–80% and a negative predictive value of 92%–96% for both ^{201}Tl and ^{99m}Tc sestamibi.

The study by Bonow et al. (714) employed 3 sets of ^{201}Tl SPECT images at peak stress, with 4-hr delay and after reinjection. Some defects that appeared to improve on 4-hr imaging actually worsened after reinjection, possibly because of ^{201}Tl kinetics in the presence of "resting ischemia." If the 4-hr images were omitted, the postreinjection study could appear to demonstrate a fixed defect. These segments could be reclaimed or found to redistribute and normalize, with evidence of viability, after 24 hr (704,707,708,714). The performance of 3 SPECT studies in a patient in a single day is impractical and puts a great burden on both patient and laboratory. Alternatively, rest and 4-hr postreinjection SPECT imaging may be followed by 24-hr delayed imaging if it is believed that further evidence of redistribution and viability would make a clinical difference.

Bax et al. (716) published a meta-analysis of 37 studies to evaluate methods to predict functional improvement after revascularization. Here, the sensitivity of the MPS was greatest, whereas low-dose dobutamine had highest specificity and overall predictive value, in spite of its high subjectivity and poor reproducibility. Is the perfusion method *too* sensitive? Beller (717) thinks not! Thallium-201 uptake marks regional viability (718). The accuracy values are compounded by the application in many studies of a fixed cutoff for the limit of scintigraphic viability, in which the relationship is rather proportional and continuous, varying from the relationship noted with the normal echocardiographic response to dobutamine. Issues of image analysis and pathophysiologic considerations are discussed later in this volume and elsewhere (719).

The method, applied with stress or as a rest–redistribution reinjection sequence, is of great value when considering the possible benefits of revascularization compared with transplantation (155,710). It is the presence of significant and preferably extensive viable myocardium in ischemic, asynergic myocardial areas that makes revascularization the intervention of choice and related to the greatest benefit, with significant potential for the restoration of resting function (692,693,714). Of course, whenever revascularization and specifically bypass surgery are recommended, even in the setting of extensive viability, the risk related to the procedure in the presence of poor left ventricular function, the likelihood of improved function in the setting of massive left ventricular dilatation and the risk related to extracardiac conditions (such as cerebrovascular disease) must be carefully considered.

Regional myocardial viability had originally been related to the presence of reversible perfusion defects (720,721). However, studies by Bonow et al. (714)

demonstrated the value of reinjection ^{201}Tl methods and established the level of tracer uptake as the marker of viability. These studies popularized the idea that viability was related to a relative regional activity level ≥50%. Others demonstrated a direct and relatively linear relationship between the level of regional activity and the likelihood of functional improvement after revascularization. Asynergic regions related to redistributing ^{201}Tl segments were more likely to demonstrate functional improvement after revascularization than those with mild-to-moderate fixed defects (79% and 30%, respectively; $P < 0.001$) (720,722). Perrone-Filardi et al. (250) studied the likelihood of functional reversibility among 40 CAD patients with LVEF <45% with dobutamine echocardiography and rest–redistribution ^{201}Tl stress MPS. The incidence of improvement of regional function after revascularization was overestimated by the visually assessed dobutamine response. However, the relative percentage of regional activity related quite linearly, at levels above and below 50%, with the likelihood of functional improvement after revascularization. Among 54 patients with an ischemic cardiomyopathy studied with dobutamine echocardiography and stress ^{201}Tl MPS, Amanullah et al. (723) found that contractile reserve was more often related to hypokinetic than akinetic or dyskinetic segments and that normal or near normal segments or reversible defects on MPS, as well as contractile reserve with gated low-dose dobutamine ^{99m}Tc sestamibi, were significantly more sensitive for the identification of functional reversibility and potential viability than was evaluation of contractile reserve alone.

Specificity of Viability Studies. No functional improvement would be expected in areas of fixed defects if they related to an admixture of necrotic and normal myocardium, as in the setting of nontransmural MI. Yet, protection against ischemia may result. However, if the finding represents an admixture of subepicardial hypoperfusion and subendocardial necrosis, incomplete redistribution may be seen but would have little implication for functional improvent, because subepicardial function contributes little to systolic motion. Longstanding hibernation may relate to irreversible ultrastructural changes and irreversible dysfunction in the setting of persistent radiotracer uptake. These, with the adequacy of revascularization (693,713) and a positive selection bias favoring intervention of "viable" segments, are some of the factors that may reduce the specificity of image findings.

Technetium-99m Sestamibi/Tetrofosmin. Technetium-99m sestamibi enters the myocardium by diffusion and is not energy dependent. Like all current perfusion agents, however, its passage and localization are dependent on the presence of an intact and viable cell membrane and intracellular structure. Technetium-99m sestamibi uptake and that of tetrofosmin are well related to regional viability. Yet, their lack of significant redistribution suggests that their absence may not exclude viability as well as that of ^{201}Tl (Fig. 98). However, Udelson et al. (446) (Fig. 99) have demonstrated that sestamibi uptake parallels that of ^{201}Tl in patients with CAD and left ventricular dysfunction. Here (446), sestamibi distribution appeared more to resemble the delayed or postreinjection pattern of ^{201}Tl distribution rather than that seen in early ^{201}Tl administration. They also have demonstrated that an increased LVEF is not the only potential benefit to revascularization (724). Other studies also have demonstrated the likelihood of restored regional function after revascularization in relation to regional uptake of ^{99m}Tc-based agents with conventional SPECT methods (444,725,726). The uptake and viability assessment of sestamibi was similar to that of ^{201}Tl at rest in patients with ischemic cardiomyopathy (727). A review article by Bisi et al. (728) supports the value and accuracy of ^{99m}Tc sestamibi for viability evaluation and demonstrates the evidence that it is every bit as accurate as ^{201}Tl. Acampa et al. (729) found differences in defect intensity and size but no difference in the evaluation of viability when ^{201}Tl, sestamibi and tetrofosmin were imaged in 17 patients.

In an effort to identify "stunned" myocardium and predict functional recovery, a prospective study in 84 patients with AMI compared LVEF measured on admission and 6 wk later, with infarct size measured on admission and discharge with ^{99m}Tc sestamibi rest imaging (730). Perfusion imaging identified stunned myocardium and predicted postinfarction functional improvement in patients with discordant left ventricular function and dysfunction beyond that explained by the size of the associated infarction. Others, with hyperkinetic ventricles and LVEF higher than expected from the related infarct size, demonstrated a fall in LVEF on late study. Predischarge perfusion imaging predicted function late after infarction. This study was reminiscent

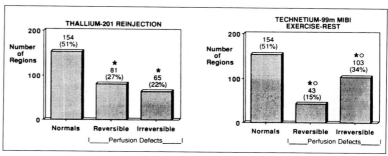

Figure 98   Thallium-201 (^{201}Tl) reinjection compared with technetium-99m (^{99m}Tc) sestamibi distribution. Shown is the distribution of findings on the segmental analysis of exercise perfusion images acquired with ^{201}Tl and the reinjection technique, left, and with ^{99m}Tc sestamibi and the exercise–rest separate 2-day protocol. In this patient population, more reversible segments were detected on ^{201}Tl reinjection imaging compared with exercise–rest ^{99m}Tc sestamibi imaging. This is 1 piece of evidence suggesting the superior viability assessment capability of ^{201}Tl methods, possibly the result of its characteristic redistribution. * = $P < 0.001$, compared with reversibility on ^{201}Tl redistribution imaging (not shown); * ° = $P < 0.01$, when ^{99m}Tc sestamibi is compared with ^{201}Tl reinjection with respect to reversibility. (Reprinted, with permission, from Cuocolo A, Pace L, Ricciardelli B, et al. Identification of viable myocardium in patients with chronic coronary artery disease: comparison of thallium-201 scintigraphy with reinjection and technetium-99m methoxyisobutyl isonitrile. *J Nucl Med* 1992;33:505–511.)

of the assessment of the "functional infarct size" in animals studied serially after AMI (458).

Nitrates. Nitroglycerin or nitrates given sublingually (731) or, more effectively, intravenously (732) appear to increase regional perfusion and radiotracer myocardial uptake in rest perfusion images by dilation of epicardial or collateral coronary vessels and increase the ability to identify the full potential of viable myocardium. Identification of viable myocardium seems to be enhanced by the administration of sublingual or transdermal nitroglycerin (282,281,733, 734). This maximizes the estimate of regional viability but may, if given with pharmacologic stress, bring an underestimation of MIR as a result of an increase in baseline epicardial or regional coronary collateral flow. Batista et al. (735) have demonstrated that the performance of nitroglycerin rest imaging increased the uptake of the radiotracer and reversible defects with exercise ^{99m}Tc sestamibi MPS among 38 patients with prior infarction. The method enhanced identification of viable segments to a level related to rest–redistribution or reinjection ^{201}Tl.

The Advantage of Gating. Technetium-99m radionuclide angiography and gated ^{99m}Tc sestamibi perfusion imaging were analyzed in the postexercise recovery period in 31 patients with severe coronary disease and exercise-induced angina. Prolonged systolic dysfunction, albeit mild, was evident even 30 min after exercise in some patients with induced angina, after documented resolution of perfusion defects. "Stunning" was documented (736). A comparison of left ventricular function on gated SPECT MPS, at rest and with stress, may also be of value in the identification of stunned myocardium (183). The addition of wall motion to perfusion data resulted in the increase in sensitivity to viable myocardium (737).

Negative Evidence. Yet not all studies support the relationship of ^{99m}Tc sestamibi uptake to regional viability. Marcassa et al. (738) studied 48 patients with chronic CAD and resting regional dysfunction. Rest sestamibi images were compared with redistribution ^{201}Tl images after rest administration, using objective,

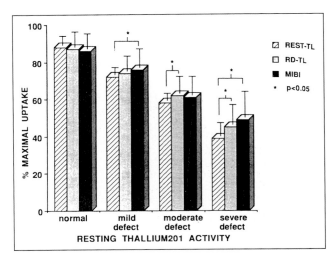

Figure 99 Thallium-201 (^{201}Tl) redistribution compared with technetium-99m (^{99m}Tc) sestamibi. Shown is a bar graph comparing initial rest ^{201}Tl activity (REST-TL), delayed rest–redistribution ^{201}Tl activity (RD-TL) and 1-hr postrest injection ^{99m}Tc sestamibi (MIBI) in akinetic or dyskinetic segments. Segments are normalized to the mean resting ^{201}Tl activity. Here, ^{99m}Tc activity was similar to that of ^{201}Tl activity. (Reprinted, with permission, from Udelson JE, Coleman PS, Metherall J, et al. Predicting recovery of severe regional dysfunction: comparison of resting scintigraphy with 201-Tl and 99m-Tc-sestamibi. *Circulation* 1994;89:2555–2561.)

quantitative methods (*738*). Uptake of the tracers was similar in normal segments and with fixed ^{201}Tl defects, but sestamibi uptake was significantly lower in segments that were reversible on delayed imaging. Also, there was a lack of correlation between ^{99m}Tc sestamibi and PET FDG uptake in 22 patients with prior infarction (*739*). FDG evidence of viability was present in 50% of 64 segments with ^{99m}Tc sestamibi activity >40%. Moderate and severe sestamibi defects underestimated viability. These findings cause concern about the underestimation of viable but dysfunctional myocardium with rest imaging using ^{99m}Tc-based agents. The relative value for viability evaluation of this and other ^{99m}Tc-based perfusion agents is still debated.

There is further skepticism from those who believe that perfusion alone, and certainly relative regional perfusion as measured in a conventional SPECT study, is not a reliable marker for viability (*715*).

The Effects of Dobutamine. Regional myocardial blood flow was quantitated with PET nitrogen-13 ammonia in 15 patients with quantitative coronary angiography during incremental dobutamine infusion (*740*). Dobutamine increased flow in good correlation with the increase in rate–pressure product (.93) and augmented flow inversely, but weakly, in proportion to the severity of regional coronary stenosis (.63). However, reduced flow augmentation in stenotic beds often overlapped the normal levels at low levels of flow increment, making differentiation of normals from stenotic beds impossible. The dobutamine-induced increase in flow generally did not reach the levels produced by coronary dilators. Dobutamine flow augmentation did not test the CFR. Although the presence and severity of coronary stenosis can still be tested with the comparison of differential flows induced, the method may lose sensitivity when the achieved double product fails to achieve a sufficient rate–pressure product. This may be especially important when evaluating a secondary ischemic end point, such as wall motion, and may be insufficient when seeking to assess the risk of high-stress noncardiac surgery. Akinetic segments probably are composed of a mixture of viable and scarred tissue. Alternatively, viable segments with significant ^{201}Tl uptake may be tethered by scarred segments and so cannot respond to revascularization. For these reasons, perhaps functional improvement after revascularization is not the best measure of either image markers of viability or the potential benefit of revascularization.

The ability to augment function in viable yet dysynergic segments appears to be flow related. When coronary flow was reduced to 50% in an animal model of low-flow ischemia, regional ^{201}Tl was >50% of peak uptake and function was reversible, yet low-dose dobutamine brought no systolic functional augmentation and no increase in the regional flow, each of which is needed for augmentation of systolic function and recruitment of functional reserve (*740*).

Lee et al. (719) found a similar insufficiency of low-dose dobutamine to augment function in 54% of dysfunctional myocardial segments in 19 study patients. Here, these segments were noted to be viable on the basis of PET FDG uptake, and flow reserve, measured quantitatively with PET oxygen-15 water, was reduced (719). With these relationships, the pathophysiologic underpinnings of the method appear insecure, and the excellent clinical abilities of the method appear quite fortuitous.

In spite of concerns to the contrary, the diagnostic and prognostic abilities of the conventional perfusion method have held up well in the post-thrombolytic era. Patients with prior thrombolysis or other forms of revascularization, as well as uninstrumented patients, are evaluated well for viability and recurrent disease, generally in the setting of recurrent symptoms.

What Are the Important End Points for Viability?

The improvement of left ventricular function and LVEF may not be the only benefits of revascularization to dysfunctional myocardium. Demonstrated improvement in regional wall motion, improved heart failure status and prolonged survival after revascularization may relate to aspects of improved myocardial dynamics and may occur even in the absence of evident improvement in LVEF. The latter may be an overemphasized and relatively superficial indicator of the benefits of revascularization in the setting of viable but dysfunctional myocardium. Although function may not be restored, revascularization may nonetheless benefit survival, reduce the detrimental effects of ventricular remodeling (724) and reduce subsequent ischemic events.

Outcomes end points are most desirable for evaluation of the prediction of regional viability. However, most studies simply assess the serial change in LVEF weeks to months after revascularization. Although an improved LVEF may relate to an improved outcome, so too may the lack of LVEF improvement. Outcome may be favorably influenced by reduced ischemia induction, prevention of remodeling or arrhythmia, reduced diastolic dysfunction or reduced likelihood of subsequent MI or death, in the absence of improved LVEF. One study demonstrated no difference in outcome after revascularization between groups with or without improvement in LVEF (741). However, 7 published studies demonstrate that viable but dysfunctional myocardium presents a high-risk substrate with a high likelihood of significant improvement in outcome when revascularized and a worsened outcome when treated medically (709,742–747). Among patients with severe left ventricular dysfunction and ischemic cardiomyopathy, the extent of PET mismatch was found to correlate directly with improvement in cardiac functional status after revascularization (748) and was found also to serve far better than traditional methods for the selection of patients who will demonstrate a survival benefit (749). Those with PET mismatch demonstrated a 97% 1-yr survival rate compared with an 11.4% in-hospital death rate and a 79% 1-yr survival in those selected for revascularization based on traditional methods (748). Similar relationships between MPS indicators of viability and outcome have been found in relation to [201]Tl (709). Are PET viability methods better than SPECT? Do results apply to those with very low LVEF or very large ventricles? How much mismatch or ^{201}Tl/^{99m}Tc uptake or how much of the left ventricle must be involved to assure a favorable result of revascularization?

Fluorodeoxyglucose Imaging and Improvement of Function After Revascularization

Metabolic activity demonstrated on PET FDG imaging in excess of perfusion in the same area, the "mismatch" pattern, remains the gold standard for viability (see *Self-Study Program III. Cardiology. Topic 3: Cardiac PET Imaging*). Early studies demonstrated the superiority of PET "mismatch" compared with conventional MPS for viability assessment. More recent work has demonstrated increased advantages to the application of convention SPECT perfusion methods (*749*). FDG uptake with a perfusion–metabolism mismatch in dysfunctional myocardial segments presents a high likelihood of improved regional and global left ventricular function after revascularization. Christian et al. (*695*) found that roughly one-third of unselected patients undergoing CABG with reduced left ventricular function improve LVEF >4% after surgery, a large group. With this, an improved heart failure classification as well as improved prognosis have been demonstrated. This has an important implication for the management of patients with congestive heart failure, among whom 80% have CAD as its basis. Perfusion measured in early studies by PET is now more often measured for this purpose with conventional SPECT methods. Because of the relative scarcity of cyclotrons and PET scanners and the cost of PET imaging where cardiac perfusion studies have now been approved for specific reimbursement, a "hybrid" SPECT perfusion/PET metabolism is often performed. Using special collimation, FDG may now itself be imaged with standard scintillation cameras (*750*). Care must be taken in the comparison of the 140-keV or 81-keV perfusion and 511-keV metabolism images for "mismatch," because attenuation in the former may masquerade as underperfusion. For this reason, a prone image should always be made when the causes of "defects" are questioned. However, assuming the questioned defect is the only defect in the perfusion study, normalization with prone imaging should not lead to PET metabolic imaging but, instead, to canceling the scheduled PET study, because here perfusion tracer uptake is a good indicator of viability needing no further adjudication.

Bax et al. (*751*) studied 55 patients with contractile dysfunction with FDG PET and ^{201}Tl perfusion SPECT. FDG uptake identified segments that improved functionally after revascularization and, when in great enough abundance (>3 of 20 segments or >15% of the ventricle) brought an improvement in LVEF and heart failure symptoms (*747*). The degree of improvement in heart failure symptoms related directly to the amount of "hibernating" myocardium evident. The greatest chance of functional improvement related to hibernation in the LAD distribution.

Patients demonstrating a significant extent of this "mismatch" pattern, but not those with a match pattern, generally improve function and have been shown to improve heart failure classification and survival after revascularization but not with medical therapy (see *Self-Study Program III. Cardiology. Topic 3: Cardiac PET Imaging*, Figs. 5A–E). Recent studies actually demonstrate an increased mortality when revascularization is performed in those with a "match" pattern (*709,710,739,747,751,752*). Those with "matched" defects generally will not improve with revascularization and may suffer. Several studies performed in >500 patients (*444,742–745,753–755*) demonstrated that the event rate is significantly higher when patients with extensive hibernation are treated medically. Deaths in these patients occurred early after hibernation was diagnosed, suggesting that revascularization should be performed early (*756*). Elseasser et al. (*757*) demonstrated 3 stages of cellular degeneration, which progress in severity over time with eventual cell death in the presence of persistent ischemia or hibernation, and related the perfusion imaging findings to the effects of revascularization. Again, the best surgical and functional results related to the least pathologic segments, indicating the need for early identification of hibernation and early intervention. This was again confirmed by Beanlands et al. (758), who noted a greater increase in LVEF after CABG performed early rather than late in patients with reduced LVEF and evidence of hibernation.

Evidence suggests that viability in dysynergic regions must involve 15%–25% of the left ventricular mass if revascularization is to yield an increased LVEF. According to pathologic studies and clinical observations (757–759), LVEF is not likely to improve, regardless of the extent of dysfunctional but viable myocardium, in the presence of fibrosis affecting >40% of the left ventricular mass. Further, massive left ventricular dilatation with proposed stretching and distortion of the relationship between contractile elements will reduce the likelihood of reversal and functional improvement with revascularization, even in the presence of apparent viability. This unfortunate circumstance may relate as well to ventricles with a very low LVEF. CABG performed in very large ventricles with very low LVEF still carries a significant risk, possibly without the great potential benefit that would accompany revascularization in the setting of viable and dysfunctional myocardium in other circumstances.

Much of the focus of studies relating levels of perfusion and metabolism and the dobutamine response to myocardial viability and functional improvement after revascularization has been on patients with LVEF >30%, without gross ventricular dilatation and in whom the primary symptom is angina. These are situations in which patients presenting primarily with heart failure or severe reduction in LVEF are underrepresented. Haas et al. (748) evaluated the results of revascularization in 35 patients with a mean LVEF of 30%, selected on the basis of clinical parameters, and 34 patients with a mean LVEF of 28%, selected on the basis of PET. There was a 10% short-term surgical risk and a poor long-term outcome in those chosen without reference to PET parameters. Although there has been no extensive evaluation of revascularization in patients with viable myocardium and a very low LVEF, Muhlbaier et al. (760) demonstrated the greatest surgical revascularization benefit in the group with the lower ejection fraction. Louie et al. (761) found that, even with adequate target vessels and extensive hibernation, an end-diastolic diameter >70 mm or an LVEF <15% brought increased complications with CABG and a low likelihood of improved LVEF. Yamaguchi et al. (762) found that, even in patients with severe angina and extensive hibernation, a left ventricular volume >100 ml/m^2 would more likely relate to worsening heart failure and an increased incidence of death than to improved LVEF after revascularization. In patients with very large left ventricles, the problem of self attenuation has been raised, making viability assessment difficult with SPECT performed in the absence of attenuation correction. In these patients, PET may be more useful than SPECT. In addition, the chance of functional and symptomatic improvement falls with the duration of heart failure. Schwartz et al. (763) demonstrated an improvement in function only when heart failure was present <50 days!

The Clinical Issue

In the United States, 4–5 million patients have congestive heart failure, amounting to 1%–2% of the population. Heart failure is the leading discharge diagnosis in patients ≥65 yr of age, accounts for 1 million hospitalizations/yr and $11 billion in direct health care costs. In a review of 13 randomized heart failure trials

(*764*), 68% of patients had CAD, with prognoses directly related to LVEF. Prognoses worsened significantly with LVEF <35%, and survival was benefited by CABG in those with reduced LVEF and multivessel disease (*36*). Although CABG was superior to medical treatment in such patients with poor left ventricular function (*36,304,310*), the risk of surgery increased proportionately and inversely to the LVEF (*304,310*), with a 60% 5-yr survival with surgical treatment of this group. Patient selection for revascularization must be optimized.

In patients with CAD and poor left ventricular function, the clinical question often arises as to whether the patient would benefit from revascularization or if cardiac transplantation would be more beneficial. In the situation in which contractile function is compromised, the myocardium may still be viable in 2 situations: (1) Myocardial stunning, which is dysfunction occurring after recent severe ischemia but persistent despite restoration of myocardial blood flow or reduced blood flow demand. Here, the delay in functional recovery varies directly with the severity of ischemic insult. (2) Myocardial hibernation, in which downregulation of cardiac function appears to relate to a chronic reduction of blood flow. However, the condition may be seen with preserved perfusion and may be related to recurrent stunning (*765,766*). Thallium-201 uptake demonstrates myocardial viability, because its uptake is an energy-requiring process related to adequate blood flow and implying an intact sarcolemmal function with maintained electrochemical gradients and preserved metabolism. However, many myocardial segments with reduced ^{201}Tl uptake with standard imaging methods will improve function after revascularization (Fig. 100). The full value of ^{201}Tl imaging is yielded only with 4- and 24-hr redistribution and postreinjection imaging. Technetium-99m sestamibi and tetrofosmin do not redistribute, and so they may suffer insensitivity to viability assessment. However, several articles support their value in this regard. Myocardial viability in dysfunctional segments using PET imaging is based on the finding of active myocellular metabolism in the presence of severely reduced perfusion. Various protocols utilizing combinations of rest, redistribution and reinjection thallium imaging have been devised, validated and compared to optimally assess the presence of dysfunctional but viable myocardium (*707,714,767*). A number of studies have demonstrated thallium protocols using either rest–redistribution or stress–redistribution reinjection protocols to be nearly as accurate as PET in assessing myocardial viability (*707,715*). These protocols all depend upon the optimal localization of the perfusion radiotracer in the myocardium and dynamic redistribution of thallium with time. Generally, stunned myocardium would be expected to have regional dysfunction in the region of normal or near-normal perfusion, whereas

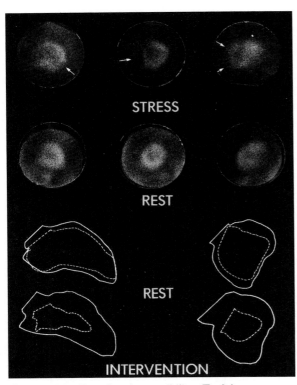

Figure 100 Functional reversibility. (Top) Large reversible abnormalities (arrows) are noted in the perfusion images. (Bottom) End-diastolic (solid lines) and end-systolic (dotted lines) outlines from the left ventriculogram of the same patient acquired at rest and after ventricular ectopy indicate reversibility of wall motion abnormalities. Normal resting perfusion indicates viability and expected reversibility of functional abnormalities with a ventricular premature contraction after nitroglycerin or after successful revascularization. (Reprinted, with permission, from Brundage BH, Massie BM, Botvinick EH, et al. Improved regional ventricular function after successful surgical revascularization. *J Am Coll Cardiol* 1984;3:902–911.)

hibernating myocardium would relate to regional dysfunction in the presence of a spectrum of scintigraphic findings that relate to viability and infarcted myocardium with rest dysfunction in a region of a fixed defect. These differ from ischemia, in which normal rest function usually relates to reversible defects.

Thus, the decision to refer the patient with dysfunctional myocardium to revascularization can be greatly assisted by the use of MPS, with which dysfunction based in viable but underperfused myocardium could well benefit from revascularization. Udelson et al. (768) reviewed the clinical importance and methods of viability evaluation, and Beller et al. (769) presented a review of the issue.

Fluorodeoxyglucose Imaging with Conventional Cameras

See *Self-Study Program III. Cardiology. Topic 3: Cardiac PET Imaging* and see *Self-Study Program III. Cardiology. Topic 5: Myocardial Perfusion Scintigraphy. Technical Aspects; 126–129.*

RISK STRATIFICATION IN THE POST-THROMBOLYTIC ERA

The Prethrombolytic Era

Many studies performed before thrombolytic therapy demonstrated the ability of exercise or pharmacologic stress MPS to identify and risk stratify CAD after infarction (316,318,474). In these and other studied noted previously, with 508 patients undergoing exercise MPS, multivessel defects identified 72% of patients with multivessel disease with a specificity of 86%. In these same studies, the sensitivity of the exercise test for multivessel disease detection was only 59%. As reviewed previously, Gibson et al. (288) demonstrated the superiority of exercise MPS with ^{201}Tl to risk stratify uncomplicated postinfarction patients 65 yr old or younger, compared with stress testing alone or even angiography (Figs. 70,71).

Conservative (Medical) Versus Aggressive (Coronary Angiography and Revascularization) Management

Although the results of early studies were ambiguous (495), MPS appears to maintain its accuracy and clinical value in the "post-thrombolytic patient" (496–498). The method of perfusion scintigraphy has been applied well and is of great value for the assessment of the benefit of thrombolysis, in many blinded studies (273–277).

However, MPS may be unnecessary if patients come to angiography regardless of stress image findings. Today, >70% of patients, with regional variation, come to angiography early after infarction (774,775). It is tempting to then intervene and open the occluded vessel or bypass the heart with 3-vessel disease. Although this is widely done, there is little data to support this practice, and an international sampling of practice demonstrates no survival benefit or improved outcome for angiography and revascularization performed routinely days after infarction (273,274,465,508,645,776,777). The TIMI Phase II clinical trial (653) demonstrated no difference in outcomes among 3339 patients with acute infarction, among whom 1681 were treated with immediate angiography and revascularization and 1658 were treated with a conservative approach. In fact, routine early angiography may increase mortality (778).

The Controversy

There remains an active ongoing controversy regarding the most clinically appropriate and most cost-effective manner of risk stratification, after thrombolytic therapy. Angiography itself is not predictive at the time of the procedure. Neither qualitative nor quantitative angiographic variables at 90 min after thrombolysis can predict subsequent coronary reocclusion (*779*). A broader question relates to the controversy regarding the most clinically appropriate and most cost-effective method to evaluate postinfarction patients in general. Should coronary angiography be routinely performed in these patients, or can it be performed selectively after risk is determined noninvasively?

Fully 70% of patients undergo angiography after MI. The cardiologist then tends to act on the findings with a high rate of PTCA, stent or CABG. However, there is no current data to justify this practice. Reports from several countries repeatedly demonstrate that uniform intervention after acute MI does not improve outcome! Although compelling evidence demonstrates the value of primary angioplasty (*517,569,570,832*), a recent summary of studies assessing the value of early intervention after MI demonstrates that the indiscriminate use of angiography and PTCA within 2–7 days of MI actually increases mortality and costs (*513,655,674,780–783*) (Figs. 101–103).

The answer to this question lies in part in the several large randomized trials that have been published and that demonstrate the value of revascularization in this acute setting, but only with the presence of clinically demonstrable MIR. Most, if not all, of these present MPS as the noninvasive method that can subset patients

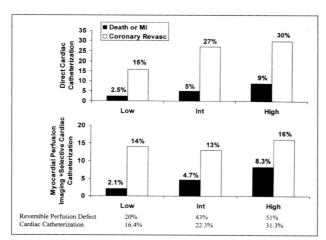

Figure 101 Event rates by pretest clinical risk subsets according to management group. "Hard and soft" event rates among those with stable angina were lower in all pretest risk subsets among those sent to angiography only after abnormal stress myocardial perfusion scintigraphy compared with those sent directly to angiography. Low = low pretest likelihood; Int = intermediate pretest likelihood; High = high pretest likelihood; MI = myocardial infarction. (Reprinted, with permission, from Shaw LJ, Hachamovitch R, Berman DS, et al. The economic consequences of available diagnostic and prognostic strategies for the evaluation of stable angina patients: an observational assessment of the value of precatheterization ischemia. For the Economics of Noninvasive Diagnosis (END) Multicenter Study Group. *J Am Coll Cardiol* 1999;33: 661–669.)

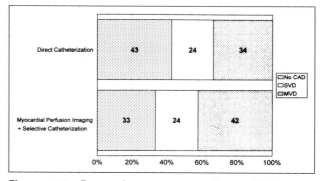

Figure 102 Extent of coronary artery disease (CAD) according to management group. The incidence of normal coronary angiograms was much lower among those sent to angiography only after abnormal stress myocardial perfusion scintigraphy (MPS). The incidence of normal angiograms among those studied first with scintigraphy was not as high, because of the selective nature of the population and the image criteria applied to recommend angiography. Of course, many more with normal stress MPS never went to angiography. MVD = multivessel coronary disease; SVD = single-vessel disease. (Reprinted, with permission, from Shaw LJ, Hachamovitch R, Berman DS, et al. The economic consequences of available diagnostic and prognostic strategies for the evaluation of stable angina patients: an observational assessment of the value of precatheterization ischemia. For the Economics of Noninvasive Diagnosis (END) Multicenter Study Group. *J Am Coll Cardiol* 1999;33:661–669.)

into those to be treated conservatively with medical management and those to be treated aggressively, catheterized and potentially revascularized (*7,36,278,279,306,464*).

Ellis et al. (*131*) could demonstrate no clinical benefit nor improvement in left ventricular function among post-thrombolysis patients with residual stenoses submitted to routine angioplasty in the absence of test evidence of MIR and evidence of ischemia on scintigraphy. Rouleau and a group of international authors (*509*) related outcomes to the frequency of angiography and revascularization in their respective countries. In the United States and Canada, there was a similar incidence of death (23% and 22%, respectively) and reinfarction (13% and 14%, respectively), although coronary angiography (68% and 35%, respectively) and revascularization (31% and 12%, respectively) were performed much more often in the United States. Similar data was generated in the postinfarction GUSTO-II study (*509,667*), in which U.S. and Canadian centers again differed in the incidence of coronary angiography (81% and 26%, respectively) and revascularization (59% and 15%, respectively) but not in mortality rate, (5.6% and 5.7%, respectively).

Patients presenting with ischemic symptoms within 4 hr of onset of infarction symptoms and with at least 1-mm ST elevation were assigned to aggressive, angiography-first (n = 1681) or conservative management (n =

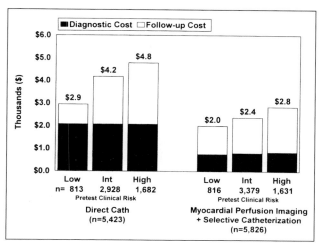

Figure 103   Cost effectiveness of myocardial perfusion scintigraphy evaluation. Shown are the overall diagnostic and follow-up costs of care for aggressive management with direct catheterization and conservative management with initial stress perfusion imaging and angiography based on the findings among 11,372 consecutive stable angina patients who were referred for stress myocardial perfusion tomography or cardiac catheterization. Diagnostic and follow-up costs of care were 30%–41% higher for patients undergoing direct cardiac catheterization. Solid bars = diagnostic cost; open bars = follow-up cost; Cath = cardiac catheterization; Low = low pretest likelihood; Int = intermediate pretest likelihood; High = high pretest likelihood. (Reprinted, with permission, from Shaw LJ, Hachamovitch R, Berman DS, et al. The economic consequences of available diagnostic and prognostic strategies for the evaluation of stable angina patients: an observational assessment of the value of precatheterization ischemia. For the Economics of Noninvasive Diagnosis (END) Multicenter Study Group. *J Am Coll Cardiol* 1999;33:661–669.)

1658) groups. The former went to immediate angiography and revascularization when appropriate anatomically. The latter were managed medically, unless evident spontaneous ischemia or ischemia on low-level stress testing brought invasive study and possible revascularization. Both management groups had the same favorable outcomes (*654*). The TIMI II trial demonstrated no benefit to an aggressive, invasive approach compared with angiography, based on ischemic risk, documented noninvasively (*387*).

In a large randomized study of 1473 patients with unstable angina or non-Q–wave MI, the event rate over the first year did not differ between those treated with aggressive and conservative management strategies (*387,388*). In the former group, immediate angiography and revascularization were applied as the primary treatment option, whereas the latter group received medical therapy unless evident recurrent or significant provoked ischemia, often identified on stress testing and MPS, justified crossover to the aggressive–invasive management group.

Non-Q–wave MIs are generally partial or "incomplete" infarctions. With the expectation that many patients with this condition are at high risk and will experience a subsequent event, they are generally managed with an invasive strategy. The VANQWISH study (*655*) randomized 920 patients with non-Q–wave infarction to either invasive management, in which patients went to coronary angiography within 72 hr after diagnosis and were managed based on the findings, or conservative management, in which medical therapy was instituted and noninvasive testing with perfusion imaging was again applied early to determine the indication for angiography. The number of hard end points (death and MI) and the number of revascularization procedures were significantly higher in the invasive strategy group at hospital discharge, at 1 mo and at 1 yr. Overall mortality did not differ between groups. Most patients with non-Q–wave infarction do not benefit from routine, early invasive management and revascularization.

The FRISC II prospective, randomized multicenter trial compared revascularization rates and outcomes, death or nonfatal infarction in 2457 patients with unstable anginal and non-Q infarction evaluated at 58 Scandinavian hospitals (784). Conclusions stated that early invasive evaluation and revascularization related to fewer events compared with angiography based on the results of stress testing. However, there was no difference in death rate between those treated invasively and based on noninvasive evaluation. The difference in infarction rate was statistically significant but marginal, representing an absolute advantage of 2%! But at what cost? If asked, the investigators could not tell their patients that early intervention would increase the length of their lives, and infarction rate was greater among women managed with early angiography than with information based on noninvasive findings. Imaging was not performed.

There is no convincing data supporting routine angiography after uncomplicated infarction, thrombolysis, non-Q–wave infarction or unstable angina. However, the presence of ventricular tachycardia or postinfarction angina is an indication for angiography.

The Thrombolytic Era

MPS Inadequate? In this post-thrombolytic era, some studies suggest the inadequacy of risk stratification by MPS. It is likely that this, in part, relates to the relatively low incidence of multivessel disease, death and total events in patients enrolled in several multicenter thrombolytic trials (278,279). These enrollees are generally younger, without prior infarction, hemodynamic instability or heart failure and with a higher rest LVEF than generally characterizes the population with acute infarction (785).

The incidence of 3-vessel CAD was only 13% among those enlisted in the GUSTO-I trial (786). Patients selected for acute PTCA of a single vessel are essentially risk stratified with the performance of the successful procedure, a beneficial method, likely superior to acute thrombolytic therapy (787,788). Thus, all methods may be hard pressed to identify, soon after revascularization, the few events that occur.

Most important, too, is that many with acute MI are not treated because of the narrow inclusion criteria of thrombolytic protocols. Designed to filter out those most likely to suffer an acute coronary occlusion and to benefit from its restored patency, these criteria often omit many others who also may benefit. A noninvasive method to so identify such patients would be desirable (789).

MPS Adequate? However, exercise perfusion imaging (217,776,777) and pharmacologic stress perfusion imaging (464,465) have demonstrated excellent risk stratification in studies performed in the "thrombolytic era" (217,464), in which the stress test without imaging is of little prognostic value (464,776,777).

The quantitative application of perfusion imaging demonstrated that the frequent spontaneous, albeit late, reperfusion of infarct-related regions is associated with significant myocardial salvage. If the method can identify the effects of spontaneous recanalization so well after infarction (790), why should it not discern improvement after thrombolysis or acute angioplasty? In fact, it does!

pretest probability, patients with an intermediate pretest probability have the greatest realization of cost effectiveness.

Several analyses of cost effectiveness were performed when MPS was relatively new and planar (632–634). They based their assumptions on then current diagnostic accuracies, costs and event rates related to a given anatomy. These studies were anatomy rather than pathophysiology based and founded on statistical assumptions rather than on actual patient outcomes as performed in later studies conducted on a pathophysiologic image-related basis with more advanced MPS methods. Patterson et al. (632) have done much work in this area (Fig. 9). They evaluated the effects of perfusion scintigraphy on pretest probability calculated by the method of Diamond and Forrester (102). The study illustrates test effectiveness in the diagnosis and exclusion of disease to be greatest when diagnosis is in doubt and the pretest probability is intermediate. They have also illustrated that test results in parallel (e.g., an abnormal scintigram supporting an abnormal stress ECG) add a degree of diagnostic security. There is a certain potential benefit in using combined tests for predictive power. Conversely, because errors related to 2 tests are additive, such assessment must be carefully applied (632–634). Another study by Patterson et al. (633) evaluated cost effectiveness in terms of dollars and cents. Here, a theoretical population of 1000 men aged 45 years was used as a model of test effectiveness for the assessment of asymptomatic CAD. By this analysis, if catheterization were performed on patients presenting with both positive stress ECG and scintigraphy, rather than on all patients with a positive stress ECG alone, costs would be halved and 85% of those asymptomatic patients with significant coronary lesions would still be identified. This excludes any benefits of eliminating the risk and discomfort of needless angiography and does not consider anatomical–pathophysiologic differences, which would add to the scintigraphic advantage. Although costs have increased since the study publication, relative values and study conclusions still appear valid. Similarly, the diagnostic accuracy of MPS has improved, bringing a probable underestimation in the findings of the study.

Patterson et al. (632–634) assessed CAD diagnosis and cost effectiveness in terms of years of life preserved in relation to 4 testing approaches (Fig. 92). The authors assessed costs in relation to disease prevalence as well. The lowest cost was seen in relation to the performance of angiography only if both stress test and scintigram were positive. On the other hand, when prevalence is plotted versus mortality, it is clear that this approach pays the greatest penalty for patient misdiagnosis in terms of mortality when both tests are required to be positive. Again, mortality was relatively low and stable at all prevalence rates, when angiography was performed on all patients. The same data were assessed, taking into account all possible factors, and the cost per patient diagnosed was calculated. This parameter, most closely related to what we could call cost effectiveness, was lowest for the approach calling for angiography but only after positive scintigraphy. The difference was most significant at low disease prevalence, yet persisted to rates >50%. When test effectiveness was assessed in terms of survival, this approach again yielded the lowest cost per year of quality life preserved. This analysis is strictly based on diagnostic costs and fails to consider advantages related to less tangible factors, which also must be factored into the cost-effectiveness equation.

This group presented a cost-effectiveness analysis for CAD diagnosis in a population of 96 patients presenting with symptoms of unknown cause (84). If stress testing, MPS and angiography were performed on all patients, no patients with disease would be missed, but the cost per patient diagnosed would be high. If angiography is omitted when both stress ECG and scintigraphy are negative, or when the history is diagnostic, again no patients are missed, but the costs fall dramatically. In addition to demonstrating cost effectiveness, this analysis also demonstrates the value of the scintigraphic method in excluding coronary disease.

Although these analyses demonstrate the interaction of tests in affecting costs, cost effectiveness must be assessed also in terms of the diagnostic sacrifices we find acceptable. These considerations are as much ethical as clinical. Patterson et al. (227) performed a more complicated analysis in seeking to estimate the cost effectiveness of screening postinfarction patients for left main and 3-vessel disease. Most cost effective was the performance of angiography in those patients with stress scintigraphic perfusion abnormalities outside the infarct zone or in those with other clinical or stress test indicators of extensive ischemia. Few patients were missed. Here, the use of all diagnostic and clinical parameters resulted in both high diagnostic and, if we recognize the poor prognosis related to the anatomy identified, outcome efficacy. Most recently, this same group analyzed diagnostic accuracies of most modalities, as well as their cost effectiveness, and found PET perfusion scintigraphy to be more cost effective than conventional scintigraphy (634). Both were more cost effective than stress echocardiography.

Shaw et al. (781) evaluated the coronary risk related to scan findings in patients with stable angina and related these findings to measures of cost effectiveness where $50,000/life saved served as the acceptable limit. The authors presented one of several studies that suggest that the application of perfusion scintigraphy to decide on coronary angiography in patients with stable angina could reduce medical costs by >30% (782,813). These workers evaluated 5821 consecutive symptomatic patients who were followed for a mean of 2.5 yr without intervention at 6 large clinical and research centers. Working with data generated in these 3620 patients, the authors analyzed stress perfusion images and the results of stress testing using the Duke Treadmill Score and related them to outcome in terms of hard event rate. Image defect size stratified outcome well among patients in each Duke Score classification, grouped as low, intermediate and high. They demonstrated a 30%–50% cost saving for the risk stratification of patients with stable angina using the pathway that selects candidates for angiography, based on the results of perfusion imaging compared with initial stratification with angiography. This analysis included initial test costs and costs of the postimage evaluation (Table 33). There was a high measure of cost effectiveness, especially in application of the method to the elderly.

Miller et al. (380) examined the financial impact of 2 management strategies, initial stress perfusion scintigraphy (n = 5826) or angiography-first (n = 5423), to document ischemia in 11,249 stable angina patients who underwent coronary angiography for clinical reasons at several community hospitals. Patients were then followed to the resultant medical management and outcomes.

Table 33

THE COST EFFECTIVENESS OF STRESS MYOCARDIAL PERFUSION SCINTIGRAPHY IN 5821 STABLE ANGINA PATIENTS

Pretest cardiac risk	Annual death rate	Cost-effective analysis* ($/life saved)	
		All	Elderly
Low (n = 826)	0.6%	$254,209	$34,650
Intermediate (n = 3388)	1.6%	$28,887	$23,310
High (n = 1607)	4.4%	$52,960	$42,737

*<$50,000/life saved = cost effective.

Adapted, with permission, from Shaw LJ, Hachamovitch R, Marwick TH, et al. Cost-effectiveness analysis of stress myocardial perfusion imaging in stable angina pectoris: influence of age and pretest risk of coronary disease [abstract]. *J Am Coll Cardiol* 1997;29:137A.

Those with initial noninvasive evaluation had a lower incidence of normal coronary angiograms (33% versus 52%), a lower incidence of revascularization (13.7% versus 26.3%) and a lower incidence of cardiac death (2.8% versus 3.3%), with a lower cost per patient studied ($4882 versus $8212). In these patients, early perfusion imaging to direct patients to invasive study was clearly cost effective.

Shaw et al. (*18*) evaluated the costs related to the evaluation of CAD by 5 different strategies (Fig. 32): (1) no evaluation, in which nothing is invested and nothing is found; (2) coronary angiography first in all patients; (3) angiography only in those suggested as high risk on the basis of clinical variables; (4) angiography only in those with a high-risk scan; (5) a more selective application of scintigraphy based on clinical variables and angiography based on image findings. The last strategy results in a more selective application of angiography, with fewer resultant revascularization procedures and no increased morbidity (*18*).

In an intense study of the cost effectiveness of diagnostic and prognostic methods, Shaw et al. (*782*) compared >11,000 patients who underwent MPS and coronary angiography with a matched group that went to angiography without MPS evaluation. Although angiography was more frequent among all CAD risk groups in the population having direct angiography and in whom revascularization was more frequent, care costs were higher but hard event rates were not different from those in the group sent to angiography based on MPS findings, in whom angiography and revascularization was less frequent and costs were much less. Similarly, Mishra et al. (*813*) demonstrated that the impact of stress SPECT MPS reduces coronary angiography and revascularization with similar hard event rates and reduced costs compared with those sent directly for angiography based on clinical and stress test results in a group of patients with an intermediate pretest CAD likelihood.

A European study that demonstrated the accuracy and cost effectiveness of stress MPS (*783*) complements a number of other studies already reviewed that testify to the cost effectiveness of MPS in a variety of patient groups (*15,17–20,308–313,319,337,338,340,341,348,593,595*). Although test cost and diagnostic accuracy are important contributors to the overall cost effectiveness, the resultant health benefits and influence on subsequent health costs are important and must also be calculated (*128,322–324*). MPS then is an excellent example of high management efficacy as well as cost effectiveness. Studies have already been noted that demonstrate the potential outcome efficacy of the method (*478,634,782,810,814*).

Two meta-analyses present a different viewpoint (*815,816*).

OTHER METHODS

Today, no methodology should be immune to extensive evaluation and review of cost effectiveness. The new high-technology modalities, such as cine computed tomography (CT) (*817*), magnetic resonance (MR) imaging and PET, as well as more established methods such as echocardiography, must be evaluated broadly and critically, as conventional scintigraphy has been evaluated (Fig. 104). Stress echocardiography has been uncritically accepted by many who perform it but has been rejected by many others who have tried it. Others are torn by related issues of economics and politics. Stress echocardiography has brought into contrast the features of scintigraphy and has ironically contributed to a strong movement of many cardiologists toward nuclear cardiology and to a growing movement to make the method their own. The

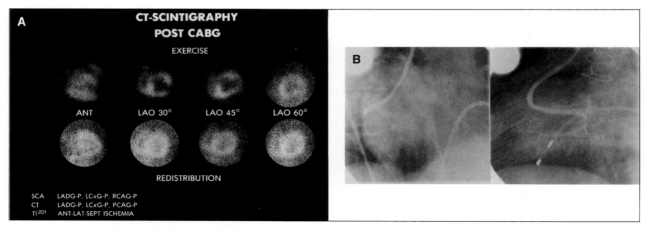

Figure 104 Computed tomography (CT) and perfusion scintigraphy. Rest CT examination of this patient with chest pain late after bypass surgery revealed flow through the left anterior descending (LAD) and circumflex (LCX) grafts and reported them both patent. (A) Scintigraphy revealed stress-induced ischemic changes in anterior, septal and lateral regions (ANT-LAT-SEPT), the distribution of both vessels. (B) Angiography (SCA) revealed stenosis at the insertion sites of both vessels. The scintigram provided pathophysiologic information, often clarifying anatomic information. CABG = coronary artery bypass graft surgery; CAG = coronary artery graft; G = graft; P = patent; R = right coronary artery; LAO = left anterior oblique. (Reprinted, with permission, from Englestad B, Wagner S, Herfkens R, et al. Evaluation of the post coronary bypass patient by myocardial perfusion scintigraphy and computed tomography. *Am J Radiol* 1983:141:507.)

search for appropriate echocardiographic stress methods and contrast agents has been problematic but promises to enhance the field (*513,514,818–821*). Although cine CT can identify coronary calcifications, relationships drawn with coronary stenoses and especially prognoses have not been firmly established. Although this method is relatively inexpensive, the cost of more physiologic stress evaluation and possibly unnecessary invasive interventions often performed for clarification, has not been measured. A recent study demonstrated no relationship between the presence and degree of coronary calcification and the findings on perfusion imaging among 204 asymptomatic subjects studied by both methods (*822*). CT "beam hardening artifacts" and other physical problems have not permitted the measurement of regional perfusion (*823–828*). However, CT angiography looks promising, may actually permit the 3-dimensional depiction of the coronary anatomy and the identification of regional coronary stenoses (*829*) and has recently been approved by the FDA (*830*). The presence of calcification as determined by this method may serve to identify patients with greatest need for risk-factor modification (*831*). The intrinsic contrast of MRI may permit imaging of the coronary anatomy, if the motion of the coronary arteries can be overcome (*828,832–836*). This method presents the capability for exquisite functional assessment, as well as the potential for perfusion analysis and noninvasive angiography. Yet, some of these applications, such as dobutamine function evaluation, can be performed more simply and cheaper by other methods. Other applications are in development, without clear evidence of widespread applicability or reproducibility and not yet supported by computer algorithms for rapid, automated analysis. Perfusion evaluation, as recommended with new echo contrast agents in development, CT or MR contrast, all look at markers of intravascular volume rather than true cellular uptake and perfusion, the scintigraphic marker.

The more expensive the modality, the greater must be its demonstrated clinical advantage in order to justify its application. In the context of these new, expensive modalities, conventional scintigraphic methods must be seen as relatively inexpensive. The clinical value and expense of these tests should be assessed in reference to the patient population and the specific clinical question being considered. Advantages of a method must be placed in the clinical context in which it is applied, and its full effect on patient outcome must be analyzed. Such outcome analysis will be emphasized in the "new health care." Then, when the situation arises, the response will be both appropriate and cost effective.

COMPARISON OF STRESS SCINTIGRAPHY WITH ECHOCARDIOGRAPHY

Introduction: Editorial Comment

In 1983, the editor of this book was the moderator of a local symposium on noninvasive methods. The guest speaker that day was (and is) the most prestigious individual in the echocardiography world and the inventor and leading advocate of stress echocardiography. He spoke as if stress echocardiography were the dominant noninvasive imaging method for CAD diagnosis, when, in fact, it was rarely applied. I asked him, "What is the state of the scintigraphic method at your institution?" He replied, "We killed the nuclear guy a long time ago!" To this the moderator replied, "I don't doubt that, but was it justifiable homicide or murder!" Surely the cardiology community had the power to figuratively "murder" nuclear cardiology and replace these methods with those that they then practiced. So, some years ago, when I was asked by the SNM Publications Committee to contribute to and edit this series, I thought that possibly, by the time it was done, there would be no one to read it. Stress echocardiography was, after all, claiming "equality," and I knew the advantages of the modality, its wide proliferation and the enthusiasm of its practitioners. In fact, I thought the echo-related method need not even be as good as the scintigraphic method, just passable, and those who used and profited from echocardiography would proclaim its replacement of scintigraphic methods justified. Some practitioners, in fact, have done exactly this! But I had faith in the method and in my cardiology colleagues. More than that, we must all have faith in the process. The truth, whatever it is, will be known. Today there may be people interested in reading these words, and nuclear cardiology has never been stronger or more a part of both nuclear medicine and cardiology.

The Reality of Basic Considerations

The effort to document the diagnostic accuracy and prognostic value of stress echocardiography simply compares echocardiographic studies with perfusion scintigrams in the same or different populations or to literature "controls." There is no credible study that demonstrates superiority of the stress echocardiographic method or a clear advantage in its application to any specific population. Rather than superiority, the advocacy and literature of stress echocardiography are unique in that they simply claim to demonstrate equality with alternative scintigraphic methods. However, it then contends that the advantages of the modality, its totally noninvasive nature, "low" cost and lack of ionizing radiation, give it superiority. The arguments are often shifted from the advantages of the method (diagnostic and prognostic accuracy, localization, etc.) to those of the modality (cost, ionizing radiation, speed, computer processing required, etc.). These are then exaggerated to favor vested interests and suggest that MPS should never be performed (Table 34). Rarely noted are the disadvantages of the analysis of poststress images and their contribution to reduced test sensitivity (Fig. 105).

Table 34
STRESS ECHOCARDIOGRAPHY AND STRESS
PERFUSION IMAGING

When evaluating the clinical method and determining its appropriate application in patients, we should consider the advantages of the method, not the modality.

Modality	Method
Noninvasive	Accuracy
Safety of the modality	Safety of the method
Personnel	Reproducibility
Equipment	Legibility
Cost	Failure rate
Radiation	Objectivity
Computer needed	Diagnostic
Speed	Prognostic (no myocardial infarction, post-myocardial infarction, postrevascularization, preoperative etc.)
	Sensitivity
	Specificity
	Predictive value of a negative test
	Localization
	Viability
	Applicability to women
	Applicability to large patients
	Use in special conditions (lung disease, unstable angina, left ventricular hypertrophy, left bundle branch blockage)
	Impact on patient management
	Ability to utilize all forms of stress
	Cost effectiveness

Cost. Cost effectiveness is erroneously reduced to the cost of the test. The test cost is taken as the patient bill, and the cost to the institution or physician group is ignored, as is its profitability. Little note is made of the high cost of each dose of echocardiographic contrast. Yet, contrary to the testimony of earlier experts in the field, this is often required to opacify the ventricular cavity, permitting wall motion assessment not otherwise possible, and has itself spawned a modest industry. Efforts to develop new methods to enhance visualization of the endocardium recognize the insufficiency of the current method but are themselves not yet established, nor will they be cost free (*837,838*) (Figs. 106–109). They will not likely present a panacea. Further, data from the quantitative prospective analysis of large populations, not available with stress echocardiography, demonstrate the cost effectiveness of stress MPS (*571,782*). The health care budget is about 15% of the U.S. gross national product. The cost of coronary disease evaluation and treatment adds about $130/yr to each health insurance premium. Not stated is that the leading cost to Medicare in 1995–1997 was echocardioraphy! Until recently, reimbursement of stress echocardiography studies was only modestly less than that for stress MPS. However, in the midst of falling reimbursements, that for echocardiographic procedures will be most affected, as if to reduce overall costs to the system. Will this further encourage its application or reduce enthusiasm on the part of those who offer it?

Radiation. Confronting the public phobia about radiation and disseminating the truth about radioactivity and radiation exposure must be primary goals of all nuclear cardiology and nuclear medicine education. Radiation has been positioned as the scourge of humankind, rather than as a benefit of the peaceful use of the atom. A radionuclide dose equal in radiation exposure to 2 posterior–anterior and lateral chest X-rays or a "flat and upright" of the abdomen now carries the perceived threat of Chernobyl or the threat of an atomic bomb. Some who hide their radiation badges to avoid evidence of overexposure while performing angiography raise anxiety about the radiation exposure at scintigraphy. Radiation exposure from high-altitude commercial flight (0.1 mrem/hr >30,000 feet) or from simply sleeping with another person

Several studies evaluating outcomes in relation to a normal stress echocardiogram have demonstrated event rates ranging from 3%–14% yr. Krivokapich et al. (*351*) followed 360 patients who had undergone exercise echocardiography and found a 9% event rate, including MI, cardiac death or revascularization. The author found a normal image result to relate to a 3% hard event rate, but this rose to 7% among those with prior infarction or revascularization and a negative test. Similar high event rates in patients with normal stress echocardiograms have been reported by other investigators (*350, 352,805,847*). Picano et al. (*353*) published the results of a large, prospective multicenter trial examining the efficacy of stress echocardiography after MI. A total of 923 patients were considered in this analysis, based upon recruitment from 11 different laboratories. Although new stress-induced wall motion abnormalities were the most powerful predictor of cardiac death, the rate of cardiac death in patients with normal scans was still 2%–3%. Thus, as in the other studies discussed, stress echocardiography failed to identify a patient cohort defined as low risk by the AHCPR guidelines that could be successfully managed without further testing (*31*). These results disqualify the use of this modality in a pathophysiologic strategy such as that outlined above.

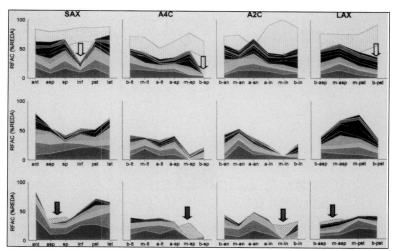

Figure 109 Color kinesis histograms: coronary artery disease. Shown are stacked color histograms of regional fractional area change obtained from images in Figure 108. The normal range of regional fractional area change shown as a stippled band in the background of the resting histograms allowed objective identification of the regional wall motion abnormalities noted in this patient at rest (top, open arrows). The resting histograms, scaled down to 60% and shown as dotted areas in the background of histograms obtained with dobutamine, allow objective detection of stress-induced wall motion abnormalities (bottom, solid arrows) in the perfusion territory of the left anterior descending coronary. Although this and other computer-derived and -displayed data will add objectivity to current subjective, visual echocardiographic assessment, what is their reproducibility and range of their normal values and to what extent will they introduce new errors? Such contrast enhances wall motion but does not approach the evaluation of perfusion. SAX = parasternal short axis; A4C = apical 4-chamber; A2C = apical 2-chamber; LAX = parasternal long axis. (Reprinted, with permission, from Koch R, Lang RM, Garcia MJ, et al. Objective evaluation of regional left ventricular wall motion during dobutamine stress echocardiographic studies using segmental analysis of color kinesis. *J Am Coll Cardiol* 1999;34:409–419.)

In 1993, Bateman et al. (*847*) studied 435 matched patients with a spectrum of pretest coronary disease likelihood who had either stress echocardiography or stress perfusion scintigraphy (Fig. 110). Followed for 1 yr, those 213 patients with a low pretest likelihood and a normal imaging study of either variety had no events, but those 222 patients with known disease or a high pretest likelihood had a 2.2% event rate with a normal stress scintigram and a 14.1% event rate with a normal stress echocardiogram! Examination of the current literature documented a significant difficulty or inability of the normal stress echocardiogram to identify populations with a low event rate, low risk and a good prognosis (*333,351–353,754,844, 846–857*). Only recently have some studies appeared to suggest a low event rate in relation to a normal stress echocardiogram. Most of these continue to select low-risk populations and are performed in a retrospective fashion (*857*).

Because of the well documented predictive value of MPS for the presence and extent of MIR for cardiac death and nonfatal infarction (*6,7,9–14,19,21, 46,66,70,116,190,194,296,417,746*), the reduced sensitivity of stress echocardiography and its variable, subjective nature raises concern for a possible

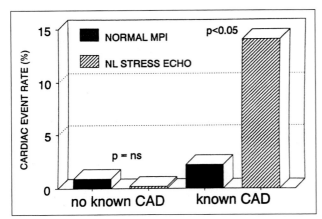

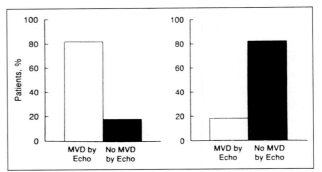

Figure 110 The predictive value of stress echocardiography compared with stress myocardial perfusion scintigraphy (MPS). Shown is the cardiac event rate in patients with normal myocardial perfusion images (MPI) or stress echocardiograms (ECHO), based on whether patients had known or no known coronary artery disease (CAD). In patients with no known CAD, the event rate was very low in both groups. However, in patients with known CAD (and a low pretest likelihood), the cardiac event rate was much higher in patients with a normal stress echocardiograms compared with those with a normal stress MPS. Do we need imaging studies in patients with low likelihood of CAD? (Reprinted, with permission, from Bateman TM, O'Keefe JH, Barnhart CS, et al. Clinical comparison of cardiac events during follow-up after ischemic exercise test suggests superiority of SPECT thallium-201 over echocardiography [abstract]. *J Am Coll Cardiol* 1993;21:67A.)

Figure 111 Exercise echocardiography for multivessel disease (MVD). Shown is the ability of exercise echocardiography (Echo) to identify patients with or without MVD by angiography according to rest ejection fraction, where those with left ventricle ejection fraction (LVEF) < 40% (11 patients) are shown at left and those with LVEF ≥ 40% (49 patients) are shown at right. It seems that exercise echocardiography adds little to the rest LVEF, and the presence of multivessel disease could be diagnosed simply from the rest LVEF in this study. (From Roger VL, Pellikka PA, OH JK, et al. Identification of multivessel coronary artery disease by exercise echocardiography. *J Am Coll Cardiol* 1994;24:109–114.)

deficiency in its ability to identify patients at risk for cardiac events. Brown's review (*14*) addressed this question. Although normal stress perfusion scintigraphy has demonstrated a low incidence of death or infarction (<1%), even in the presence of known CAD in the year after a normal exercise stress imaging study (*14,223*), a review of the 15 current published stress echocardiographic studies that address risk stratification reveals an alarmingly high event rate (9%–15%) in the presence of a normal stress echocardiogram. Although many stress echocardiographic studies demonstrate a higher event rate among those with positive compared with negative tests (*11,351,848–850*), this is not always the case. Even when the method does so differentiate populations according to risk, those with "low risk" may be higher than acceptable. Quintana et al. (*848*) found an event rate of 5% among those with normal stress echocardiograms. Excluding studies evaluating only patients with prior infarction, wall motion abnormalities or a high pretest coronary likelihood, the 9 remaining studies demonstrated a hard event rate of 6%/yr among 751 normal stress echocardiograms, a rate too high to justify conservative management. Further, this event rate was no different from the 8%/yr rate among patients with known CAD and abnormal stress echocardiograms. The 2 largest studies of the prognosis of stress echocardiography (*848,851*) demonstrate no difference between normal and abnormal stress echocardiograms. Poldermans et al. (*848*) studied 430 patients and found no difference in the hard event rate among those with a negative or positive dobutamine stress echocardiographic study. This value was most prominent among those 207 with prior infarction, where the event rate in both groups was 9%. In a large study by Sciara et al. (*851*) of 778 patients undergoing postinfarction risk stratification with dobutamine–atropine stress echocardiography, the risk of subsequent infarction or cardiac death was 5% in patients with both positive and negative stress echocardiograms. Among 9 studies (*351,848–855*), 6 with dobutamine and 3 with exercise stress, that reported specific figures related to the hard end points of death or nonfatal infarction and the related incidence of ischemia, the annualized rate of death and nonfatal MI in 751 patients with known CAD and a negative stress echocardiogram was 6%/yr. This would actually qualify as a high event rate in the The Unstable Angina Guidelines of the AHCPR and was not different from the hard event rate in the same studies among patients with known CAD and a positive stress test (8%). It far exceeds the hard event rate in patients with a negative stress perfusion scintigram (*14,333*), even in the presence of known CAD (*344,845,850*).

In an article not included in the Brown review, Marcovitz et al. (*858*) studied the prognosis over a mean of 15 mo after the performance of clinically requested ("indicated") dobutamine stress echocardiography to a maximum 40 μg/kg/min dose. Although an abnormal response related to a 7.9 odds ratio for hard cardiac events and the fixed response (a rest wall motion abnormality unchanged with dobutamine) had a 6.1 odds ratio compared with the normal response, multivariate analysis revealed only a "mixed" or biphasic functional response (increased wall motion at low dose and decreased motion at high dose) to be statistically significantly related ($P = 0.03$) to hard events in the follow-up period. Of course, 185 among 291 study patients had rest wall motion abnormalities, with 23 of 29 hard events occurring in those with rest abnormalities, which themselves were predictive of events! As is generally the case, no evidence of study reproducibility was offered, and studies were stopped at peak dose (90% of predicted rate), with new wall motion abnormalities, typical angina, hypotension or arrhythmia. In another study, Chuah et al. (*329*) identified the number of abnormal segments at peak stress and stress-induced left ventricular dilation as the 2 stress echocardiographic markers of prognostic risk. However, again 558 (65%) among those studied had rest wall motion abnormalities, which, at least in part, contributed to the prognostic measure. Although event-free survival was lower in those with normal stress studies compared with abnormal, and the event rate in normal responders approached that seen for scintigraphy, no statistical difference in the subsequent event rate could be identified between normal and abnormal ischemic responders. Interesting was the extreme reproducibility documented here: a 96% agreement in the scoring (from 1–5) of 480 segments at rest and 90% at stress in 30 selected patients, and a 100% agreement in the subjective interpretation of the left ventricular volume response to stress with an apparent appreciation of volume changes <5 ml! Although some studies appear to demonstrate the prognostic value of the echocardiographic method, closer analysis reveals difficulties (*859*).

Some recent studies appear to attest to the high predictive value of a negative stress echocardiogram. Although 2 of the 5 show a relatively low event rate in association with a normal stress echocardiogram (*860,861*), the other 3 (*351,603,862*) have event rates of 1.6%–3%/yr, well above the 1% value generally taken as the upper limit of the low-risk subgroup. These have an 8-fold or more hard event rate compared with SPECT perfusion studies published in the same time frame (*21,128*), in spite of the selection of much lower risk study cohorts. Further, the total event rates are much greater in the echocardiographic studies, strongly suggesting that progressive CAD is clearly missed. Other studies, performed with the same methodology as previous studies and generally in select populations, present a response to the extensive data that suggest a strong predictive value of a normal stress MPS (*857,863*). Other recent studies demonstrate the continued insufficiency of a negative stress echocardiogram and the misleading methods applied to its evaluation (*857,860,864*).

The ability of MPS to identify this low-risk population, even in the presence of CAD, has placed it in this role with a strong and appropriate impact on the performance of coronary angiography and revascularization. The image abnormalities can be quantified and related to outcome in a graduated fashion. A recent study and much data presented here have shown that the degree of image abnormality provides important data that appropriately directs coronary patients to medical or revascularization therapy. MPS image findings clearly influence the performance of coronary angiography and revascularization. Scintigraphy clearly serves as the "gatekeeper" for these next-most expensive and dangerous steps, in those with a normal stress scintigram who have a 1%–3% rate of coronary angiography even in the presence of a high clinical disease likelihood (*16,32,223,318, 336,645,648,651,652*). The current data support this application of scintigraphy. Although such data, demonstrating the influence of study results on angiographic rates, are not available for stress echocardiography, the high event rate related to a negative test does not support a similar use for stress echocardiography. To do so would burden the patient with an unacceptably high event rate.

Specificity and Sensitivity. Many studies performed by echocardiography advocates using a variety of stress techniques nonetheless demonstrate the higher sensitivity of the scintigraphic method with the extremely high specificity of the stress echocardiographic method (*122,602,848,865–870*). It is often claimed that such accuracy relates only to single-vessel disease and that the specificity of stress echocardiography is equal or superior to that of the scintigraphic method for identification of multivessel CAD. Of course, less sensitive tests may see disease more specifically with more extensive and severe involvement. Also, populations generally studied with stress echocardiography are younger and with a lower CAD likelihood. The stress echocardiographic method has less impact on management of patients studied, and so positive tests, influenced by the pretest likelihood and presentation, are less frequent and less readily discovered Yet, the literature strongly demonstrates the superior sensitivity of the scintigraphic method for the identification of multivessel, high-risk disease in ~66%–72% of such patients, compared with 50% by stress echocardiography (*512*). Beyond intrinsic abilities of the scintigraphic method, such sensitivity may relate as well to the use of the method in selection of patients for coronary angiography.

Certainly the most important element in testing to identify extensive high-risk CAD is not to miss it! MPS appears better correlated with true pathology where scintigraphic image infarct size, based in perfusion and measured in patients before heart transplantation (*443*), appears better correlated with pathologic measures than echocardiographic infarct size, based in wall motion. Attention must also be given to methods of studies claiming diagnostic or prognostic advantage. Sensitivity must be assessed with reference to the population studied and the methods applied. MPS has been evaluated in patients with and without prior infarction, in those with known CAD and in those in whom the condition is not suspected. It has been tested with every radionuclide and protocol. Many echocardiographic studies fail to emphasize such details and the ways in which they might influence test sensitivity and specificity. Of course, test sensitivity will soar among populations with prior infarction, and the estimate of multivessel disease will increase in the setting of rest wall motion abnormalities. The study by Roger et al. (*871*) seems to demonstrate the value of stress echocardiography for the identification of multivessel CAD, but the diagnosis actually relates as well to the rest ejection fraction (Fig. 111). Here, a rest LVEF <40% was well correlated with multivessel disease, whereas an LVEF >40% was related to the absence of multivessel disease: the stress study was unnecessary for this differentiation! This study indicates the extreme difficulty of the echocardiographic diagnosis of multivessel CAD in the presence of normal wall motion, a difficulty compounded by the general rule to stop the stress test with the appearance of the first new wall motion abnormality. The study is interesting in other ways, because the LVEF was, as in all such echocardiographic studies, not calculated with the stress study. Yet, the earlier experience with stress blood pool scintigraphy demonstrated great diagnostic and prognostic value of the peak stress LVEF, which we still seek to capture with first-pass analysis of perfusion data. Further, blood pool analysis of wall motion was objectified by the functional stroke volume, phase and ejection fraction images, not available to the echocardiographic method. Early stress echocardiographic studies tried unsuccessfully to analyze the rest and stress LVEF, ventricular volumes and Doppler flow measurements. This likely relates to the inability of the method to identify the endocardium in many stress segments and is a reason why the method has remained, as opposed to scintigraphy, entirely qualitative and subjective. What is the implication of a method that claims highest sensitivity based on qualitative, subjective measurements and discards quantitative measures proven previously to be of great diagnostic and prognostic value?

This now appears to be well recognized by workers in the field who have introduced and advocated the application of some objective aid in stress echocardiographic interpretation. Studies now applying echocardiographic tissue Doppler imaging, harmonic imaging and color kinesis, among others, seek to demonstrate accuracy and reliability in stress protocols by enhancement of the endocardium (*837,838*). Contrast to enhance the cavity will also aid endocardial tracking. Many advocates have moved away from the subjective evaluation of wall motion and realize that objective tools are needed to aid reproducibility and sensitivity. One study demonstrated a marked increase in sensitivity, from 53% to 76%, with the application of color kinesis (*837*) (Figs. 106–109). However, although evolving, these methods require new expensive equipment and complex methodology and have not been disseminated. Will they prove valuable and practical? What credibility should be applied to stress echocardiographic studies performed without these aids? Even the inventor of the stress echocardiographic method has been forced to alter his methodology to counter ambiguities and errors (*842*). Sampling errors are minimized by the analysis of multiple cycle "loops," and ambiguities in wall motion analysis related to cardiac motion are addressed by alignment with a mitral valve reference point (*872*). Do most cardiologists know of these changes? Can they implement them on their instrumentation? Although these enhancement methods address problems, they do not solve them. These and other problems are not addressed by the several endocardial enhancement methods.

Studies Comparing the Two Methods. Some studies compare the methods in the same population (*125,865–870*). At least 5 of these studies (*125,602,867, 869,870*), including the oft-quoted study by Quinones et al. (*122*), demonstrate the same reading of normal, stress-induced or fixed abnormalities in a large majority of segments by both methods. However, not emphasized is the impressively greater ability of the scintigraphic method to identify MIR, with the preponderance of reversible, ischemic abnormalities on the perfusion study occurring in segments related to coronary lesions subtending segments with normal wall motion or unchanging abnormalities of wall motion and functional evidence of scar. In these studies involving >500 patients, stress scintigraphy consistently identified 30% more ischemia on segmental or per-patient evaluation, and patients with extensive 3-vessel disease were not missed. Further, 20%–46% of segments that demonstrated jeopardized myocardium on scintigraphy were normal or scarred on stress echocardiography (*122,651,869*). These findings belie the concern that the relative nature of MPS will too often produce a normal pattern in the setting of homogeneous underperfusion, as does the high sensitivity of the SPECT method in those with severe 3-vessel disease and the excellent prognosis of a normal perfusion scintigram in patients with CAD (*14*). Of course, most recently SPECT perfusion images with technetium-based radiotracers have been applied routinely to the concomitant evaluation of left ventricular function by both first-pass and gated poststress methods. Perfusion scintigraphy remains the only clinically applicable noninvasive method that permits evaluation of both myocardial perfusion and function. Although the Unstable Angina Guidelines (*31*) support stress MPS and stress echocardiography as equally accurate options, there is far more evidence supporting the greater risk stratification of the former. A recent article applied exercise echocardiography to more than 200 patients with unstable angina and found that the risk stratification ability of the method was no better than that of the stress ECG (*406*). Although the 2 methods may sometimes be combined to yield greater sensitivity, such efforts too often bring confusion and gain needless exposure for the weaker method (*873*) and simply expose the weakness of the established method and modality.

One editorial approaches the choice of a method for pharmacologic stress testing as an athletic (boxing) competition (*874*). However, dobutamine stress itself is too often suboptimal, and the echocardiographic method is difficult to apply and has poor reproducibility. After early contact, with perfusion scintigraphy on the ropes, pharmacologic stress MPS has fought back strongly, and the echocardiographic method has not been able to deal the "knock-out" punch (*874,875*). Other methods of MRI assess regional perfusion and CFR (*876*).

Meta-Analysis. Studies are sometimes packaged as meta-analyses. Shaw et al. (*803*) performed a meta-analysis of 10 dipyridamole scintigraphic studies with 1994 patients and 5 dobutamine echocardiographic studies with 445 patients (see *Self-Study Program III. Cardiology. Topic 2: Pharmacologic Stress*). None of the original participating dobutamine echocardiography studies had sufficient patient numbers to satisfactorily differentiate high from low prognostic subgroups, whereas 4 scintigraphic studies had sufficient sample sizes. The scintigraphic values were influenced strongly by a single large study with negative results. Among those undergoing dipyridamole scintigraphy there were more canceled operations, preoperative coronary angiography, pre- and postoperative revascularization, ischemia, hard and soft cardiac events and heart failure. Yet, evidence presented suggests there were comparable method accuracies, and the echocardiographic method demonstrated a greater event odds ratio when positive. Because of the lower numbers of patients studied, this finding was related to a much wider range of statistical uncertainty than that related to MPS. Another meta-analysis by Fleischmann et al. (*331*) evaluated 44 "comparable" stress (exercise) echocardiographic (2637 patients) and

SPECT (3237 patients) studies, many performed by the same group and with omission of much recent data. Sensitivities were similar but the specificity of exercise echocardiography was higher than that of stress scintigraphy. However, as in all such analyses, the studies applied varying forms of exercise, varying criteria for abnormal, varying imaging protocols and varying radionuclides in populations with little control over case mix. Although an attempt was made to identify post-test referral bias, it is difficult to prospectively assess this activity and impossible from an article not delineating bias on a case-by-case basis. From data specifically dealing with this factor and applied with greater confidence by the user, it seems likely that this bias is far greater for the scintigraphic method. As with all meta-analyses, publication alone is too often a criterion of inclusion and study quality is not, and we are forced to consume with a single swallow a host of data, some generated from poorly prepared articles previously unheard of and published in lesser journals. Never noted is the number of uninterpretable echocardiograms or segments unseen, the objectivity of interpretation, the blinded (or not) nature of the readings, their reproducibility, the fact that several current individual scintigraphic studies themselves present analysis of large patient numbers as large as the compilation here presented or the high and graded prognostic value of perfusion scintigraphic studies noted above. Another meta-analysis (330) purports to evaluate the methods as applied in women. It is guilty of all the previously noted deficiencies in presenting data from a selective compilation of stress echocardiographic and scintigraphic studies, many of relative obscurity. The compilation is based primarily on planar thallium studies without significant input from the recent MPS literature. The studies noted here simply add the pooled results of the individual studies statistically but do little to discern the value of the studies reported. The last 2 analyses were compiled and authored by attending physicians in a large academic echocardiography laboratory, with no experience in current scintigraphic methods and with vested and possibly conflicting interests. Of course, many studies in the literature, on both sides of the issue, bear similar potential biases. Such bias may be subtle or unseen and often unintentional, but nonetheless influential in forming the results and affecting as well the meta-analysis.

What does this all mean? When done properly and with adequate included studies, application of the principle of meta-analysis may yield additional data beyond the study components. However, this seems to be the exception. To the editor, meta-analysis is the academic journal article correlate of condensing your bad debts into one whopper! They are by nature selective and, although they claim to be analytic, present no new data. They simply add numbers in an attempt to reach statistical significance where none exists and do not necessarily shed light or expose great truths. Individual study weaknesses persist but may now be obscured. In studies presented, the reader must not attribute more to the sum than to each included study.

And why does echocardiography appear less sensitive and more specific with a higher event rate among normal studies? The latter could relate to a greater population subjected to a post-test referral bias because of the greater impact of MPS findings on management decisions. All could potentially be explained by the scintigraphic identification of limited stenoses, not angiographically significant. Their relationship to events increases sensitivity. Their failure to correlate with obvious anatomic lesions reduces specificity. However, other reasons also apply.

Reproducibility. Reproducibility, even among expert readers in stationary dobutamine studies, is poor (877) and compares poorly with that of stress perfusion

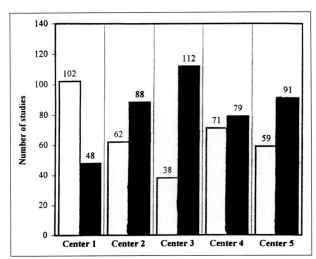

Figure 112 Interobserver variability: dobutamine stress echocardiography. Negativity (solid bars) versus positivity (open bars) for the 150 dobutamine stress echocardiograms by institution. Because of the nature of the intervention, there was little effect related to patient motion, respiratory artifact or other factors related to exercise stress. Nonetheless, note the wide variability in agreement among blinded expert readers at different institutions. These are related to the method but relate in a major way to subjective reading of the modality. Number above bars = number of patients. (Reprinted, with permission, from Hoffmann R, Lethen H, Kleinhaus E, et al. Comparative evaluation of bicycle and dobutamine stress echocardiography with perfusion scintigraphy and bicycle electrocardiogram for identification of coronary artery disease. *Am J Cardiol* 1993;72:555–559.)

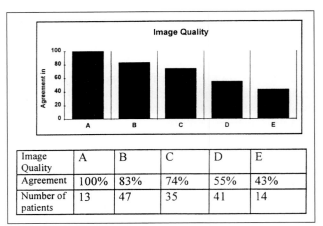

Image Quality	A	B	C	D	E
Agreement	100%	83%	74%	55%	43%
Number of patients	13	47	35	41	14

Figure 113 Interobserver variability: the effects of image quality. Shown is the extent of majority (not total) interinstitutional agreement in relation to the assessed image quality of dobutamine stress echocardiograms. Majority agreement could mean that 3 of 5 institutions (A–E) agreed. Regardless of the form and even if the bar graph plotted "full agreement," there is no way to avoid losses of image quality in large numbers of cases with current methods of echocardiographic acquisition, processing and display, when applied to unselected populations. (Reprinted, with permission, from Hoffmann R, Lethen H, Kleinhaus E, et al. Comparative evaluation of bicycle and dobutamine stress echocardiography with perfusion scintigraphy and bicycle electrocardiogram for identification of coronary artery disease. *Am J Cardiol* 1993;72:555–559.)

scintigraphy (Figs. 112,113). Quantitation is subjective, has not been submitted to critical analysis and in-depth assessment of reproducibility and is rarely performed clinically. In contrast to MPS, in which defect size and density form a basis for clinical management, this deeply restricts the ability of the echocardiographic method to address risk stratification. Only recently has a qualitative, visual impression of a stress-induced increase in end-systolic volume been reported to relate to a poor prognosis (*329*). The subjective echocardiographic reading of wall motion remains quite variable and, in the absence of objective analytic criteria, often belongs to the individual who yells the loudest.

Other Considerations. There is no comparison of echocardiographic findings with a normal data base. Although there is much comment relating to photon attenuation and the difficulty it presents to interpretation, there is no recognition of the attenuation of ultrasound. There is also no consideration of the effect of nonvisualized wall segments, the selective nature of the data placed in cine review, its limited frame rate, the general lack of blinded interpretation, the postexercise and less sensitive nature of treadmill exercise echocardiography, the limited choices of pharmacologic echocardiographic stress methods, the loss of sensitivity with an insufficient double product at exercise with dobutamine or with delay in image acquisition after exercise. The insufficiencies and cost of the dobutamine study must also be noted. Dobutamine is contraindicated in known severe coronary disease and unstable angina and has a high relative risk (*878*) and a long half-life relative to stage duration. The dobutamine protocol is lengthy and requires a trained nurse infusionist. It frequently induces paradoxical hypotension or bradycardia, amounting to 53% of 860 patients studied including 33% without new or worsening wall motion abnormalities (*329*), and frequently needs supplementation of its effects with handgrip, increased time per stage, increased dose, added dipyridamole and most commonly atropine. The recent commercial attempt to develop a new sympathomimetic agent with more vigorous and reliable effects than dobutamine, testifies to the insufficiencies of the current method and the perceived profit related to its improved replacement.

Echocardiographic Contrast. Current echocardiographic contrast agents generally seek to opacify the cavity and improve wall motion analysis at a high cost. This, when generic dipyridamole and competition between manufacturers of scintigraphic perfusion agents is driving down costs of MPS. All clearly realize the advantages of tests based in the perfusion-related ischemic end point rather than the wall motion endpoint (see *Self-Study Program III. Cardiology. Topic 2: Pharmacologic Stress*). For this reason, a significant effort is now underway to develop a perfusion tracer that will survive transit through the pulmonary capillary bed and permit the evaluation of myocardial perfusion. New methods of echocardiographic image processing may enhance the abilities of echo contrast to visualize coronary arteries or coronary perfusion (*879*). Yet, again, the project resembles in its zeal and method the United States effort to go to the moon. Whether the effort will succeed will depend on the science. However, large amounts of capital are being invested with the knowledge that current stress echocardiographic methods are insufficient and only an ultrasound-based perfusion agent, as good as current scintigraphic agents, will succeed in capturing the entire field. However, it is the delay in the development of such methods and the superiority of the scintigraphic perfusion-based study compared with the wall motion-based echocardiographic stress evaluation that is motivating the movement of cardiologists toward scintigraphic methods and supporting a renewed growth in nuclear cardiology.

Technical Considerations. Often the difficulties of the subjective evaluation are compounded by the definition of normal. Assessments are variable as to whether augmentation of or failure to decrement wall motion represents a normal exercise response or whether the biphasic response is applied to the identification of dobutamine-induced ischemia. Of course, recent advances in the scintigraphic approach to attenuation, motion and other artifacts, the near obsessive analytic nature of scan interpretation and the related improvement in specificity, well documented in the literature, are never quoted as the early comparison data ages. The advantages of the graded scintigraphic compared with the dichotomous echocardiographic response, so important for risk stratification as well as viability evaluation, are never mentioned (*250*). Sometimes, prestigious physician groups setting guidelines, such as those relating to noninvasive testing methods in unstable angina, equate stress echocardiographic with scintigraphic methods, although there is much data documenting the risk-stratifying ability of the latter but not the former! Such abusive practice is too often expanded to other issues in which, with increasing frequency, diagnostic or prognostic advantages of the scintigraphic method are erroneously adapted by or ascribed to the echocardiographic method, with the idea that the 2 are "the same."

Current Status. If stress echocardiography has such advantages as a method to compound with its advantages as a modality, why then is anyone still doing MPS? More important than the literature is the experience and response of the readership, the practicing physician. Early in the introduction of stress echocardiography, the method was largely ignored, and much credibility was lost as the advocates preached application of an unsupportable method based in review of lengthy videos evaluated serially. With introduction of digital techniques, the method became feasible and was implemented with enthusiasm, which increased with financial needs. Lately, nuclear cardiology has demonstrated impressive staying power with increasing volume, involvement by cardiologists, high equipment sales rates and the clinical influence of MPS.

An obvious indicator of the validity and acceptance of any clinical method is its influence on clinical decision making. Here, the impact of scintigraphy has been widely documented, but the impact of stress echocardiography is less apparent (*642*). Never noted is the relative stress echocardiographic or scintigraphic study volume performed at institutions that claim, in publications, superior echocardiographic ability. Has the nuclear cardiology laboratory or the practice of Dr. Verani (*122*) suffered since the publication of the comparison study? If not, why not? What does this have to say about the data in this and other studies proclaiming the end of nuclear cardiology? Similarly, nuclear cardiology is the actual current major activity of some open-minded practitioners who have published and spoken widely regarding the virtues of stress echocardiography. These facts indicate that there is more to these methods than some of the literature reports. After an often intense but unfulfilling experience with stress echocardiography, and in spite of the extreme cost, inconvenience and time, cardiologists are putting in the 500 hr of didactic training and case work demanded by the Nuclear Regulatory Commission (NRC) to qualify for the clinical use of radionuclides in order to do nuclear cardiology. Scintillation camera sales are on the increase again, largely as a result of the surge in sales of dedicated cardiac devices. Study numbers project a 15% increase in 1998, with 4.2 million perfusion studies compared with 2 million stress echocardiograms. Why would this occur when all the cardiologist needs to do is buy the echocardiographic acquisition and display equipment, attend a brief course on the subject, stock the schedule with their own patients and bill? There is only 1 logical reason for these events: the clinical value and superiority of the scintigraphic method with the proven advantages listed in Table 7.

A sample size of 40,000 patients was needed in the GUSTO trial to demonstrate that thrombolytic therapy saves lives. The ability of MPS to measure salvage of myocardium appears to be a highly reproducible and cost-efficient surrogate for the "hard end points." It is for these and reasons of reproducibility, objectivity, overall cost effectiveness and its quantifiable and prognostic nature that the perfusion imaging method was utilized in the earlier thrombolytic trials as a current surrogate for hard outcomes and permitted documentation of method value in only limited patient numbers.

It is also for these reasons too that perfusion studies are used with regularity as the standard for documentation of the effect of new surgical methods to revascularize the myocardium (*282*) and pharmacologic (*283*) or mechanical methods (*284*) to grow collateral vessels or relieve ischemia in other ways.

Electrophysiology and nuclear cardiology are now the 2 most sought after skills by cardiology groups seeking an additional member. There is now a large, 3000-member international group, the American Society of Nuclear Cardiology (ASNC), advocating the method, defending the rights of those who apply it, seeking the highest standards of practice, guiding development and progress in the field and fostering education of both user and practitioner. Intensive courses in technical and clinical areas are offered in preparation for the Nuclear Cardiology Certifying Exam, a vehicle that promises access to the field for all qualified practitioners.

Recently, and largely as a result of the combined efforts and urging of nuclear physicians and cardiologists, the NRC has agreed to lower required didactic hours from a restrictive and unnecessary 1200 hr. Completion of the "Nuclear Cardiology Report Card," an analysis of and standard for nuclear cardiology laboratory performance, is now being offered by ASNC on a voluntary basis. It clearly will be the way of the future, not only for nuclear cardiology but for echocardiography and other labs. Although adding a layer of bureaucracy, this system will force the objective demonstration of the accuracy and efficacy of all methods in individual laboratories. This can only be a beneficial step for the field of nuclear cardiology.

In an editorial, Feigenbaum (*880*) observed, "A good nuclear study will always be better than a poor echo study and a good echo study will always be better than a poor nuclear study." To this we must ask, "Which method would be best employed when both are good?" Clearly, the practitioner must strive to make them both their best and answer this question for themselves. However, we must not be content to use the method that is available. If the desired equipment or expertise is not available for the desired imaging application, import it or develop it—but see that your patients get what they need.

SUMMARY STRATEGY

Extensive published work (*6,7,9–14,19,21,47,68,72,119,198,202,307,429,782*) demonstrates the diagnostic and prognostic value of MPS and its comparison with stress testing alone and with other methods. Analysis of these findings (*128*) presents a rationale for the application of the method, for diagnostic or prognostic purposes, over the spectrum of patients with known or suspected CAD (Figs. 33–36,88–91,114). These findings suggest that stress testing alone is an adequate method of CAD evaluation for diagnostic indications in those with a normal resting ECG and a low pretest CAD likelihood. Those with low post-test CAD likelihood may then be followed or treated medically, those with high post-test CAD likelihood may be treated medically or sent to angiography and those with an intermediate post-test likelihood are best evaluated with stress MPS. Because a normal stress test would not bring post-test likelihood to levels low enough to justify the practical exclusion of CAD, these latter patients may be best studied initially with stress MPS. Although those with a normal resting ECG and an intermediate or high pretest CAD likelihood may be evaluated similarly when prognosis is the study indication, a normal stress test alone would not bring the post-test likelihood to levels low enough to justify the practical exclusion of risk from CAD nor provide the risk stratification of MPS, and these patients are best studied initially by stress MPS. Although those with a low pretest CAD likelihood and even those with a low post-test likelihood may be risk stratified better by MPS than stress testing alone, the yield would be extremely low and cost effectiveness low as well. Of course, those with an abnormal rest and uninterpretable stress ECG must be evaluated initially by stress MPS, regardless of the indication. Maddahi and Gambhir (*881*) present a mathematical model for the cost-effective application of perfusion imaging for the diagnosis of coronary disease and its prognostic assessment. Here, clinical effectiveness was based on the percentage of correct coronary diagnosis, whereas the cost was expressed in terms of the medical expenditure. The authors compared 6 competing evaluation strategies in patient subgroups with varying pretest coronary likelihoods. For diagnosis, the scintigraphic method was most cost effective in the group with intermediate disease likelihood or in those with a low disease likelihood but an abnormal rest ECG. Those with a low likelihood and normal

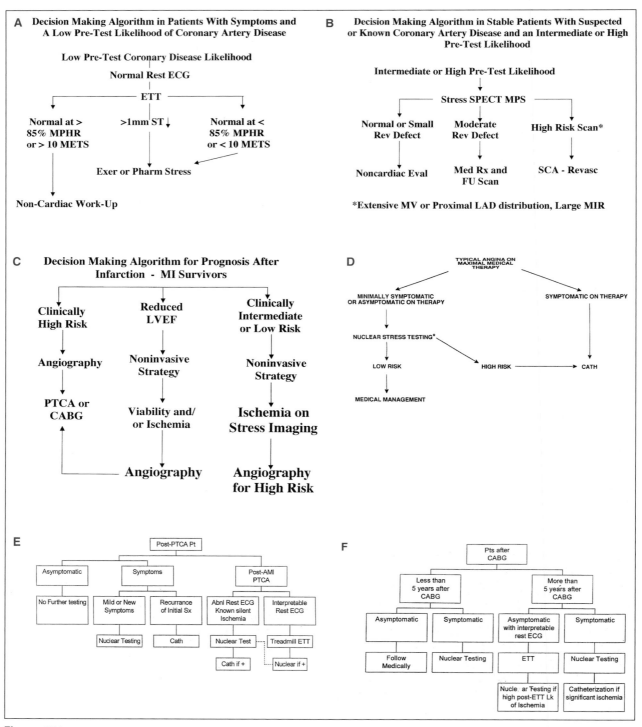

A Decision Making Algorithm in Patients With Symptoms and A Low Pre-Test Likelihood of Coronary Artery Disease

Low Pre-Test Coronary Disease Likelihood

Normal Rest ECG

ETT

Normal at > 85% MPHR or > 10 METS   >1mm ST↓   Normal at < 85% MPHR or < 10 METS

Exer or Pharm Stress

Non-Cardiac Work-Up

B Decision Making Algorithm in Stable Patients With Suspected or Known Coronary Artery Disease and an Intermediate or High Pre-Test Likelihood

Intermediate or High Pre-Test Likelihood

Stress SPECT MPS

Normal or Small Rev Defect   Moderate Rev Defect   High Risk Scan*

Noncardiac Eval   Med Rx and FU Scan   SCA - Revasc

*Extensive MV or Proximal LAD distribution, Large MIR

C Decision Making Algorithm for Prognosis After Infarction - MI Survivors

Clinically High Risk   Reduced LVEF   Clinically Intermediate or Low Risk

Angiography   Noninvasive Strategy   Noninvasive Strategy

PTCA or CABG   Viability and/ or Ischemia   Ischemia on Stress Imaging

Angiography   Angiography for High Risk

D

TYPICAL ANGINA ON MAXIMAL MEDICAL THERAPY

MINIMALLY SYMPTOMATIC OR ASYMPTOMATIC ON THERAPY   SYMPTOMATIC ON THERAPY

NUCLEAR STRESS TESTING*

LOW RISK   HIGH RISK   CATH

MEDICAL MANAGEMENT

E

Post-PTCA Pt

Asymptomatic   Symptoms   Post-AMI PTCA

No Further testing   Mild or New Symptoms   Recurrance of Initial Sx   Abnl Rest ECG Known silent Ischemia   Interpretable Rest ECG

Nuclear Testing   Cath   Nuclear Test   Treadmill ETT

Cath if +   Nuclear if +

F

Pts after CABG

Less than 5 years after CABG   More than 5 years after CABG

Asymptomatic   Symptomatic   Asymptomatic with interpretable rest ECG   Symptomatic

Follow Medically   Nuclear Testing   ETT   Nuclear Testing

Nuclear Testing if high post-ETT Lk of Ischemia   Catheterization if significant ischemia

Figure 114

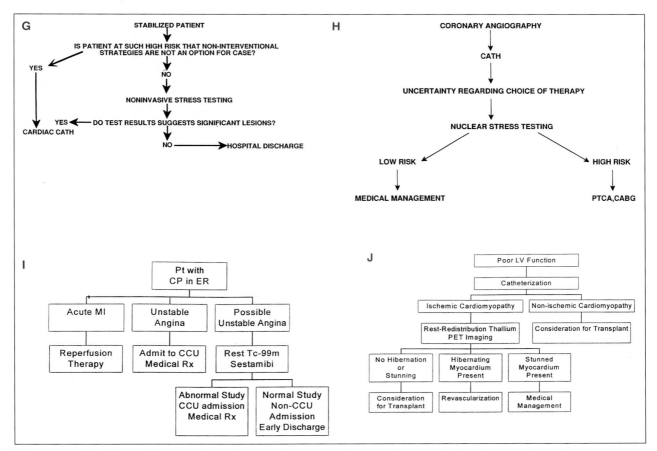

Figure 114   Decision-making algorithms. Presented are general approaches to patients with a spectrum of coronary syndromes. Of course, they must be individualized for the specific patient. (A) In symptomatic patients with a low pretest likelihood of coronary artery disease (CAD) and a normal rest electrocardiogram (ECG); (B) in symptomatic patients with an intermediate or high pretest CAD likelihood; (C) in survivors of an acute myocardial infarction (AMI); (D) in patients with typical angina on maximal medical therapy; (E) after angioplasty/stent; (F) after coronary artery bypass graft (CABG); (G) in the stabilized patient with unstable angina; (H) in the patient with an ambiguous coronary angiogram (cath); (I) in patients presenting to the emergency room (ER); and (J) in patients with reduced left ventricular (LV) function. CP = chest pain; ETT = treadmill test; Eval = evaluation; Lk = likelihood; MV = multivessel CAD; MIR = myocardium at ischemic risk; Pts = patients; Rev = reversible; Revasc = revascularization; Rx = treatment; SCA = selective coronary angioplasty; Sx = symptoms; CCU = coronary care unit; PTCA = percutaneous transluminal coronary angiography; LVEF = left ventricular ejection fraction; LAD = left anterior descending coronary artery. (A–C adapted, with permission, from Beller GA. Paper presented at Nuclear Cardiology Symposium, Toronto, Canada, 1998. ; D–I adapted, with permission, from Hachamovitch R. Myocardial perfusion imaging for risk stratification in CAD. Extracting all the information. Patient selection for nuclear cardiology procedures: meeting the demands of the cardiologist in 1998. Paper presented at the annual meeting of the American Society of Nuclear Cardiology, Atlanta, GA, 1998. J adapted from Hachamovitch R, Berman DS, Kiat H, et al. What drives post-nuclear testing management in patients with known coronary artery disease [abstract]? *Circulation* 1995;92:I–438.)

baseline ECG required only a stress test. In those with a high pretest likelihood, direct referral to coronary angiography was the most cost-effective diagnostic step. However, generally angiography should best be reserved for those in whom myocardial revascularization is considered, because of the high risk of medical therapy. Because perfusion imaging presents incremental prognostic value compared with other methods, scintigraphy should be appropriately applied for risk stratification to determine those who would benefit most from intervention. In those with a normal rest ECG and low pretest coronary likelihood, the risk of events is also low, and neither angiography nor scintigraphy are indicated. Here, in most cases, stress testing without imaging will suffice. For diagnosis, those with an intermediate pretest disease likelihood should get stress testing with imaging of those with an abnormal, ambiguous, uninterpretable or insufficient test. In those with an intermediate or high pretest disease likelihood, the high rate of abnormal images and the high potential event rate makes stress perfusion imaging again the initial prognostic study of choice. Angiography would again be based on image findings. An abnormal or uninterpretable baseline ECG would make stress scintigraphy requisite in any population requiring stress testing, in which subsequent evaluation and management would be based on image findings. In any group needing stress evaluation but unable to exercise adequately, pharmacologic stress with a coronary dilator would be the appropriate choice.

In light of these results and all previously presented, a strategy for CAD diagnosis and risk stratification is recommended combining the use of clinical information, exercise testing and, in some patient subsets, scintigraphy (Fig. 115). With this approach, patients with an interpretable ECG and low pretest likelihood of CAD have an extremely low event rate on follow-up and should be studied initially with stress testing. If abnormal and with intermediate-to-high post-test CAD likelihood, they should be re-evaluated by stress MPS unless risk appears prohibitive (*674*), in which case they should go to angiography. In patients with interpretable ECGs and intermediate-to-high pretest CAD likelihood, the first test ordered should be an exercise MPS. Whether studied for diagnosis or prognosis, patients with an intermediate-to-high pretest likelihood of CAD and an uninterpretable (stress) ECG, as well as those unable to exercise satisfactorily, would be referred directly to MPS. Those unable to exercise would be studied with pharmacologic stress testing. Those patients with abnormal scans would then be considered candidates for aggressive medical management or referral to catheterization, based on image

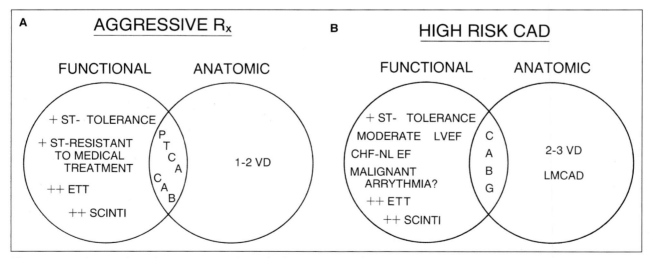

Figure 115 Approach to the coronary patient: the interaction of clinical, pathophysiology and anatomy. Shown are diagrams that summarize the generic approach to the stable coronary patient with (A) limited 1- or 2-vessel disease (1-2 VD) or (B) extensive 2- or 3-vessel (2-3 VD) or left main (LM) coronary artery disease (CAD). In each case, it is the interaction of the clinical presentation, exercise tolerance, the presence of heart failure (CHF) with the results of functional and pathophysiologic testing, left ventricular ejection fraction (LVEF), ST depression(+), a markedly abnormal stress test (++ETT) or a markedly abnormal stress scintigram (++scinti) that will determine the pattern of clinical management, medical treatment, angioplasty/stent (percutaneous transluminal coronary angioplasty [PTCA]) or coronary bypass graft surgery (CABG). Scintigraphy has demonstrated an expanded role in this decision-making algorithm. The presentation does not pretend to be all inclusive.

findings, whereas those patients with normal scans can be safely considered to be low risk and not in need of further testing unless otherwise recommended by clinical factors. As reviewed above, the safety and efficacy of this approach has now been established in patients with known CAD, as well as in the elderly, in women and in relation to pharmacologic stress testing and with all agents and imaging protocols (Fig. 116).

Current and Future Research

Previous research efforts in the field of medical- and catheter-based revascularization have employed MPS as the "surrogate" to the survival end point. Here, reduced perfusion defects in those having thrombolytic therapy or acute angioplasty demonstrated evidence of myocardial salvage. Recent developments in the area of methods of "medical revascularization" have placed MPS in a prominent new light. Here, research to document the benefit of mechanical efforts, such as enhanced external counterpulsation, and pharmacologic methods, with the infusion of VegF, fGF (282–284) and other agents and methods (504), are based in no small part in evidence of revascularization presented by MPS. It is the relative objectivity, reproducibility and clear relation of the method to regional myocardial perfusion that permits this application in costly, multicenter trials to establish the value of an important new line of potential coronary disease therapy. Beyond this, the role of perfusion scintigraphy in guiding medical management has not been fully investigated. Is it reliable enough to apply even in groups in whom management has apparently been well established: those with single- or 3-vessel disease? No prospective multicenter trial has applied perfusion imaging to a revascularization-versus-medical management decision process. The full complementary contribution of function evaluation to perfusion image findings has not yet been fully established, and the methodology of gated SPECT is still in development. The utility of the method in the evaluation of patients with ventricular dysfunction or heart failure has not yet been fully established. Given the value of perfusion imaging, the frequency at which it should be repeated in follow-up is not established. The cost effectiveness of the method has not been well or fairly assessed in light of its current documented value for risk stratification. New radionuclides, imaging protocols and processing methods are on the horizon, supported by ever stronger and less expensive hardware. Attenuation and scatter correction methods, PET SPECT and other innovations will strongly advance the field. The method has expanded to serve a range of patient and clinical categories, including patients acutely ill from coronary as well as noncardiac conditions. Patients and the method would be much benefited by the introduction of a portable scintillation camera based in SPECT technology. The full and fair comparison of stress perfusion and echocardiographic methods has not been done. The influence of vested interests and personal financial considerations play too great a role in the support of each method.

Nuclear cardiology is strong and a growing partner of both nuclear medicine and cardiology specialists. ASNC is initiating new methods to raise the quality of practice and supporting innovations in the field (882). This is only a partial list and much remains to be done.

When Is Perfusion Imaging Cost Effective for Diagnosis/Prognosis?
Extensive population study data indicates that myocardial perfusion scintigraphy is generally of value and cost effective for coronary disease DIAGNOSIS in the presence of an intermediate pretest likelihood, or with an abnormal baseline ECG and for coronary disease PROGNOSIS in the presence of intermediate or high pretest disease likelihood and in association with pharmacologic stress.

Figure 116

ANNOTATED REFERENCES

1. Botvinick EH, Taradash MR, Shames DM, et al. Thallium-201 myocardial perfusion scintigraphy for the clinical clarification of normal, abnormal and equivocal electrocardiographic stress tests. *Am J Cardiol* 1978;41:43–49.

(This early effort demonstrated the diagnostic superiority of planar stress perfusion scintigraphy compared with stress electrocardiography [ECG] and stress testing. It was especially advantageous when the stress ECG was equivocal, as in the setting of left ventricular hypertrophy, resulting from resting ST-T abnormalities, and with suboptimal stress levels.)

2. Hamilton GW, Trobaugh GNB, Ritchie JL, et al. Myocardial imaging with Tl-201: an analysis of clinical usefulness based on Bayes' theorem. *Semin Nucl Med* 1978;8: 358–370.

(The utility of the method, and possibly its accuracy, will vary with the frequency of the condition in the population studied. In this early test of the diagnostic accuracy of myocardial perfusion scintigraphy, the method discriminates between those with and without coronary artery better than does stress electrocardiography [see *101–103*].)

3. Berman DS, Garcia EV, Maddahi J. Thallium-201 scintigraphy in the detection and evaluation of coronary artery disease. In: Berman DS, Mason, DT. *Clinical Nuclear Cardiology*. New York, NY: Grune & Stratton; 1980.

(This is an early review of the myocardial perfusion scintigraphy method.)

4. Hlatky M, Botvinick E, Brundage B. The independent value of exercise thallium scintigraphy to physicians. *Circulation* 1982;66:953–959.

(A consecutive group of actual clinical cases of patients presenting for evaluation of symptoms of possible coronary disease was summarized and given to a large group of collaborating board-certified cardiologists. Each patient had stress planar perfusion scintigraphy as part of his or her evaluation. Initially, cardiologists were asked to estimate the likelihood of coronary disease given the clinical presentation, including the stress test result. Next, they were asked how they would manage the patient. Finally, they were told the findings of scintigraphy and again asked their estimated likelihood of coronary disease and management. Scintigraphic findings strongly affected the diagnosis and management, with an increased tendency toward angiography in the setting of an abnormal scintigram and a shift toward conservative therapy with the finding of a normal or benign scintigram. Myocardial perfusion scintigraphy influenced the cardiologists' diagnoses and did so significantly in the direction of angiographic findings, this with planar images and no quantitation. These biases were supported by the angiographic findings, demonstrating an appropriate utilization of image findings. Today, this reliance on SPECT scintigraphic data is even stronger and probably more justified.)

5. Melin JA, Wijns W, Vanbursele RJ, et al. Alternative diagnostic strategies for coronary artery disease in women: demonstration of the usefulness and efficiency of probability analysis. *Circulation* 1985;71:535–543.

(This article reviews diagnostic methods for coronary disease in reference to the incidence of disease in the population. Given the lower incidence of disease in younger women, these considerations have specific relevance in this population. Alternative strategies for the diagnosis of coronary artery disease were studied in 93 infarct-free women presenting with chest pain and in 42 consecutive women prospectively analyzed. Strategies were derived based on the findings. If the history and stress electrocardiography were initially applied and stress myocardial perfusion scintigraphy [MPS] applied if the poststress likelihood was 10%–90%, 1/3 of stress MPS could be avoided and angiography reduced by 50% without loss of accuracy. Of course, prognostic value was not considered. When the female population evaluated is appropriate for study, they will benefit, as do men, from both the diagnostic and prognostic advantages of the scintigraphic method.)

6. Kotler TS, Diamond GA. Exercise thallium-201 scintigraphy in the diagnosis and prognosis of coronary artery disease. *Ann Int Med* 1990;113:684–702.

(In this pooled analysis, 122 articles reporting both the sensitivity and specificity of thallium-201 myocardial perfusion scintigraphy were assessed. The method was found to be valuable in coronary artery disease [CAD] diagnosis, especially with an abnormal resting electrocardiogram, limited exercise tolerance and intermediate disease likelihood and for prognostic evaluation of those with known or suspected CAD.)

7. Brown KA, Boucher CA, Okada RD, et al. Prognostic value of exercise Tl-201 imaging in patients presenting for evaluation of chest pain. *J Am Coll Cardiol* 1983;1: 994–1001.

(The prognostic value of exercise myocardial perfusion scintigraphy [MPS] was evaluated in 139 consecutive nonrevascularized patients followed for 3–5 yr. Among 100 patients without prior myocardial infarction, the number of reversible segments on planar exercise MPS was the best predictor of events, whereas in those with prior MI, left ventricular ejection fraction [LVEF] on angiography was the best predictor. SPECT provides greater ability to quantitate defect size and clinical risk.

This study applied multivariate analysis and found that death correlated best with the number of reversible segmental defects. Next most prognostic was the total perfusion image defect size followed by the number of diseased vessels. After these values were extracted, the number of fixed defects, the LVEF, the positive stress electrocardiogram and other stress testing variables studied were not contributory.)

8. Canhasi B, Dae M, Botvinick E, et al. Interaction of "supplementary" scintigraphic indicators and stress electrocardiography in the diagnosis of multi-vessel coronary disease. *J Am Coll Cardiol* 1985;6:581–587.

(This article presents the concept of "nonperfusion indicators" of ischemia. Here, the presence of lung uptake, cavitary dilation or basal uptake added to the likelihood of extensive coronary disease and made likely more extensive disease than that manifested by simple analysis of perfusion defects. Lung uptake appears to relate to increased transit time through the lungs and correlates with elevated pulmonary venous pressure and congestive heart failure. Cavitary dilation relates to the production of regional or global ischemia or regional underperfusion. Basal uptake, the least applied of the 3 signs, indicates reduced distal myocardial perfusion of a large scale, with relatively increased uptake at the base, producing a "filling in" of the usually open basal region. The presence of any of these findings in the setting of regional perfusion defects suggests more extensive disease than that delineated by the perfusion defects themselves.

Lung uptake, cavitary dilation and basal myocardial uptake were demonstrated to supplement the extent of abnormalities on stress myocardial perfusion scintigraphy and even the presence of a markedly positive stress test in the identification of patients with extensive, high-risk coronary artery disease. Today, in many cases, we relate image abnormalities to their related risk rather than to associated anatomy.)

9. Staniloff HM, Forrester JS, Berman DS, Swan HJC. Prediction of death, myocardial infarction, and worsening chest pain using thallium scintigraphy and exercise electrocardiography. *J Nucl Med* 1986;27:1842–1848.

(The prognostic power of myocardial perfusion scintigraphy during 1-yr follow-up in patients without myocardial infarction was assessed in a group of 819 patients. This article demonstrates the excellent prognostic value of scintigraphy, where worsening scintigraphic findings, taken in relation to the related stress, correlated well with events.)

10. Ladenheim M, Pollock BH, Rozanski A, et al. Extent and severity of myocardial hypoperfusion as predictors of prognosis in patients with suspected coronary artery disease. *J Am Coll Cardiol* 1986;7:464–471.

(The incremental ability of the clinical history, exercise electrocardiography and myocardial perfusion scintigraphy to identify coronary events in the year after testing was assessed in 1659 patients with symptoms suggesting coronary artery disease but without prior myocardial infarction, percutaneous transluminal coronary angioplasty or coronary artery bypass graft. Prognostic power was quantified in terms of the area under the receiver operating characteristic curve in this population with 74 hard events. Stepwise logistic regression analysis identified the number of reversible defects, defect severity and the achieved heart rate. Defect extent and severity related exponentially to prognosis, whereas rate related inversely and linearly to event rate. Low heart rate shifted upward the relationships between defect size and severity with event rate. Compared with coronary angiography, which could stratify risk over a 3-fold range from roughly 3%–10%, these variables could substratify risk from 2%–80% event likelihood and approached the aim of risk stratification to move from group stratification to a specific patient prognosis. We want to say to our patients "This is your prognosis," not "You belong to a group with this prognosis.")

11. Ladenheim M, Kotler T, Pollock B, et al. Incremental prognostic power of clinical history, exercise electrocardiography and myocardial perfusion scintigraphy in suspected coronary artery disease. *Am J Cardiol* 1987;59:270–277.

    (The incremental ability of the clinical history, exercise electrocardiography [ECG] and myocardial perfusion scintigraphy [MPS] to identify coronary events in the year after testing was assessed in the same 1659 patients with symptoms suggesting coronary artery disease noted in reference *10*. Prognostic power was quantified in terms of the area under the receiver operating characteristic curve in this population with 74 hard events. In 1451 patients with a normal rest ECG, the clinical history was the best prognostic variable, with improved prognostication [by 5%] only with inclusion of MPS results. In 208 patients with an abnormal rest ECG, stress MPS added significantly and equally to risk stratification beyond the stress ECG. Application of these findings to the development of a strategic model increased the ability to stratify risk with the development of very low- and very high-risk groups, impossible with the stress ECG alone.)

12. Younis LT, Byers S, Shaw LJ, et al. Prognostic importance of silent myocardial ischemia detected by intravenous dipyridamole thallium myocardial imaging in asymptomatic patients with coronary artery disease. *J Am Coll Cardiol* 1989;14:1635–1641.

    (The study analyzed image variables among 107 asymptomatic patients studied with dipyridamole stress myocardial perfusion scintigraphy. Stepwise logistic regression analysis selected a reversible thallium-201 defect, which was present in 12 of the 13 patients who died or had nonfatal acute myocardial infarctions, as the only significant predictor of events. An induced defect in these patients does likely represent clinical asymptomatic ischemia.)

13. Hendel RC, Layden JJ, Leppo JA. Prognostic value of dipyridamole thallium scintigraphy for evaluation of ischemic heart disease. *J Am Coll Cardiol* 1990;15: 109–116.

    (Dipyridamole myocardial perfusion scintigraphy demonstrated prognostic value in a large unselected population of 516 patients and appears to be an adequate alternative to physiologic exercise testing in the evaluation of coronary artery disease.)

14. Brown KA. Do stress echocardiography and myocardial perfusion imaging have the same ability to identify the low-risk patient with known or suspected coronary artery disease? *Am J Cardiol* 1998;81:1050–1053.

    (Although both stress myocardial perfusion scintigraphy [MPS] and stress echocardiography appear to have prognostic value, the annual death and acute myocardial infarction rates appear to be much higher among patients with negative stress echocardiograms compared with negative stress MPS. The event rate with the former, but not the latter, limits its ability to serve as the "gatekeeper" for additional invasive studies and interventions.)

15. Berman DS, Kiat H, Friedman JD, Diamond GA. Clinical applications of exercise nuclear cardiology studies in the era of healthcare reform. *Am J Cardiol* 1995;75: 3D–13D.

(This is a focused review of the clinical applications of nuclear cardiology in the current environment of medical practice. The reproducible and objective nature of the data, its accuracy and prognostic value are even more important and valued advantages in modern medicine.)

16. Bateman TM, O'Keefe JH Jr, Dong VM, et al. Coronary angiographic rates after stress single-photon emission computed tomographic scintigraphy. *J Nucl Cardiol* 1995;2:217–223.

(This large retrospective study of rates of coronary angiography was performed in 4162 patients who underwent perfusion scintigraphy and were followed for a 26-mo period. Sixty percent of those studied had reversible defects. Thirty-two percent of those with reversible defects, compared with only 3.5 of those with normal scans [n = 1663], went to angiography within 3 mo of study. Among those with "high-risk" patterns of reversibility [left anterior descending coronary artery or multivessel disease and/or abnormal lung uptake] [n = 1141], 60% went to angiography, compared with only 9% of those with mild to moderate defects [n = 1358]. Reversibility and "high-risk" reversibility were the strongest predictors of angiography. The data in these images are utilized to a high degree. Further, after 3 yr, the hard event rate among those with normal scans or those with mild defects was only 3%, so these patients should be treated medically.)

17. Shaw LJ, Hachamovitch R, Eisenstein E, et al. and the Economics of Noninvasive Diagnosis Multicenter and Duke Noninvasive Research Working Groups. Biostatistic and economic principles for diagnostic and prognostic modeling in nuclear cardiology: part I. *J Nucl Cardiol* 1996;3:538–545.

(The authors present an overview of noninvasive prognostic methods in coronary artery disease with focus on the diagnostic and prognostic value of stress myocardial perfusion scintigraphy. Part II presents an outline for the integration of economic evaluation into clinical decision making.)

18. Shaw LJ, Kesler KL, Eisenstein EL, et al. A multicenter study of 11,372 patients to examine cost-effective strategies for diagnosis of coronary artery disease. Decision analysis: utilization of tests, procedures for 5 strategies in 100 patients [abstract]. *J Am Coll Cardiol* 1996;27:286A.

(Patients were prospectively enrolled and studied with the gamut of stress methods and radiopharmaceuticals. The diagnostic yield for catheterization after appropriate suggestive perfusion imaging study was superior to that of direct angiography [$P < 0.001$]. At all clinical risk levels, cost was incrementally higher for direct angiography. Stress perfusion imaging minimizes cost and maximizes diagnostic yield for patients at risk for coronary disease. Similarly, the ratio of outcomes/cost effectiveness and cost/life saved are lowest for catheterization after appropriate suggestive perfusion imaging strategy [see *674,781*].)

19. Hachamovitch R, Berman DS, Kiat H, et al. Comparison of incremental prognostic value, risk stratification and cost effectiveness of rest/exercise Tl-201/Tc-99m sestamibi SPECT in women and men. *J Am Coll Cardiol* 1996;28:34–44.

(This study analyzes 2592 patients of both sexes, who came to diagnostic evaluation for possible coronary artery disease [CAD]. All underwent scintigraphy and were otherwise treated based on clinical findings. Patients were divided on the basis of the pretest likelihood of CAD. Large reversible defects in the absence of fixed defects or smaller reversible defects in the presence of a large fixed defect, indicating a large prior myocardial infarction, indicated a high event rate. Patient management was clearly influenced by scintigraphic findings, in which the larger the reversible defect, the more likely was angiography. Both women and men with an interpretable stress electrocardiogram and an intermediate or high post-exercise test likelihood of CAD, as well as all those with an uninterpretable stress electro-cardiograph demonstrated a significant risk stratification benefit from scintigraphic study. MPS appears to be well utilized to identify patients at greatest risk, with excellent correlation to subsequent anatomy. Hard events, cardiac death, infarction, and remote revascularization during the 2 mo after MPS were well predicted in these groups on the basis of image findings. Scintigraphic prognoses were much better defined and prognostic subgroups better separated in females, where scinti-graphic abnormalities were weighted more heavily toward a poor prognosis and a higher event rate. Therefore, contrary to popular belief, perfusion scintigraphy better stratifies coronary risk in females, and the same scintigraphic abnormality appears to relate to a worse prognosis than in males.)

20. Berman DS, Hachamovitch R. Risk assessment in patients with stable coronary artery disease: incremental value of nuclear imaging. *J Nucl Cardiol* 1997;3:S41–S49.
      (This is a thorough review of the subject.)

21. Hachamovitch R, Berman DS, Shaw LJ, et al. Incremental prognostic value of myo-cardial perfusion single photon emission computed tomography for the prediction of cardiac death: differential stratification for risk of cardiac death and myocardial infarction. *Circulation* 1998;97:535–543.
      (This study analyzed the incremental value of exercise SPECT myocardial per-fusion scintigraphy [MPS] for the prediction of individual hard end points and its implications for risk stratification in a group of 5183 consecutive patients, followed for 642 ± 226 days after SPECT MPS. The event rate related to a normal scan was 0.5%. The frequency of both cardiac death and nonfatal infarction increased with worsening scan defects. Risk stratification was based on scan find-ings within groups determined by their prescan coronary artery disease [CAD] likelihood. Those one-third of patients with a low pretest likelihood of CAD had a very low event rate, with cardiac death or nonfatal infarction less than 1% and so did not require image evaluation for prognosis, unless quality of life issues were considered. Further analysis identified a patient cohort with mildly abnormal scans, who are severely threatened by infarction but not by cardiac death. Such patients would probably not benefit from revascularization, not proven to prevent infarction, unless refractory symptoms are present. Instead, they could perhaps be treated medically with a noninvasive strategy and aggressive risk factor reduction and may not require coronary angiography. Those with moderate-to-severely-abnormal scans were at high risk of cardiac death and, according to this study, should be treated aggressively with angiography and appropriate revasculariza-tion. These findings were consistent for patients having either pharmacological or exercise stress MPS and were confirmed by the subsequent retrospective analysis of patients at the same institution. These findings have significant implications for the use of MPS in the guidance of post-test patient management and the decision to refer to catheterization or treat medically. This could result in significant cost savings without change in outcomes. Of note is the fact that the incremental myo-cardial infarction rate paralleled defect size and density and, so, indirectly support the relationship between the severity of coronary stenosis and the occurrence of subsequent infarction [see *593*]. The strong prognostic relationship between im-age findings and outcomes in this and other studies again supports the relation-ship, albeit sometimes indirectly, between the severity of coronary stenoses and outcomes.)

22. Snader CE, Marwick TH, Pashkow FJ, et al. Importance of estimated functional capacity as a predictor of all-cause mortality among patients referred for exercise thallium single photon emission computed tomography: report of 3400 patients from a single center. *J Am Coll Cardiol* 1997;30:641–648.
      (These workers analyzed "all-cause" mortality compared with image findings and workload achieved at exercise in metabolic equivalents [METs] in an overall low-risk population. Those who achieved >6 METs had a mortality <3% over a

2.5-yr follow-up, whereas those with workload <6 METS, had a 6% mortality over this same period. Perfusion image findings were independent predictors of mortality.)

23. Lauer MS, Okin PM, Larsen, et al. Impaired heart rate response to graded exercise. Prognostic implications of chronotropic incompetence in the Framingham Heart Study. *Circulation* 1996;93:1520–1526.

(Here, the cumulative mortality of a large study group related well to the achieved double product. Those who reached the predicted rate for their age had a 2% mortality over 8 yr, whereas those who did not reach this level had a 6% mortality over this same time period.)

24. Gianrossi R, Detrano R, Mulvihill D, et al. Exercise-induced ST depression in the diagnosis of coronary artery disease: a meta-analysis. *Circulation* 1989;80:87–98.

(This meta-analysis of 147 consecutive publications comparing exercise-induced ST changes with coronary angiography involved 24,074 patients, who were included in both tests. Like all meta-analyses, this is no better than the data included. Here, that data is relatively unselected and massive. There was a wide variability in diagnostic accuracies [sensitivities, 23%–100%; specificities, 17%–100%] among studies, unexplained by information reported in the medical literature.)

25. Sansoy V, Watson DD, Beller GA. Significance of slow upsloping ST-segment depression on exercise stress testing. *Am J Cardiol* 1997;79:709–712.

(If horizontal ST depression was the lone electrocardiographic criterion for ischemia, then sensitivity, specificity and positive and negative predictive values were 49%, 84%, 64% and 74%, respectively. If 1 mm of upsloping ST depression was also added as an ischemic criterion, these values were 71%, 56%, 49% and 77%, respectively, gaining sensitivity at the cost of specificity and positive predictive value.)

26. Miller TD, Christian TF, Taliercio CP, et al. Severe exercise-induced ischemia does not identify high risk patients with normal left ventricular function and 1 or 2 vessel coronary artery disease. *J Am Coll Cardiol* 1994;23:219–224.

(The study demonstrated an inability to risk stratify between those with or without evidence of severe exercise-induced ischemia, based on stress testing and stress electrocardiographic parameters.)

27. Bogaty P, Guimond J, Robitaille NM, et al. A reappraisal of exercise electrocardiographic indexes of the severity of ischemic heart disease: angiographic and scintigraphic correlates. *J Am Coll Cardiol* 1997;29:1497–1504.

(Stress electrocardiographic indices of high-risk coronary artery disease, including early, deep, prolonged, downsloping and horizontal ST depression occurring at a low achieved double-product disease, failed to correlate with either the extent of coronary involvement or the extent of perfusion defect in 66 consecutive patients with stable angina and 70% stenosis of 1 or more coronary arteries. There was no correlation in this study between the extent of ST depression and the extent of induced perfusion defect, a more direct index of myocardium at ischemic risk.)

28. Taylor AJ, Sackett MC, Beller GA. The degree of ST-segment depression on symptom-limited exercise testing: relation to the myocardial ischemic burden as determined by thallium-201 scintigraphy. *Am J Cardiol* 1995;75:228–231.

(The correlation between exercise-induced ST depression and myocardium at ischemic risk on related quantitative SPECT thallium-201 perfusion imaging was evaluated in 144 patients. Overall, there was a poor correlation between the extent of induced ST depression and image abnormalities. The study found no difference in the amount of induced perfusion defect and total extent of image defects between those with exercise-induced ST depression ≥ or < 2 mm. Only the group with ST depression >2 mm demonstrated a comparably greater amount of ischemic myocardium. As shown elsewhere, even deep, early ST depression may be misleading in appropriate clinical company. The article considers the issue of "ischemic burden.")

29. Mark DB, Shaw L, Harrell FE, et al. Prognostic value of a treadmill exercise score in outpatients with suspected coronary artery disease. *N Engl J Med* 1991;325:849–853.

   (The Duke Treadmill Score is an index derived from elements of exercise test performance, including treadmill time or metabolic equivalents [METs; energy] achieved and amount of induced ST depression and severity of angina, to evolve a single value related to the likelihood and risk [and outcome] of coronary artery disease [CAD]. It has been applied as a noninvasive method of CAD risk stratification in the Unstable Angina Guidelines [see *31*] and others. Myocardial perfusion scintigraphy has been shown to substratify risk well among Duke score responses [see *32,33*].)

30. Shaw LJ, Peterson ED, Shaw LK, et al. Use of a prognostic treadmill score in identifying diagnostic coronary disease subgroups. *Circulation* 1998;98:1622–1630.

   (This study analyzed the Duke Treadmill Score as a diagnostic and risk stratification method in coronary artery disease [CAD]. The composite Duke score provided excellent diagnostic and prognostic information in symptomatic patients suspected of having CAD. Stress myocardial perfusion scintigraphy has been shown to risk stratify within groups stratified as low, intermediate or high risk based on the Duke Treadmill Score [see *32,33,349*].)

31. Agency for Healthcare Policy and Research. *Unstable Angina: Diagnosis and Management.* Clinical practice guideline No. 10. AHCPR publication number 94-0602. Washington, DC: U.S. Department of Health and Human Services; 1994.

   (These guidelines serve as general boundaries governing application of the methods. They are governed by the literature as well as political and economic factors and do not consider the contribution of experience. They are definitely not binding on clinical practice, in which the individual physician governs management largely based on experience and the tools available.)

32. Hachamovitch R, Berman DS, Kiat H, et al. Exercise myocardial perfusion SPECT in patients without known coronary artery disease: incremental prognostic value and impact on subsequent patient management. *Circulation* 1996;93:905–914.

   (This was an extensive prospective study of the incremental prognostic value, role in risk stratification and impact on patient management of SPECT myocardial perfusion scintigraphy in 2203 consecutive patients without history of coronary disease or previous infarction, catheterization or revascularization, who were followed for 566 days. Multiple logistic regression analysis and calculation of the global χ^2 revealed that scan data contributed 95% of the information [global $\chi^2 = 169$] that brought patients to angiography and 5% was contributed by historic and stress test findings [global $\chi^2 = 31$]! The scan results substratified risk well among all groups, based on their pretest coronary disease likelihood, in which normal scans were low risk in all groups and risk increased with worsening scan findings. Referring physicians used this test to determine management, and early postscan referral rates to angiography and revascularization paralleled the hard event rates in each category, which directly related to each category of scan result. There were very low referral rates when the scan was normal or probably normal, with increasing rates with worsening scan findings. Scan findings paralleled event rates in all scan categories.

   Nor did the findings on exercise variables, such as the Duke Treadmill Score, pretest coronary disease likelihood, symptoms, sex or age, eliminate the incremental prognostic value of scintigraphic findings. Scintigraphic findings brought further risk stratification, even after consideration of presenting symptoms, age, sex, disease likelihood and the Duke Treadmill Score, a well-accepted quantitative treadmill test scoring system based on electrocardiographic [ECG] findings and stress test parameters. Both the "hard" event rate and the catheterization rate were well stratified on the basis of scintigraphic findings within patient groups demonstrating low, intermediate and high Duke Treadmill Scores. It was the image defect score, rather than the ECG and stress test parameters, that related to event rate and determined management! The hard event rate was 0.4% among those with an intermediate-risk Duke classification but a normal scan. Scintigraphic risk stratification was beneficial among those with interpretable stress ECGs and intermediate-to-high postexercise test coronary disease likelihood or in those with an uninterpretable rest ECG, regardless of pretest likelihood.

When subdivided into groups based on sex, image findings stratified event rates well among both men and women. However, the risk related to a severe image defect in women far exceeded the risk of such an image in men [19.2% versus 6.3%]. Although the catheterization rate increased with the severity of scan findings, the catheterization rate in women was similar to that in men for all ranges of scan defect. Perhaps it should be higher in women with severe defects.

In a patient population without previous coronary history and low coronary-related risk, SPECT perfusion imaging adds incremental prognostic information and risk stratifies patients even after historic, clinical and exercise information is known. The scintigraphic method is used generally and appropriately in determining further evaluation and treatment.)

33. Shaw LJ, Hachamovitch R, Iskandrian AE. Treadmill test scores: attributes and limitations [editorial]. *J Nucl Cardiol* 1997;4:74–78.
   (This article provides excellent evidence of the risk stratification ability of myocardial perfusion scintigraphy and its superiority to the best stress-testing index, the Duke Treadmill Score. However, as presented here, test superiority depends on the nature of the population studied.)

34. Detry J-MR, Kapita BM, Cosyns J, et al. Diagnostic value of history and maximal exercise electrocardiography in men and women suspected of coronary artery heart disease. *Circulation* 1977;56:756–761.
   (This serves as a historical record of stress testing.)

35. Guiteras VP, Chaitman RR, Waters DD, et al. Diagnostic accuracy of exercise ECG lead systems in subsets of women. *Circulation* 1977;65:1465–1474.
   (ST segment depression only with exercise and not in recovery was associated with a 23% specificity. Overall sensitivity was 79%, and specificity was 66%.)

36. Weiner DA, Ryan TJ, McCabe CH, et al. Correlations among history of angina, ST segment response and prevalence of coronary artery disease in the Coronary Artery Surgery Study (CASS). *N Engl J Med* 1979;301:230–235.
   (The CASS results demonstrated a 92% survival rate in patients with a normal left ventricular ejection fraction [LVEF] treated medically but survival of only 83% and 57% among those with LVEF of 35%–49% and <35%, respectively, who were treated medically.)

37. Gibbons RF. Electrocardiography testing with and without radionuclide studies. In: Wenger NK, Speroff L, Packard B, eds. *Cardiovascular Health and Disease in Women.* Greenwich, CT: Lejaq Communications; 1993:73–88.
   (The advantages of exercise myocardial perfusion scintigraphy compared with exercise testing without imaging are reviewed.)

38. Alexander KP, Shaw LJ, DeLong ER, et al. Value of exercise treadmill testing in women. *J Am Coll Cardiol* 1998;32:1657–1664.
   (In an extensive recent study, the Duke Treadmill Score was applied to the diagnosis and prognosis of coronary artery disease [CAD] in 976 women and 2249 men with histories of symptoms, known or suspected disease and coronary angiography. Although the score differed between men and women, as did CAD prevalence and mortality, the score was equally predictive of the diagnosis and risk related to CAD, beyond clinical indicators, in both sexes. The method was better at accurately excluding the possibility of disease in women.)

39. Chaitman BR, Bourassa MG, Lam J. Noninvasive diagnosis of coronary heart disease in women. In Eaher ED, Packard B, Wenger NK, et al., eds. *Coronary Heart Disease in Women.* New York, NY: Haymarket Daymon; 1987:222–228.
   (A thorough but relatively early review of the field. Considered are hormonal effects and other aspects of coronary disease specific to women.)

40. Hlatky MA, Pryor DB, Harrell FL et al. Factors affecting sensitivity and specificity of exercise electrocardiography. *Am J Med* 1984;77:64–71.
(This is a thoughtful and thorough analysis of the subject.)

41. Ellestadt MH. *Stress Testing: Principles and Practice.* 4th ed. Philadelphia, PA: FA Davis Co.; 1996.
(This is an excellent text on stress testing.)

42. Esquivel L, Pollock SG, Beller GA, et al. Effect of the degree of effort on the sensitivity of the exercise thallium-201 stress test in symptomatic coronary artery disease. *Am J Cardiol* 1989;63:160–165.
(The article demonstrates the relationship of the workload and, more appropriately, the achieved double product to the sensitivity of stress myocardial perfusion scintigraphy. Without an appropriate augmentation of the coronary flow demands and a strong test of the coronary flow reserve, negative tests may be false negatives and sensitivity will suffer.)

43. Iskandrian AS, Ghods M, Helfeld H, et al. The treadmill exercise score revisited: coronary arteriographic and thallium perfusion correlates. *Am Heart J* 1992;124: 1581–1586.
(A treadmill score based in ST depression, anginal and exercise duration was compared with thallium-201 myocardial perfusion scintigraphy findings in 834 patients with known coronary anatomy. Perfusion image defects correlated better with anatomy than did the treadmill score.)

44. Iskandrian AS, Heo J, Lemick J, Ogilby JD. Identification of high risk patients with left main and three-vessel coronary disease using stepwise discriminant analysis of clinical, exercise and tomographic thallium data. *Am Heart J* 1993;125:221–225.

(These authors demonstrated that the results of exercise perfusion imaging predicted well the presence of extensive coronary artery disease [CAD], when compared with exercise-induced ST depression or any other clinical factors in 834 patients, including 217 women. They found that the presence of a multivessel defect was a far better predictor of ischemia and CAD [$\chi^2 = 107$] than were exercise heart rate achieved [$\chi^2 = 27$] or ST depression [$\chi^2 = 8$]. Specificity was somewhat reduced in women, probably a result of confusion of breast attenuation with perfusion defects in this relatively early SPECT study.)

45. Rozanski A, Diamond GA, Bergman D, et al. The declining specificity of exercise radionuclide ventriculography. *N Engl J Med* 1983;309:518–522.
(This classic evaluation reveals a truth that affects the diagnostic specificity of all methods that are themselves used to determine which patients will be evaluated by the "gold standard method," here coronary angiography. To the degree that only those with abnormal perfusion images will be sent to angiography and because method sensitivity is apparently high, the number of patients with negative angiograms will be small and the fraction of patients with false-positive angiograms will approach 100%. Such a selection process would send the test specificity to 0! Of course, this is not accurate. This is proven in early studies before scintigraphy was used to select patients for angiography and by the high normalcy rate determined independently from the selection process. Because of this same selection process, method sensitivity is also probably not as high as calculated. Yet, because of the known excellent prognosis associated with a normal [or probably normal] perfusion scintigram, the method is not missing many patients with coronary disease and certainly not many with severe disease. Because of the reliance on scintigraphic studies for patient management decisions, it is not likely that a control group will be evaluated for its true specificity. Surely 1 reason that a method may appear to have greater diagnostic specificity than another is the fact that it is not as heavily used in patient management decisions or, alternatively, that it has a lower sensitivity.)

46. Detrano R, Janosi A, Lyons KP, et al. Factors affecting sensitivity and specificity of a diagnostic test: the exercise thallium scintigram. *Am J Med* 1988;84:699–708.

(The authors analyze the accuracy of stress perfusion scintigraphy and the factors that affect diagnostic accuracy. Major among these is the nature of the populations analyzed, as, for example, with or without previous infarction. Although those with prior infarction would be expected to have a higher sensitivity for coronary diagnosis, that diagnosis would be least helpful in that group, among whom the diagnosis is already known. Some early articles dealing with this method and many early studies of the diagnostic accuracy of stress echocardiography fail to note the effect of the population studied on the study results. Of course, a high sensitivity, demonstrable only in those with previous infarction, is not as good as it would appear. A testimonial to the scintigraphic method is that sensitivities remain high in the absence of infarction and that some studies, even multicenter studies, present equally high diagnostic sensitivities in the presence or absence of previous infarction.)

47. Dash H, Massie BM, Botvinick EH, et al. The noninvasive identification of left main and three-vessel coronary artery disease by myocardial stress perfusion scintigraphy and treadmill exercise electrocardiography. *Circulation* 1979;60:276–284.

(This early article seeks to determine the ability of scintigraphy to specifically identify multivessel coronary disease. The presence and distribution of perfusion scintigraphic defects is compared with the distribution of coronary disease and with findings on stress testing and stress electrocardiography. This analysis was performed with early planar methods and before the recognition of the importance of "nonperfusion" indicators of ischemia, such as lung uptake. Defects, mostly reversible, were evident in the distribution of multiple coronary vessels in ~45% of patients with multivessel, "high-risk" disease. This was not much greater than the 35%–40% of markedly positive stress tests, with >2 mm horizontal ST depression within the first 2 stages [6 minutes] of a Bruce Protocol or induced hypotension. It is interesting that either a markedly positive stress test or scintigram identified more than two-thirds of such patients. The addition of washout, quantitation, SPECT and nonperfusion indicators has raised recognition of such high-risk anatomy on the basis of scintigraphic findings to ≥70% in some studies, with a sensitivity to coronary diagnosis ≥95%. Of course, the implications of a negative image or an image that greatly underestimates the degree of anatomic involvement are unclear and must be approached with clinical judgment in the face of the great known favorable prognostic value of a negative test, even in the presence of coronary disease. Although the results of stress testing should not be ignored but used in association with the scintigraphic findings, the application of SPECT imaging has demonstrated the ability of the method to clarify the clinical significance of even the markedly positive stress test when coronary disease diagnosis remains in doubt.)

48. Berman DS, Kiat H, Cohen I, et al. Incremental prognostic value of Tc-99m sestamibi myocardial perfusion SPECT in patients without prior myocardial infarction [abstract]. *J Nucl Med* 1994;35:59P.

(This study demonstrates the independent prognostic value of perfusion scintigraphic data and its incremental and complementary nature compared with the quantitative analysis of stress test and clinical variables in a large group of patients with no previous infarction. An exception is the generally low event rate in those with a low pretest probability, regardless of scintigraphic findings. However, intermediate- and high-likelihood groups benefit greatly from scintigraphic risk stratification. In addition, the high negative predictive value of a normal exercise technetium-99m sestamibi study has been demonstrated in a large population, regardless of the pretest likelihood based on clinical and exercise variables.

Their prognostic value and the relationships developed between stress test and scintigraphic findings suggest that their combination can be applied well to risk stratification in patients without known coronary disease and with intermediate or high likelihood of disease.)

49. Diamond GA. Reverend Bayes' silent majority. An alternative factor affecting sensitivity and specificity of exercise electrocardiography. *Am J Cardiol* 1986;57: 1175–1180.

(The authors present a method of correction of data for referral bias.)

50. Roger VL, Pellikka PA, Bell MR, et al. Sex and test verification bias. Impact on the diagnostic value of exercise echocardiography. *Circulation* 1997;95:405–410.

(As a result of the presence of a post-test referral bias, true scintigraphic sensitivity is probably lower and true specificity much higher than calculated in clinical data sets in which angiography is the "gold standard." Although similar considerations apply to other stress imaging methods, their accuracy will be affected only in relation to the confidence the public places in these methods and in proportion to the frequency with which positive tests lead to angiography. This study demonstrates that stress echocardiography, in fact, has little influence on patient management! In addition, the study demonstrated the reduced sensitivity and positive predictive value of the method in women compared with men.)

51. Maddahi J, Garcia EV, Berman DS, et al. Improved noninvasive assessment of coronary artery disease by quantitative analysis of regional stress myocardial distribution and washout of Tl-201. *Circulation* 1981;164:924–933.

52. Van Train KF, Berman DS, Garcia EV, et al. Quantitative analysis of stress Tl-201 myocardial scintigrams. A multicenter trial. *J Nucl Med* 1986;27:1726–1734.

(51,52: These articles present the most widely applied method for quantitation of myocardial perfusion images. When applied to a patient population with known anatomy, the diagnostic specificity may be reduced as a result of a post-test referral bias. For this reason, normalcy values have been derived [see *Self-Study Program III. Cardiology. Topic 5: Myocardial Perfusion Scintigraphy. Technical Aspects*].)

53. Albro PC, Gould KL, Westcott RJ, et al. Noninvasive assessment of coronary stenoses by myocardial imaging during pharmacologic coronary vasodilatation. III. Clinical trial. *Am J Cardiol* 1978;42:751–760.

(In this classic article, the authors established the rationale for stress perfusion imaging [see *Self-Study Program III. Cardiology. Topic 2: Pharmacologic Stress*].)

54. Leppo J, Boucher CA, Okada RD, et al. Serial Tl-201 myocardial imaging after dipyridamole infusion: diagnostic utility in detecting coronary stenoses and relationship to regional wall motion. *Circulation* 1982;66:649–656.

55. Taillefer R, Lette J, Phaneuft DC, et al. Tl-201 myocardial imaging during pharmacologic coronary vasodilation: comparison of oral and intravenous administration of dipyridamole. *J Am Coll Cardiol* 1986;8:76–84.

56. Ruddy TD, Dighero HR, Newell JB, et al. Quantitative analysis of dipyridamole-thallium images for the detection of coronary artery disease. *J Am Coll Cardiol* 1987;10:142–150.

(53–56: The authors of these articles present the initial calculated values for diagnostic accuracy of planar perfusion scintigraphy with dipyridamole pharmacologic stress.)

57. Ritchie JL, Trobaugh GB, Hamilton GW, et al. Myocardial imaging with thallium at rest and during exercise: comparison with coronary angiography and resting and stress electrocardiography. *Circulation* 1977;56:66–73.

(57–97: These articles are summarized after reference 97.)

58. Bailey IK, Griffith SC, Rouleau J, et al. Tl-201 myocardial perfusion imaging at rest and during exercise: comparative sensitivity to electrocardiography in coronary artery disease. *Circulation* 1977;55:79–86.

59. Rosenblatt A, Lowenstein JM, Kerth W, et al. Post-exercise Tl-201 myocardial scanning: a clinical appraisal. *Am Heart J* 1977;94:63–72.

60. Lenaers A, Block P, Van Thiel E, et al. Segmental analysis of Tl-201 stress myocardial scintigraphy. *J Nucl Med* 1977;18:509–518.

61. Verani MS, Marcus ML, Razzak MA. Sensitivity and specificity of Tl-201 perfusion scintigrams under exercise in the diagnosis of coronary artery disease. *J Nucl Med.* 1978;19:773–781.

62. Ritchie JL, Zaret BL, Strauss HW, et al. Myocardial imaging with Tl-201: a multicenter study in patients with angina pectoris or acute myocardial infarction. *Am J Cardiol* 1978;42:345–351.

63. Turner DA, Battle WE, Deshmukh H, et al. The predictive value of myocardial perfusion scintigraphy after stress in patients without previous myocardial infarction. *J Nucl Med* 1978;19:249–257.

64. Blood DK, McCarthy DM, Sciacca RR, et al. Comparison of single-dose and double-dose Tl-201 myocardial perfusion scintigraphy for the detection of coronary artery disease and prior myocardial infarction. *Circulation* 1978;58:777–786.

65. Carrillo AP, Marks DS, Pickard SD, et al. Correlation of exercise Tl-201 myocardial scan with coronary arteriograms and the maximal exercise test. *Chest* 1978;73:321–328.

66. Maisey MN, Lowry A, Bischof-Delaloye A, et al. European multicenter comparison of thallium-201 and technetium-99m methoxyisobutylisonitrile in ischemic heart disease. *Eur J Nucl Med* 1990;16:869–877.

67. Vogel RA, Kirch DL, LeFree MT, et al. Tl-201 myocardial perfusion scintigraphy: results of standard and multi-pinhole tomographic techniques. *Am J Cardiol* 1979;43:787–796.

68. Massie BM, Botvinick EH, Brundage BH. Correlation of Tl-201 scintigrams with coronary anatomy: factors affecting region-by-region sensitivity. *Am J Cardiol* 1979;44:616–624.

    (This is an early review of factors influencing interpretive accuracy of myocardial perfusion scintigraphy. This analysis presents a perspective worth considering even now.)

69. McKillop HJ, Murray RG, Turner JG, et al. Can the extent of coronary artery disease be predicted from Tl-201 myocardial images? *J Nucl Med* 1979;20:715–723.

70. McCarthy DM, Blood DK, Sciacca RR, Cannon PJ. Single-dose myocardial perfusion imaging with Tl-201: application in patients with nondiagnostic electrocardiographic stress tests. *Am J Cardiol* 1979;43:899–906.

71. Caralis DG, Bailey L, Kennedy HL, et al. Tl-201 myocardial imaging in evaluation of asymptomatic individuals with ischemic ST-segment depression on exercise electrocardiogram. *Br Heart J* 1979;42:562–569.

72. Silber S, Fleck E, Klein U, et al. Wertigkeir der Tl-201 belastungselektrokardiographie bie patienten mit koronarer herzerkrankung ohne myokardinfarkt. *Herz* 1979; 4:359–366.

73. Jengo JA, Freeman R, Brizendine M, et al. Detection of coronary artery disease: comparison of exercise stress radionuclide angiocardiography and thallium stress perfusion scanning. *Am J Cardiol* 1980;45:535–541.

74. Rigo P, Bailey IK, Griffith LSC, et al. Value and limitation of segmental analysis of stress thallium myocardial imaging for localization of coronary artery disease. *Circulation* 1980;61:973–982.

75. Caldwell JH, Ha GW, Sorenson SG, et al. The detection of coronary artery disease with radionuclide techniques: a comparison of rest–exercise thallium imaging and ejection fraction response. *Circulation* 1980;46:189–196.

76. Boucher CA, Zir LM, Beller GA, et al. Increased lung uptake of Tl-201 during exercise myocardial imaging. Clinical hemodynamic and angiographic implications in patients with coronary artery disease. *Am J Cardiol* 1980;46:189–198.

77. Iskandrian AS, Mintz GS, Croll MN, et al. Exercise Tl-201 myocardial scintigraphy: advantages and limitations. *Cardiology* 1980;65:136–144.

78. Iskandrian AS, Segal BL, Haaz W, et al. Effects of coronary artery narrowing, collaterals, and left ventricular function on the pattern of myocardial perfusion. *Cathet Cardiovasc Diagn* 1980;6:159–167.

79. Schicha H, Rentrop P, Facorro L, et al. Results of quantitative myocardial scintigraphy with Tl-201 at rest and after maximum exercise-critical analysis of predictive value and clinical application [in German]. *Z Kardiol* 1980;69:31–37.

80. Elkayam U, Weinstein M, Berman DS, et al. Stress thallium-201 myocardial scintigraphy and exercise technetium ventriculography in the detection and location of chronic coronary artery disease: comparison of sensitivity and specificity of these noninvasive tests alone and in combination. *Am Heart J* 1981;101:657–666.

(At the time this article was written, there was some doubt about the relative advantages of these methods. With SPECT; multiheaded cameras; technetium-99m–based perfusion agents; easy accurate pharmacologic stress; objective, reproducible, quantitative interpretation with diagnostic accuracy; prognostic superiority and cost effectiveness, myocardial perfusion scintigraphy and its ability to look at the primary ischemic event took overwhelming dominance.

81. Uhl GS, Kay TN, Hickman JR. Computer-enhanced thallium scintigrams in asymptomatic men with abnormal exercise tests. *Am J Cardiol* 1981;48:1037–1045.

(The diagnostic accuracy of computer-enhanced exercise thallium-201 myocardial perfusion scintigraphy [MPS] was assessed in 191 asymptomatic aircrewmen who had positive stress electrocardiograms. There were only 4 false-positive and 2 false-negative MPSs in the presence of 56 with angiographically significant disease. Enhanced stress MPS was effective in identifying asymptomatic subjects with coronary artery disease and myocardium at ischemic risk. Such sensitivity and specificity is unusual among a low likelihood population.

The results in this article demonstrate the prognostic value of dipyridamole perfusion scintigraphy in the setting of noncardiac, nonvascular surgery. It also emphasizes a multifactorial approach to risk assessment and the importance of quantitating image abnormalities as well as the compounding effect of other clinical factors.)

82. Guiney TE, Pohost GM, McKusick KA, et al. Differentiation of false- from true-positive ECG responses to exercise stress by Tl-201 perfusion imaging. *Chest* 1981;80:4–11.

83. Melin JA, Piret LJ, Vanbutsele RJM, et al. Diagnostic value of exercise electrocardiography and thallium myocardial scintigraphy in patients without previous myocardial infarction: a Bayesian approach. *Circulation* 1981;64:1019–1027.

84. Patterson RE, Horowitz SF, Eng C, et al. Can exercise electrocardiography and Tl-201 myocardial imaging exclude the diagnosis of coronary artery disease? Bayesian analysis of the clinical limits of exclusion and indications for coronary angiography. *Am J Cardiol* 1982;49:1127–1135.

(The authors make practical assumptions about test accuracy, test cost and the frequency of conditions generally to determine prognostic and clinical abilities of each method.)

85. Faris JV, Burt RW, Graham MC, et al. Tl-201 myocardial scintigraphy: improved sensitivity, specificity, and predictive accuracy by application of a statistical image analysis algorithm. *Am J Cardiol* 1982;49:733–743.

86. Kambara H, Kawashita K, Yoshida A, et al. Identification of patients with coronary artery disease using a scoring system of coronary risk factors, electrocardiography, and myocardial perfusion imaging (prospective and retrospective). *Jpn Circ J* 1982;46:235–243.

87. Cinotti L, Meignan M, Usdin JP, et al. Diagnostic value of image processing in myocardial scintigraphy. *J Nucl Med* 1983;24:768–775.

88. Patterson RE, Kirk ES. Coronary steal mechanisms in dogs with one-vessel occlusion and other arteries normal. *Circulation* 1983;67:1009–1016.

89. Chaitman BR, Brevers G, Dupras G, et al. Fluoroscopy when the exercise ECG is strongly positive. *Am Heart J* 1984;108:260–267.

90. Osbakken MD, Okada RD, Boucher CA, et al. Comparison of exercise perfusion and ventricular function imaging: an analysis of factors affecting the diagnostic accuracy of each technique. *J Am Coll Cardiol* 1984;3:272–281.

91. Hung J, Chaitman BR, Lam J, et al. Noninvasive diagnostic test for the evaluation of coronary artery disease in women. A multivariate comparison of cardiac fluoroscopy, exercise electrocardiography, and exercise thallium myocardial perfusion scintigraphy. *J Am Coll Cardiol* 1984;4:8–14.

92. Burke JF, Morganroth J, Soffer J, et al. The cardiokymography exercise test in the diagnosis of coronary artery disease. *Am Heart J* 1984;107:718–725.

93. Del Rio-Meraza A, Vilapando-Gutierrez J, Nava-Lopez G, et al. Correlation between exercise electrocardiographic test, myocardial perfusion test with Tl-201, and contrast coronary arteriography in patients with ischemic heart disease. *Arch Invest Med* 1985;16:175–184.

94. Hung J, Chaitman BR, Lam J, et al. A logistic regression analysis of multiple noninvasive tests for the prediction of the presence and extent of coronary artery disease in men. *Am Heart J* 1985;110:460–469.

    (The incremental diagnostic yield of clinical data, the stress electrocardiogram [ECG], stress thallium myocardial perfusion scintigraphy [MPS] and calcium on cardiac fluoroscopy in 171 symptomatic men was investigated. Multiple logistic regression analysis resolved a quantitative model confirming that optimal diagnostic efficacy is obtained when noninvasive tests are ordered sequentially. Cardiac fluoroscopy, which sought information similar to cine CT but in a qualitative manner, was far less effective than the stress test ECG and MPS.)

95. Rothendler JA, Okada RD, Wilson RA, et al. Effect of a delay in commencing imaging on the ability to detect transient thallium defects. *J Nucl Med* 1985;26:880–887.

96. Weiner DA. Accuracy of cardiokymography during exercise resting. Results of a multicenter study. *J Am Coll Cardiol* 1985;6:502–510.

97. Amor M, Verdaguer M, Karcher G, et al. Les examens isotopiques a l'effort dans l'insuffisance coronaire. *Arch Mal Coeur* 1985;78:55–63.

    (57–97: These references deal with the evaluation of diagnostic accuracy of stress planar myocardial perfusion scintigraphy compared with stress electrocardiography, other scintigraphic agents and/or coronary angiography from 1977 through 1994. The sensitivities and specificities quoted in the text represent a mean value and do not reflect the variety of techniques employed, population studied, developing experience with and insight into the method or the range of abilities applied. Although introducing a range of variability to the results, it also makes them even more impressive for their extent and range of participants. No other stress imaging method has been so widely investigated and critically analyzed as perfusion scintigraphy.)

98. Machencourt J, Denis B, Wolf JE, et al. Sensitivity and specificity of myocardial scintigraphy after exercise injection of thallium-201 and after rest injection of dipyramidole: cardiographic comparison of 70 subjects [in French]. *Arch Mal Coeur* 1981;74:147–156.

99. Narita M, Kurihara T, Usami M. Noninvasive detection of coronary artery disease by myocardial imaging with thallium-201: the significance of pharmacologic interventions. *Jpn Circ J* 1981;45:127–136.

100. Timmis AD, Lutkin JE, Fenney LJ, et al. Comparison of dipyridamole and treadmill exercise for enhancing thallium-201 perfusion defects in patients with coronary artery disease. *Eur Heart J* 1980;1:275–286.

101. Wilde P, Walker P, Watt I, et al. Thallium-201 myocardial imaging: recent experience using a coronary vasodilator. *Clin Radiol* 1982;33:43–52.

(97–101: The authors of these articles compare the results of perfusion scintigraphy acquired in association with dynamic and pharmacologic stress methods.)

102. Diamond GA, Forrester JS. Analysis of probability as an aid to the clinical diagnosis of coronary artery disease. *N Engl J Med* 1979;300:1350–1358.

103. Diamond GA, Forrester JS, Hirsch M, et al. Application of conditional probability analysis to the clinical diagnosis of coronary artery disease. *J Clin Invest* 1980;65:1210–1217.

(102,103: Because diagnostic likelihood varies among different population subgroups and because prognostic value varies in these groups in relation to their diagnostic likelihood, populations must be grouped according to disease likelihood before analysis of test value in any given population. These classic articles form the basis for the determination of the "pretest probability" of coronary disease. Here, large populations were analyzed by age, gender and the presence and character of symptoms and probabilities of coronary disease determined on the basis of related angiographic findings. This classification and others like it form the basis of population analysis, in which the value of a given diagnostic or prognostic method is tested in a given patient population.)

104. Kaul S. Technical, economic, interpretive, and outcomes issues regarding utilization of cardiac imaging techniques in patients with known or suspected coronary artery disease. *Am J Cardiol* 1995;75:18D–24D.

(This is an excellent and thorough analysis of technical and economic issues related to the application of any diagnostic method, with specific relevance to scintigraphic and other imaging methods in coronary disease. The clinical value and application of diagnostic methods are analyzed, with consideration of statistical matters that determine diagnostic accuracy, prognostic value and clinical applications based on cost effectiveness and "outcomes" issues.)

105. Dans PE, Weiner JP, Melin JA, et al. Conditional probability in the diagnosis of coronary artery disease: a future tool for eliminating unnecessary testing. *South Med J* 1983;76:1118–1126.

(103–105: These authors analyze the relationships among the post-test likelihood of disease, the sensitivity of the test and the incidence of disease in the population being evaluated. The appropriateness of test application may be determined with these facts in mind. No method has been more thoroughly analyzed in this regard, than perfusion scintigraphy.)

106. Froelicher VF, Thompson AJ, Wolthuis R, et al. Angiographic findings in asymptomatic aircrewmen with electrocardiographic abnormalities. *Am J Cardiol* 1977;39:32–39.

(Coronary angiography performed in 298 asymptomatic, healthy airmen with electrocardiographic [ECG] abnormalities and abnormal exercise tests was normal in 60%. Abnormalities on ECG have a lower specificity for coronary artery disease in healthy subjects.)

107. Watson DD. Quantitative SPECT techniques. *Semin Nucl Med* 1999;29:192–203.
   (This is a current review of methods of SPECT quantitation and image interpretation [see *119,338,357*].)

108. Najm YC, Timmis AD, Maisey MN, et al. The evaluation of ventricular function using gated myocardial imaging with Tc-99m sestamibi. *Eur Heart J* 1989;10:142–148.
   (This is 1 of the early papers that demonstrated the accuracy of the method and the advantages of combined function and perfusion data available from gated technetium-99m sestamibi imaging. Unlike the first-pass method, the gated method reflects function at the time of imaging, not the time of injection. Imaging first-pass function at the time of injection reflects function at peak intervention.)

109. Smith WH, Watson DD. Technical aspects of myocardial planar imaging with technetium-99m sestamibi. *Am J Cardiol* 1990;66:16E–22E.

110. Sinusas AJ, Beller GA, Smith WH, et al. Quantitative planar imaging with technetium-99m methoxy isobutyl isonitrile: comparison of uptake patterns with thallium-201. *J Nucl Med* 1989;30:1456–1463.

111. Koster K, Wackers FJTh, Mattera JA, Fetterman RC. Quantitative analysis of planar technetium-99m sestamibi myocardial perfusion images using modified background subtraction. *J Nucl Med* 1989;31:1400–1408.

112. Kiat H, Maddahi J, Roy LT, et al. Comparison of technetium-99m methoxy isobutyl isonitrile and thallium-201 for evaluation of coronary artery disease by planar and tomographic methods. *Am Heart J* 1989;117:1–11.

113. Wackers FJTh, Berman DS, Maddahi J, et al. Technetium-99m hexakis 2-methoxy-isobutyl isonitrile: human biodistribution, dosimetry, safety, and preliminary comparison to thallium-201 for myocardial perfusion imaging (phase I and phase II studies). *J Nucl Med* 1989;30:301–311.

114. Taillefer R, Lambert R, Dupras G, et al. Clinical comparison between thallium-201 and Tc-99m-methoxy isobutyl isonitrile (hexamibi) myocardial perfusion imaging for detection of coronary artery disease. *Eur J Nucl Med* 1989;15:280–288.

115. Watson DD, Smith WH, Beller GA, et al. Blinded evaluation of planar technetium-99m-sestamibi myocardial perfusion studies. *J Nucl Med* 1992;33:668–675.

116. Najm C, Maisey MN, Clarke SM, et al. Exercise myocardial perfusion scintigraphy with technetium-99m methoxy isobutylisonitrile: a comparative study with thallium-201. *Int J Cardiol* 1990;26:93–102.

117. Taillefer R, Dupras G, Sporn V, et al. Myocardial perfusion imaging with a new radiotracer technetium-99m-hexamibi (methoxy isobutyl isonitrile): comparison with thallium-201 imaging. *Clin Nucl Med* 1989;14:89–96.
   (This initial comparison study demostrated that myocardial perfusion scintigraphy with technetium-99m sestamibi is at least as accurate as thallium-201.)

118. Maddahi J, Kiat H, Friedman JP, et al. Tc-99m sestamibi myocardial perfusion imaging for evaluation of coronary disease: results of the North American Phase III Multicenter Clinical Trial. In: Zaret B, Beller G, eds. *Nuclear Cardiology*. St. Louis, MO: C.V. Mosby; 1992.
   (In this study, there was a diagnostic concordance of 94% between 4622 planar image segments studied with the 2 agents. Although planar imaging of both technetium-99m [^{99m}Tc] sestamibi and thallium-201 [^{201}Tl] demonstrated an incremental sensitivity for coronary diagnosis in the presence of 3-vessel disease [92% and 95%, respectively], compared with single-vessel disease [73% and 77%, respectively], SPECT image analysis demonstrated similar sensitivities for each agent in the presence of

both single- [90% and 90%, respectively] and 3-vessel disease [98% and 96%, respectively]. Interesting was the fact that the accuracies of the 2 agents analyzed by experienced readers were similar in all categories except diagnostic specificity, in which that of ^{99m}Tc sestamibi, at 95%, far exceeded that of ^{201}Tl, at 55%.

108–118: The authors of these studies and review articles present the results of quantitative analysis of planar and SPECT perfusion imaging.)

119. De Pasquale EE, Nody AC, DePuey E, et al. Quantitative rotational Tl-201 tomography for identifying and localizing coronary artery disease. *Circulation* 1988;77:316–317.

120. Fintel DJ, Links JM, Brinker JA, et al. Improved diagnostic performance of exercise Tl-201 single-photon emission computed tomography over planar imaging in the diagnosis of coronary artery disease: a receiver operating characteristic analysis. *J Am Coll Cardiol* 1989;13:650–658.

121. Mahmarian JJ, Boyce TM, Goldberg RK, et al. Quantitative exercise thallium-201 single-photon emission computed tomography for the enhanced diagnosis of ischemic heart disease. *J Am Coll Cardiol* 1990;15:318–326.

122. Quinones MA, Verani MS, Hiachin RM, et al. Exercise echocardiography versus 201-Tl single-photon emission computed tomography in evaluation of coronary artery disease: analysis of 292 patients. *Circulation* 1992;85:1026–1034.

123. Tamaki N, Yonekura Y, Mukai T, et al. Stress Tl-201 transaxial emission computed tomography: quantitative vs qualitative analysis for evaluation of coronary artery disease. *J Am Coll Cardiol* 1984;4:1213–1221.

(119–123: These authors report the diagnostic sensitivity and specificity of SPECT myocardial perfusion imaging in 2818 patients determined by qualitative visual analysis. The authors of reference *121* report the diagnostic sensitivity and specificity of SPECT myocardial perfusion imaging in patients determined by objective, quantitative computer analyses of digitized images. This study contributed to the determination of the normalcy rate as well.)

124. Heo J, Iskandrian AS. Technetium-labeled myocardial perfusion agents. Nuclear Cardiology Symposium. *Cardiol Clin* 1994;12:187–198.

(This is an extensive review of technetium-99m–based myocardial perfusion imaging agents, their physical and biologic properties, the technical aspects of their imaging and their clinical value. Planar sestamibi imaging and gating of both planar and SPECT sestamibi images are considered.)

125. Maisey MN, Mistry R, Sowton E. Planar imaging techniques used with technetium-99m sestamibi to evaluate chronic myocardial ischemia. Symposium: technetium-99m myocardial perfusion imaging agents. *Am J Cardiol* 1990;66:47E–54E.

(The authors review the technical features and diagnostic value of planar perfusion imaging with technetium-99m sestamibi, including the method and clinical value of gated planar acquisition.)

126. Hachamovitch R, Berman DS, Kiat H, et al. What drives post-nuclear testing management in patients with known coronary artery disease [abstract]. *Circulation* 1995;92:I-438.

(The authors analyze a large number of patients of both sexes, who came to diagnostic evaluation for possible coronary disease. All underwent scintigraphy and were otherwise treated based on clinical findings. Patients were divided on the basis of the pretest likelihood of coronary disease. Large reversible defects in the absence of fixed defects, or smaller reversible defects in the presence of a large fixed defect, indicating a large previous infarction, indicated a high event rate. Patient management was clearly influenced by scintigraphic findings: the larger the reversible defect, the more likely was angiography. Those with intermediate and high likelihood, as well as those with low likelihood and an uninterpretable stress electrocardiogram, demonstrated significant prognostic benefit from scintigraphy findings. The perfusion scintigram appears to be well utilized to identify patients at greatest risk, with excellent correlation to subsequent anatomy. Hard events, cardiac death, infarction and remote revascularization during 2 mo after scintigraphy were predicted well in these groups on the basis of image findings. Scintigraphic prognosis was much better defined and prognostic subgroups better separated in females, in whom scintigraphic abnormalities were weighted more heavily toward a poor prognosis and a higher event rate. Therefore, and contrary to popular belief, perfusion scintigraphy better stratifies coronary risk in females, in whom the same scintigraphic abnormality appears to relate to a worse prognosis than in males.)

127. Heller GV, Herman SD, Travin MI, et al. Independent prognostic value of intravenous dipyridamole with technetium-99m sestamibi tomographic imaging in predicting cardiac events and cardiac-related hospital admissions. *J Am Coll Cardiol* 1995;26:1202–1208.

    (Performed in consecutive patients studied for clinical reasons with dipyridamole stress technetium-99m sestamibi imaging, this study demonstrates the excellent ability of the method to risk stratify patients in terms of both hard cardiac events and subsequent cardiac-related hospital admissions, based on the size of evident image defects. The study demonstrates the reliance on the method to determine patient hospitalization and management and, based on the related hard event rates, it would appear, appropriately so! Most of the patients in the study were females, again demonstrating the value of the method in women.)

128. Berman DS, Hachamovitch R, Kiat H, et al. Incremental value of prognostic testing in patients with known or suspected ischemic heart disease: a basis for optimal utilization of exercise technetium-99m sestamibi myocardial perfusion single-photon emission computed tomography. *J Am Coll Cardiol* 1995;26:639–647.

    (The study determined the added prognostic ability, beyond classification based on clinical and exercise electrocardiographic [ECG] criteria, of normal and probably normal or "equivocal" stress perfusion studies among patients presenting for a diagnostic scintigraphic evaluation, including its effect on management and costs. Normal and probably normal scintigrams were associated with a benign prognosis in all patient groups, even those with a high coronary likelihood.

    The authors studied 1702 patients referred for exercise technetium-99m sestamibi SPECT study without revascularization, who were followed for a mean of 20 ± 5 mo. Cardiac death and nonfatal infarction were considered "hard" events, whereas revascularization >60 days after study was a "soft" event. Image findings stratified risk well among patients with low, intermediate and high pre-stress-test coronary artery disease likelihood, regardless of stress test result [normal, abnormal or uninterpretable]. Hard events and rates of referral to angiography were similarly low in those with normal and probably normal scans, regardless of whether these were associated with a low [<.15], intermediate [.15 to .85] or high [>.85] post-exercise-test coronary disease likelihood! For example, the event rate was 0.4% among 440 patients with normal scans, and an intermediate pretest disease likelihood compared with an event rate of 7.9% among the 266 patients with the same pretest clinical coronary disease likelihood but abnormal scans! Again, those with normal scans and high prescan likelihood of coronary disease had no events! The referral to angiography also was very low in all clinical subgroups when the image was normal. However, equivocal scans were related to a moderate increase in the incidence of angiography and subsequent revascularization. SPECT provided "incremental prognostic value in all subgroups analyzed." Normal scans related to a 0.2% hard and 0.7% soft event rate among 1131 patients, whereas abnormal scans related to a 7.5% hard and 7.4% soft event rate among 571 patient studies. The normal image had a generally low hard event rate, even when clinical- and exercise-related findings suggested a high likelihood of coronary disease. However, the overall event rate rose when the stress ECG was abnormal in patients with a high pretest likelihood, regardless of scan results. The scan was most clearly cost effective in those with uninterpretable stress tests or interpretable tests with intermediate and high pre-exercise test likelihood of coronary disease.)

129. Mahmarian JJ, Verani MS. Exercise thallium-201 perfusion scintigraphy in the assessment of coronary artery disease. Symposium on Nuclear Cardiology. *Am J Cardiol* 1991;67:2D–12D.

    (This is an excellent review of the field [at that time] in all its variations.)

130. Ellis SG, Mooney MR, George BJ, et al. Randomized trial of late elective angioplasty versus conservative management of patients with residual stenoses after thrombolytic treatment of myocardial infarction. Treatment of Post-Thrombolytic Stenoses (TOPS) Study Group. *Circulation* 1992;86:1400–1406.

    (No apparent benefit was noted from delayed percutaneous transluminal coronary angioplasty [4–14 days] after immediate thrombolytic therapy in this relatively low-risk group of 87 patients.)

131. Van Train K, Maddahi J, Berman D, et al. Quantitative analysis of tomographic stress thallium-201 myocardial scintigrams: a multicenter trial. *J Nucl Med* 1990;31:1168–1176.

    (This multicenter trial established the excellent diagnostic accuracy of perfusion scintigraphy as well as a high normalcy rate.)

132. Borges-Neto S, Mahmarian JJ, Jain A, et al. Quantitative thallium-201 single-photon emission computed tomography after oral dipyridamole for assessing the presence, anatomic location and severity of coronary artery disease. *J Am Coll Cardiol* 1988;11:962–970.

133. Iskandrian AS, Heo J, Kong B, et al. Effect of exercise level on the ability of thallium-201 tomographic imaging in detecting coronary artery disease: analysis of 461 patients. *J Am Coll Cardiol* 1989;14:1477–1485.

134. Maddahi J, Van Train KF, Prigent F, et al. Quantitative single-photon emission computerized thallium-201 tomography for detection and localization of coronary artery disease: optimization and prospective validation of a new technique. *J Am Coll Cardiol* 1989;114:1689–1697.

    (131–134: These authors and those of reference *121* report the diagnostic sensitivity and specificity of SPECT myocardial perfusion imaging in 1627 patients determined by objective, quantitative computer analysis of digitized images. These studies contributed to the determination of the normalcy rate as well.)

135. Maddahi J. Myocardial perfusion imaging for the detection and evaluation of coronary artery disease. In: Marcus ML, ed. *Cardiac Imaging: A Companion to Braunwald EB, Heart Disease.* Philadelphia, PA: W.B. Saunders; 1996:971–995.

    (This chapter contains the nuclear cardiology section presented in association with a major cardiology textbook and provides a limited amount of data regarding diagnostic accuracy of myocardial perfusion scintigraphy.)

136. Cullom SJ, Galt JR, Maddahi J, et al. Scatter and attenuation correction of SPECT Tc-99m sestamibi myocardial distributions: experimental validation of the effect on uniformity and contrast. *J Nucl Med* 1991;32:1067–1076.

137. Maddahi J, Prigent F, Garcia E, et al. Validation of newly developed attenuation and scatter correction methods for quantitating myocardial perfusion by Tc-99m sestamibi SPECT [abstract]. *Circulation* 1990;82:III-64.

    (136,137: These 2 early efforts present methods to correct for attenuation and scatter correction in SPECT perfusion images. The perfection and dissemination of such methods will do much to improve and further image specificity.)

138. Glover DK, Ruiz M, Edwards NC, et al. Comparison between Tl-201 and Tc-99m sestamibi uptake during adenosine-induced vasodilation as a function of coronary stenosis severity. *Circulation* 1995;91:813–820.

    (In this study of myocardial radionuclide uptake in dogs with adenosine coronary vasodilation in the presence of variable left anterior descending coronary artery stenoses, flow augmentation and the disparity between stenotic and normal perfusion beds were significantly underestimated by both radionuclides. The degree of underestimation was greatest with sestamibi, likely as a result of its earlier deviation from linearity with flow compared with thallium-201.)

139. Maddahi J, Kiat H, Van Train K, et al. Myocardial perfusion imaging with technetium-99m sestamibi SPECT in the evaluation of coronary artery disease. *Am J Cardiol* 1990;66:55E–62E.

(The authors of this article report findings in a large multicenter comparison of both planar and SPECT thallium-201 sestamibi imaging. The planar method may not be optimal for the technetium-based radionuclide, as its higher energy may "shine through" an overlying defect and obscure it.)

140. Kahn J, McGhie I, Akers M, et al. Quantitative rotational tomography with Tl-201 and Tc-99m 2-methoxy-isobutyl-isonitrile. A direct comparison in normal individuals and patients with coronary artery disease. *Circulation* 1989;79:1282–1293.

(132,140: The authors of these studies compared the relative accuracies of thallium-201 and technetium-99m sestamibi protocols for detection of disease in individual coronary arteries and for the diagnosis of coronary disease overall [see references *112–114*].)

141. Azzarelli S, Galassi AR, Foti R, et al. Wintergreen panel summaries. Accuracy of Tc-99m tetrofosmin myocardial tomography in the evaluation of coronary artery disease. *J Nucl Cardiol* 1999;6:183–189.

(The authors evaluated the accuracy of technetium-99m tetrofosmin as presented in the literature. They specifically evaluated accuracy in 235 consecutive patients, mostly men, who underwent stress tetrofosmin myocardial perfusion scintigraphy for clinical indications. The method was highly accurate and similar to image data acquired with sestamibi, with a sensitivity of 95% and normalcy of 91%. Sensitivity was 71% for the left anterior descending artery, 73% for the right coronary artery and 61% for the left circumflex artery territories, with per-vessel specificities of 94%, 91% and 96%, respectively. See Table 6D and reference *916*.)

142. Kapur A, Latus A, Davies G, et al. The robust study: a randomized comparison of three tracers for myocardial perfusion scintigraphy [abstract]. *J Nucl Med* 1999;40:85P.

(The study reports the findings related to image characteristics among 2540 randomized patients with suspected coronary artery disease studied by thallium-201 [^{201}Tl], technetium-99m [^{99m}Tc] tetrofosmin or sestamibi stress myocardial perfusion scintigraphy. Risk factors and proportions of abnormal studies were similar among the groups. Technetium-99m–based images were of higher quality and demonstrated less attenuation artifact but had greater subdiaphragmatic background, which did not differ between ^{99m}Tc-based agents. Heart/liver count ratios were lowest for sestamibi, and defect intensity was greatest for ^{201}Tl. There were no differences in diagnostic sensitivity or specificity.)

143. Nicolai E, Cuocolo A, Acampa W, et al. Exercise/rest Tc-99m tetrofosmin SPECT in patients with chronic ischemic left ventricular dysfunction: direct comparison with Tl-201 reinjection. *J Nucl Cardiol* 1999;6:270–277.

(Perfusion and viability information were the same when evaluated by quantitative exercise SPECT myocardial perfusion scintigraphy performed with technetium-99m tetrofosmin and thallium-201 reinjection methods in 33 patients with left ventricular dysfunction. In this study, the 2 methods appeared to provide similar information.)

144. Taillefer R, Soman P, DePuey EG, et al. Detection of mild to moderate coronary artery disease: comparison between Tc-99m sestamibi and Tc-99m tetrofosmin SPECT imaging with dipyridamole [abstract]. *J Nucl Med* 1999;40:86P.

(Dipyridamole stress technetium-99m sestamibi and tetrofosmin images were prospectively compared in 72 patients with mild-to-moderate coronary artery disease studied serially at 2 centers within 1 wk using same-day or 2-day stress/rest protocols and waiting 60 min after injection before imaging. Angiography was performed in all patients without intervening events within 2 mo of imaging. Images were then sent to 2 other centers, where they were read for the number, extent and severity of defects. All patients, none with previous infarction, had mild-to-moderate disease severity: 1 vessel with 70%–90% stenosis or 2-vessel disease with only 1 vessel narrowed 70% or more. Agents were applied in random order and submitted to blinded analysis, where rest and stress studies were read in random order and analyzed for quality and defect extent in a 17-segment model in 3 short-axis and 1 vertical-long-axis slice. Sestamibi sensitivity was higher and defect size was greater with sestamibi. Some physical differences between agents appear to have clinical implications.)

145. Soman P, Taillefer R, DePuey G, et al. Enhanced detection of reversible perfusion defects by Tc-99m sestamibi compared to Tc-99m tetrofosmin during vasodilator stress SPECT imaging in mild-to-moderate coronary artery disease. *J Am Coll Cardiol* 2001;37:458–462.

(Here, sestamibi, read quantitatively in 81 patients, detected greater defect extent [15% versus 125%], severity [0.6 versus 0.73 normal/defect] and reversibility [363 versus 285 segments] than did quantitated tetrofosmin among studies performed in the same patients in random order and read by an expert panel who was blinded to the radionuclide. Sestamibi detected 48% of those with mild multivessel disease as opposed to 24% with tetrofosmin, a difference that could affect risk stratification.)

146. Travin MI, Malkin RD, Garber CE, et al. Prevalence of right ventricular perfusion defects after inferior myocardial infarction assessed by low level exercise with technetium-99m sestamibi tomographic myocardial imaging. *Am Heart J* 1994; 127:797–804.

(Another advantage of technetium-99m based agents is their potential to assess right ventricular perfusion, size and function. In this study, right ventricular defects were sought and often found on stress sestamibi studies after inferior infarctions.)

147. Pereira N, Klutz WS, Fox RE, et al. Identification of severe right ventricular dysfunction by technetium-99m sestamibi gated SPECT imaging. *J Nucl Med* 1997; 38:254–256.

(Sestamibi imaging demonstrated right heart enlargement in this case report of an elderly man evaluated for chest pain and found to have multiple pulmonary emboli with acute pulmonary hypertension.)

148. Arora R, Zhao QH, Guguchev PA, et al. Identification of severe right ventricular dysfunction and pressure overload by stress radionuclide myocardial perfusion SPECT imaging with gating. *J Nucl Cardiol* 1999;6:375–376.

(The authors demonstrate the value of the gated perfusion method for the identification of right ventricular disease.)

149. Taillefer R, DePuey EG, Udelson JE, et al. Comparative diagnostic accuracy of Tl-201 and Tc-99m sestamibi SPECT imaging: perfusion and ECG-gated SPECT in detecting coronary disease in women. *J Am Coll Cardiol* 1997;29:69–77.

(This prospective study was conducted in 85 consecutive female patients and 30 volunteers with a low likelihood of coronary disease. The overall sensitivities for the diagnosis of coronary stenoses >50% and >70% with stress imaging performed in the same patients with each radionuclide were uniformly high: 75% and 84%, respectively, for thallium-201 [201Tl] and 72% and 81%, respectively, for technetium-99m [99mTc] sestamibi. In this study, sensitivity did not differ between agents and was not influenced by gating. However, specificities for stenoses >50% were 62% for 201Tl and 86% for 99mTc sestamibi [$P < 0.03$], whereas specificities for stenoses >70% were 59% for 201Tl and 83% for 99mTc sestamibi [$P < 0.02$]. When gated wall motion and thickening were added, the specificity of 99mTc sestamibi images was >92%.)

150. Rothbart R, Beller G, Watson D, et al. Diagnostic accuracy and prognostic significance of quantitative thallium-201 scintigraphy in patients with left bundle branch block. *Am J Noninv Cardiol* 1987;1:197–205.

151. Larcos G, Gibbons RJ, Brown ML. Diagnostic accuracy of exercise thallium-201 single-photon emission computed tomography in patients with left bundle branch block. *Am J Cardiol* 1991;88:756–760.

152. Tawarahara K, Kurata C, Taguchi T, et al. Exercise testing and thallium-201 emission computed tomography in patients with intraventricular conduction disturbances. *Am J Cardiol* 1992;69:97–102.

153. Matzer L, Kiat H, Friedman JD, et al. A new approach to the assessment of tomographic thallium-201 scintigraphy in patients with left bundle branch block. *J Am Coll Cardiol* 1991;17:1309–1317.

154. Krishnan R, Lu J, Zhu YY, et al. Myocardial perfusion scintigraphy in LBBB. A perspective on the issue from image analysis in a clinical context. *Am Heart J* 1993;128:578–586.

(Stress myocardial perfusion scintigraphy [MPS] was evaluated in 69 consecutive patients with left bundle branch block [LBBB]. Among 32 with coronary angiography, the overall and per-vessel sensitivity and specificity for right and left cirumflex coronary arteries were similar to those studied without LBBB. However, overall sensitivity and specificity for left anterior descending coronary artery [LAD] disease were reduced. Nonetheless, the predictive value of a positive test remained high [83%], as a result of the relatively low angiography rate in patients with minimally abnormal scans. Specificity also may be adversely affected by the presence of cardiomyopathy in some with LBBB and the bias toward catheterization in those with LAD disease. This diagnostic difficulty related to studies performed with exercise stress. Pharmacologic, dipyridamole MPS was related to specificities equal to those without LBBB.)

155. Burns RJ, Galligan L, Wright LM, et al. Improved specificity of myocardial thallium-201 single-photon emission computed tomography in patients with left bundle branch block by dipyridamole. *Am J Cardiol* 1991;68:504–508.

(Exercise stress myocardial perfusion scintigraphy [MPS] demonstrated reduced sensitivity and specificity for left anterior descending coronary artery disease, but pharmacologic, dipyridamole MPS was related to specificities equal to those without left bundle branch block.)

156. O'Keefe JH Jr, Bateman TM, Barnhart CS. Adenosine thallium-201 is superior to exercise thallium-201 for detecting coronary artery disease in patients with left bundle branch block. *J Am Coll Cardiol* 1993;21:1332–1338.

(As with dipyridamole, adenosine myocardial perfusion scintigraphy was related to specificities equal to those without left bundle branch block and superior compared with exercise imaging in this population.)

157. Wagdy HM, Hodge D, Christian TF, et al. Prognostic value of vasodilator myocardial perfusion imaging in patients with left bundle-branch block. *Circulation* 1998;97:1563–1570.

(The prognostic value of stress myocardial perfusion scintigraphy in the setting of left bundle branch block [LBBB] is demonstrated. Prognostic value was demonstrated among 245 patients with LBBB studied with dipyridamole [n = 173] or adenosine [n = 92]. Those with normal images had a 1-yr [soft] event rate of 3%, with no myocardial infarction [MI] or deaths, whereas an abnormal image related to a 1-yr event rate of 42%, with 11% having MIs and 8% dying.

150–157: Several studies have indicated the lack of specificity of myocardial perfusion scintigraphy compared with coronary angiography, in the setting of LBBB. This does not appear to be a significant factor in relation to vasodilator pharmacologic stress imaging. Here, the diagnostic specificity for coronary artery disease is maintained in the presence of LBBB, with agents such as dipyridamole or adenosine, which primarily test the coronary flow reserve and do not greatly augment heart rate and the double product. Still, some studies [*154*] indicate a preserved predictive value of a positive test, where even with exercise testing the majority of induced defects, even in the septum, will relate to coronary lesions. Although a number of these patients have a noncoronary cardiomyopathy and some defects appear better related to attenuation effects than LBBB, this does not appear to explain the lack of specificity. Nor does defect extension to the apex or its reversible nature resolve the interpretive ambiguity [see *Self-Study Program III. Cardiology. Topic 2: Pharmacologic Stress*].)

158. Johnson DL, Scanlon PD, Hodges DO, et al. Pulmonary function monitoring during adenosine myocardial perfusion scintigraphy in patients with chronic obstructive pulmonary disease. *Mayo Clin Proc* 1999;74:339–346.

(Vasodilator pharmacologic stress testing is safe in patients with chronic obstructive pulmonary disease [COPD] in the absence of bronchospasm. It is also safe in the presence of historic but medically controlled bronchospasm. It presents increased risks if performed in the presence of active bronchospasm. These authors examined pulmonary function in patients with COPD during adenosine infusion.)

159. Chikamori T, Doi YL, Yonezawa Y, et al. Value of dipyridamole thallium-201 imaging noninvasive differentiation of idiopathic dilated cardiomyopathy from coronary artery disease with left ventricular dysfunction. *Am J Cardiol* 1992;69:650–653.

(In this comparison of dipyridamole stress perfusion scintigraphic findings between 77 patients with coronary and 55 patients with noncoronary dilated cardiomyopathy, the absence of defects, the presence of small or multiple defects and lack of defect reversibility and less severe defects suggested a noncoronary etiology, whereas large, dense and reversible defects were more likely coronary related. However, limited reversible defects may yet be the marker for more extensive coronary artery disease [CAD] and extensive viable, but dysfunctional, "hibernating" myocardium. So, when we evaluate the perfusion pattern of a dilated and dysfunctional ventricle and find it most suggestive of a noncoronary cardiomyopathy, the pattern of relatively preserved uptake in a dilated ventricle, if actually associated with extensive CAD, may rarely indicate extensive viability in a ventricle with extensive "hibernation," which, in fact, needs revascularization. Alternatively, evidence of limited ischemia and associated CAD may be present in a cardiomyopathic ventricle with a noncoronary cause.)

160. Tauberg SG, Orie JE, Bartlett BE, et al. Usefulness of thallium-201 for distinction of ischemic from idiopathic dilated cardiomyopathy. *Am J Cardiol* 1993;71:674–680.

(The diagnostic image parameters for coronary artery disease [CAD] were studied in 51 patients undergoing coronary angiography for evaluation of a dilated cardiomyopathy, all with LVEF >35%. Multivariate analysis identified lung uptake, severe and large defects as the only independent predictors of CAD. Large defects had a 97% predictive value for CAD, whereas the absence of large defects was 94% predictive of nonischemic cardiomyopathy [see *154*].)

161. Ritchie JL, Bateman TM, Bonow RO, et al. Guidelines for clinical use of cardiac radionuclide imaging. Report of the American College of Cardiology/American Heart Association Task Force on Assessment of Diagnostic and Therapeutic Cardiovascular Procedures (Committee on Radionuclide Imaging), developed in collaboration with the American Society of Nuclear Cardiology. *J Am Coll Cardiol* 1995;25:521–547.

(Guidelines have been devised for the appropriate application of nuclear cardiology methods. These have expanded as data has accumulated, particularly in the area of outcomes research. However, these are only guidelines. The proper application must be determined by the clinician.)

162. Segall GM, Atwood JE, Botvinick EH, et al. Variability of normal coronary anatomy: implications for the interpretation of thallium SPECT myocardial perfusion images in single vessel disease. *J Nucl Med* 1995;36:944–951.

(The authors of this careful study correlated the location of stress-induced scintigraphic defects with angiographic anatomy in patients with single-vessel coronary disease. The findings reveal the spectrum of possible induced image abnormalities as a result of disease in a given distribution.)

163. Verani MS, Jeroudi MO, Mahmarian JJ, et al. Quantification of myocardial infarction during coronary occlusion and myocardial salvage after reperfusion using cardiac imaging with technetium-99m hexakis 2 methoxyisobutyl isonitrile. *J Am Coll Cardiol* 1988;12:1573–1581.

(The authors of this study demonstrated that the coronary anatomy correlates variably and poorly with the extent of myocardium at ischemic risk. They evaluated the risk area with technetium-99m [^{99m}Tc] sestamibi administration during coronary occlusion in dogs. With serial ^{99m}Tc sestamibi imaging, they localized and quantitated the infarct produced with permanent balloon coronary occlusion [n = 16], as well as the improvement with timely reperfusion after 2 hr of occlusion [n = 15]. The final SPECT defect size correlated well with the pathologic infarct size. In addition to the excellent correlation between triphenyltetrazolium-chloride–stained pathologic infarct size measured post mortem and SPECT defect size measured in vivo, specific patterns of defect distribution were related to the site of coronary occlusion. Improved perfusion with reduced defect size noted 48 hr after reperfusion correlated with measured regional flow, and localization of defect correlated well with known anatomy. The variable extent of the region at risk from vessel to vessel and with lesions at similar locations of the same vessel was demonstrated, graphically indicating the inability of anatomic angiography to determine this risk region. Myocardial perfusion scintigraphy permits reliable demonstration and localization of acute myocardial infarction, measurement of myocardial infarction size and quantification of salvaged myocardium. Clinical studies confirm these findings in patients [see *164*].)

164. Mahmarian JJ, Pratt CM, Boyce TM, et al. The variable extent of jeopardized myocardium in patients with single vessel coronary artery disease: quantification by thallium-201 single photon emission computed tomography. *J Am Coll Cardiol* 1991;17:355–362.

(SPECT myocardial perfusion scintigraphy [MPS] was performed and quantitated in 158 consecutive patients with single-vessel coronary artery disease. Patients with only a moderate stenosis tended to have only small defects, whereas defects measuring >10% of the left ventricle were generally related to a stenosis >70%. However, the correlation between stenosis severity and defect extent was only modest [r = 0.38]. Lesions of the left anterior descending coronary artery [LAD] generally related to the largest regional perfusion, and MPS defects and proximal LAD lesions yielded defects more than twice the size of proximal right coronary artery or left circumflex coronary artery lesions. However, there was marked heterogeneity in defect size among all vessels, regardless of lesion severity and even lesion location. Myocardium at ischemic risk could be roughly predicted only by anatomic parameters of lesion severity and location.)

165. McLaughlin PR, Martin RP, Doherty P, et al. Reproducibility of Tl-201 myocardial imaging. *Circulation* 1977;55:497–507.

166. Rehn T, Griffith LSC, Aschuff SC, et al. Exercise Tl-201 myocardial imaging in left main coronary artery disease: sensitive but not specific. *Am J Cardiol* 1981;48:217–226.

(165,166: The authors of these articles analyze the diagnostic sensitivity and specificity of planar perfusion scintigraphy for the diagnosis of specific coronary vessels.)

167. Alazraki NP, Krawczynska EG, DePuey EG, et al. Reproducibility of thallium-201 exercise SPECT studies. *J Nucl Med* 1994;35:8–14.

(In this in-depth evaluation of reproducibility, 16 of 20 patients studied serially with exercise thallium-201 perfusion imaging underwent reproducible stress testing. Fifteen of these 16 revealed identical image findings on serial study [94%], with an interobserver reproducibility of 95%.)

168. Maddahi J, Van Train K, Wong C, et al. Comparison of Tl-201 SPECT and planar imaging for evaluation of coronary artery disease. *J Nucl Med* 1986;27:999–1008.

(This and other articles suggest that SPECT presents a minor superiority compared with planar imaging, with the only clearly superior diagnostic sensitivity falling in the left circumflex distribution. Although this may be true in the hands of experts, several other facts suggest a greater SPECT advantage compared with the planar method. These include its lack of regional overlap and improved contrast resolution. The reduced concern regarding possible balanced ischemia, a normal image in the presence of generalized ischemia and the nearly total abandonment of washout analysis speak to the superiority of SPECT image sensitivity. In spite of its computer-reliant nature and the possibility of artifacts of motion and processing, the SPECT method has attracted many new enthusiasts to the field, who relate with increased comfort to image interpretation. The SPECT method, in fact, reduces evident attenuation artifact and displays and orients the full myocardial mass along the ventricular axes in each case. These are other features that add to its ease of interpretation and provide a reason that the method has yielded the highest achieved levels of diagnostic accuracy.)

169. Kiat H, Van Train KF, Maddahi J, et al. Development and prospective application of quantitative 2-day stress rest Tc-99m methoxy isobutyl isonitrile SPECT for the diagnosis of coronary artery disease. *Am Heart J* 1990;129:1255–1266.

170. Iskandrian AS, Heo J, Kong B, et al. Use of technetium-99m isonitrile in assessing left ventricular perfusion and function at rest and during exercise in coronary disease, and comparison with coronary angiography and exercise thallium-201 SPECT imaging. *Am J Cardiol* 1989;64:270–275.

(169,170: Four early studies [see references *108,112,140*] comparing exercise SPECT thallium-201 myocardial perfusion scintigraphy with SPECT technetium-99m [99mTc] sestamibi demonstrated increased sensitivity [83% versus 90%] and specificity [93% versus 80%] with SPECT 99mTc sestamibi. Such values are approached by no other method or modality.)

171. Multicenter Postinfarction Research Group. The combined evaluation of ventricular function and perfusion. Risk stratification and survival after myocardial infarction. *N Engl J Med* 1983;309:331–336.

(The role of physiologic measurements in predicting mortality after acute infarction was evaluated in 866 patients. Mortality progressively increased as left ventricular ejection fraction [LVEF] fell under 40% during the first postinfarction year. LVEF, frequent ventricular ectopy and evidence of heart failure were each independent predictors of mortality.)

172. Harris PJ, Harrell FE Jr, Lee KL, et al. Survival in medically treated coronary artery disease. *Circulation* 1979;60:1259–1269.

(The oft-cited Duke data base, demonstrating the exponential rise in postinfarction mortality, as left ventricular ejection fraction [LVEF] fell below 35%.

171,172: There is a strong relationship between LVEF and mortality in the postinfarction patient. The Duke data base and several longitudinal population studies demonstrated the direct curvilinear relationship between depression of the LVEF and survival, with an almost exponential curve describing a rapidly increasing death rate as LVEF falls below 35%.)

173. Berman DS, Germano G, Kiat H, Friedman J. Simultaneous perfusion/function imaging [editorial]. *J Nucl Cardiol* 1995;2:271–273.

(This editorial reviews the literature and laboratory experience of this prominent group with first-pass and gated sestamibi function evaluation. Gated and first-pass studies "increased our confidence in diagnosis and risk stratification and significantly augment the impact of myocardial perfusion SPECT." It is expected that quantitative wall motion, wall thickening and left ventricular ejection fraction will be a standard aspect of perfusion acquisition with technetium-99m–based radiotracers. They will add to diagnostic accuracy, prognostic value and viability evaluation. First-pass radionuclide angiography will be of added value when, after SPECT perfusion imaging, there is likely to be a persistent intermediate likelihood of coronary disease, an intermediate prognostic risk or insecurity in interpretation as a result of motion or attenuation.)

174. Cooke CD, Garcia EV, Cullom SJ, et al. Determining the accuracy of calculating systolic wall thickening using a fast Fourier transform approximation: a simulation study based on canine and patient data. *J Nucl Med* 1994;35:1185–1192.

(A method of calculating wall thickening from gated myocardial perfusion scintigraphy is presented.)

175. Benari B, Kiat H, Erel J, et al. Repeatability of treadmill exercise ejection fraction and wall motion using technetium-99m-labeled sestamibi first-pass radionuclide ventriculography. *J Nucl Cardiol* 1995;2:478–484.

(The reproducibility and repeatability of first-pass blood-pool imaging was determined in 27 patients undergoing treadmill stress perfusion imaging with first-pass evaluation, serially. There were excellent correlations between the 2 related left ventricular ejection fractions, both intraobserver [r = 0.92] and interobserver [r = 0.99]. Segmental visual score agreement for the 2 tests varied from 93% for the apical and distal inferior walls to 67% for the basal inferior wall. The method is highly reproducible and should be applicable to serial studies.)

176. Nichols K, Rozanski A, Salensky H, DePuey EG. Accuracy and reproducibility of automated tomographic ventricular function measurements [abstract]. *J Am Coll Cardiol* 1996;27:215A.

(Ventricular function evaluated from gated SPECT sestamibi images in 145 patients demonstrated great interobserver agreement, a <10% need to alter automated parameters and calculate a manual left ventricular ejection fraction [LVEF] and a strong correlation of automated LVEF and first-pass ejection fraction [r = 0.87].)

177. Klodas E, Rogers PJ, Sinak LJ, et al. Quantitation of ejection fractions using gated tomographic imaging with Tc-99m-sestamibi [abstract]. *J Am Coll Cardiol* 1996;27:215A.

(Gated SPECT sestamibi images can be analyzed to yield accurate regional ejection fractions that correlate well with regional wall motion by the same method and with the subjective assessment of echocardiography.)

178. Vacearino RA, Johnson LL, Antunes ML, et al. Thallium-201 lung uptake and peak treadmill exercise first-pass ejection fraction. *Am Heart J* 1995;129:320–329.

(The authors studied 70 consecutive patients with similar angiographic anatomy with exercise stress thallium-201 perfusion and technetium-99m [99mTc] sestamibi imaging. Demonstrated was the incremental diagnostic value of first-pass ejection fraction acquired during dynamic exercise with 99mTc sestamibi.)

179. Chua CT, Germano G, Maurer G, et al. Gated Tc-99m sestamibi for simultaneous assessment of stress myocardial perfusion, postexercise regional ventricular function and myocardial viability. Correlation with echocardiography and rest Tl-201 scintigraphy. *J Am Coll Cardiol* 1994;23:1107–1114.

(The authors support the hypothesis that wall motion on gated poststress sestamibi images predicts viability and reversibility. Thus, there may be no need for rest or redistribution images to determine viability, because viability may be discerned from perfusion-related function. However, function or apparent function evaluation is imperfect and is influenced by other factors. Function may not be evaluated well in the presence of dense defects, although such evaluation is performed objectively, and, generally, wall motion is seen even in the presence of many dense perfusion defects.)

180. Faber TL, Cooke CD, Folks RD, et al. An integrated processing program for analysis of left ventricular ejection function and perfusion. *Comput Cardiol* 1997;24:697–700.

(Faber et al. validated this method in 80 patients studied with first-pass technique [r = .82; SEE = 8.5%]. Further, these same workers demonstrated the relative reproducibility of the left ventricular ejection fraction [LVEF] by this method and the stability of the calculation with varying assumed wall thickness, where the assumption of a 1.5-cm end-diastolic wall thickness brought only a 6% [relative] error in calculated LVEF.)

181. Faber TL, Cooke CD, Peifer JW, et al. Three-dimensional displays of the left ventricular epicardial surface from standard single photon computed tomographic (SPECT) perfusion quantification techniques. *J Nucl Med* 1995;36:697–703.

(The method also has been well correlated with left ventricular volumes and mass calculated from gated MRI studies.)

182. Tadamura E, Kudoh T, Matooka M, et al. Assessment of regional and global left ventricular function by reinjection Tl-201 and rest Tc-99m sestamibi ECG-gated SPECT. *Am J Cardiol* 1999;33:991–997.

(Gated thallium-201 reinjection and stress sestamibi gated SPECT were applied to the calculation of left ventricular ejection fraction, end-diastolic and end-systolic volumes, regional wall thickening and wall motion and compared with these same parameters calculated from 3-dimensional MRI in 20 patients with coronary artery disease. The agreement was excellent and, with perfusion data, promises improved diagnostic and prognostic accuracy without an increase in cost or radiation exposure.)

183. Bateman TM, Magalski A, Barnhart C, et al. Global left ventricular function assessment using gated SPECT-201: comparison with echocardiography [abstract]. *J Am Coll Cardiol* 1998;31:441A

(Left ventricular ejection fraction [LVEF], end-diastolic and end-systolic volumes were calculated from gated sestamibi studies. They compared well, over a broad range of normal and abnormal, with these same measures on echocardiography. Quantitative volumes may be determined for the rest thallium-201 [^{201}Tl] study and the technetium-99m stress study of the dual-isotope protocol. In the analysis of 783 consecutive studies, gated ^{201}Tl EF at rest and stress were compared. Approximately 3.5% of studies demonstrated a fall of LVEF $\geq 10\%$. This finding was correlated with a 33% incidence of lung uptake, 89% incidence of cavitary dilation and a 40% incidence of multivessel coronary disease.)

184. Nichols K, DePuey EG, Rozanski A. Automation of gated tomographic left ventricular ejection fraction. *J Nucl Med* 1996;36:475–482.

185. Germano G, Kavanagh PB, Su HT, et al. Automatic reorientation of 3-dimensional transaxial myocardial perfusion SPECT images. *J Nucl Med* 1995;36:1107–1114.

186. Germano G, Kiat H, Kavanagh PB, et al. Automatic quantification of ejection fraction from gated myocardial perfusion single photon emission computed tomography (SPECT). *J Nucl Med* 1995;36:2138–2147.

(180–186: These are a few of the articles that helped establish the automated calculation of left ventricular ejection fraction from gated SPECT myocardial perfusion scintigraphy.)

187. Smith WH, Kastner RJ, Calnon DA, et al. Quantitative gated single photon emission computed tomography imaging: a counts-based method for display and measurement of regional and global ventricular systolic function. *Nucl Cardiol* 1997;4:451–463.

188. Calnon DA, Kastner RJ, Smith WH, et al. Validation of a new counts-based gated single photon emission computed tomography method for quantifying left ventricular systolic function: comparison with equilibrium radionuclide angiography. *J Nucl Cardiol* 1997;4:464–471.

(187,188: The authors of these articles demonstrate the methodology and accuracy of gated SPECT myocardial perfusion scintigraphy for the evaluation of systolic left ventricular function.)

189. Williams KA, Taillon LA. Gated planar technetium-99m labeled sestamibi myocardial perfusion image inversion for quantitative scintigraphic assessment of left ventricular function. *J Nucl Cardiol* 1995;2:285–295.

(Here, planar images are presented as white-on-black displays, and the intensity of "cavitary activity" is measured in diastolic and systolic frames of the gated planar images and equated to cavitary volume. In vivo and patient studies demonstrated the value of the image inversion method and its high correlation with left ventricular ejection fraction [LVEF] calculated by established methods. Although the LVEF calculated from gated planar perfusion images may correlate with other methods, this is likely a fortuitous effect of related physical factors and does not relate to actual measures of ventricular cavity size or prognostic measures reliably related to it. Although gating may be applied to planar studies, the intensity of the overlying wall likely influences apparent cavitary size more than does ventricular function. The LVEF calculated from gated planar images has been shown to correlate with other methods. In this study, intensities were inverted and the low-intensity central region of the planar perfusion image was given an inversely high intensity. This was then taken as the cavity [it is, in fact the overlying myocardial wall] and analyzed as the blood pool, where counts [intensity] are proportional to volume. In fact, these intensities bear no relation to volume and there is no counts marker here. Nonetheless, the method results in an LVEF calculation that correlates with proven methods. Dilated ventricles with thin and often poorly perfused walls will demonstrate high counts and volumes in the display of inverse intensities. The thin overlying wall will change little in systole, giving the impression of a low LVEF. The relationship should deteriorate when intensity characteristics of the blood pool do not correlate with those of the overlying myocardium. This could occur when viewing a large, poorly contracting cavity in a scarred cardiomyopathic ventricle, through a normally perfused and contracting wall in the presence of segmental coronary disease. The converse, viewing the cavity through a limited scar in a ventricle with a normal volume and minor reduction in LVEF, would also bring disagreement and error.)

190. Johnson LL, Verdesca SA, Aude WY, et al. Postischemic stunning can affect left ventricular ejection fraction and regional wall motion on post-stress gated sestamibi tomograms. *J Am Coll Cardiol* 1997;30:1641–1648.

    (Left ventricular ejection fraction [LVEF] was calculated from rest gated sestamibi studies acquired in 81 sequential patients who were noted to have a defect on the initial gated stress study imaged with a 2-day stress–rest sestamibi protocol. LVEF was >5% less than that seen at rest in 22 [36%] patients, suggesting poststress stunning in these cases.)

191. Bateman TM, Case JA, Cullom SJ, et al. Myocardial stunning detected by exercise gated SPECT Tl-201: a new scintigraphic marker of severe extensive coronary artery disease [abstract]. *J Am Coll Cardiol* 1998;31:441A.

    (In the analysis of 783 consecutive studies, gated thallium-201 ejection fraction at rest and stress were compared. Approximately 3.5% of studies demonstrated a fall of left ventricular ejection fraction ≥10%. This evidence of stunning late after the intervention suggests a more advanced level of ischemic disease. This finding was correlated with a 33% incidence of lung uptake, 89% incidence of cavitary dilation and a 40% incidence of multivessel coronary disease. Interesting was the fact that it was seen as often in association with coronary dilator as with exercise stress.)

192. Bateman TM, Case JA, Moutray KL, et al. Is there clinical value in measuring LVEF both post-stress and at rest during ECG-gated myocardial perfusion SPECT scintigraphy [abstract]. *J Am Coll Cardiol* 1999;33:482A.

    (The summed segmental difference score [SDS] calculated from a 20-segment model and representing a measure of myocardium at ischemic risk [MIR] was related to the presence and degree of reduced left ventricular ejection fraction [LVEF] when poststress LVEF was compared with that at rest. Both the exercise- and adenosine-related falls in LVEF correlated with the presence of an SDS ≥ 8, the limit of a large perfusion defect. The relationship with the adenosine-related fall in LVEF was surprising. This may be more apparent than real and relate to subendocardial ischemia and evident cavitary dilation. Nevertheless, the fall in LVEF appears related to MIR.)

193. DePuey EG, Parmett S, Ghesani M, et al. Comparison of Tc-99m sestamibi and Tl-201 gated perfusion SPECT. *J Nucl Cardiol* 1993;3:278–285.

(The authors demonstrate the weakness of thallium-201 (^{201}Tl) for gated images. Reduced data density in each image frame brings poor image quality and related interobserver variability, reduced reproducibility and accuracy of the evaluation of left ventricular function with gated ^{201}Tl images.)

194. Sciagraa R, Bisi G, Santoro GM, et al. Evaluation of coronary artery disease using technetium-99m sestamibi first-pass and perfusion imaging with dipyridamole infusion. *J Nucl Med* 1994;35:1254–1264.

(The authors studied the contribution of first-pass stress left ventricular ejection fraction to coronary artery disease [CAD] diagnosis. Both perfusion and quantitative first-pass imaging were accurate for CAD detection, but perfusion imaging was more sensitive. Although 17 patients had previous infarctions, the analysis was performed in regions outside any infarct perfusion zone and so was a pure study of induced ventricular dysfunction.)

195. Iskandrian AE, Kegel JG, Tecce MA, et al. Simultaneous assessment of left ventricular perfusion and function with technetium-99m sestamibi after coronary artery bypass grafting. *Am Heart J* 1993;126:1199–1203.

(Gating has been applied to the evaluation of the results of coronary artery bypass graft. Abnormal perfusion images were not uncommonly detected in the presence of normal left ventricular function and ejection fraction. Yet, the combination of perfusion and function, here as elsewhere, promises augmented clinical value.)

196. Borges-Neto S, Shaw LJ, Kesler KL, et al. Prediction of severe coronary artery disease with Tc-99m sestamibi perfusion and function studies: a comparison with clinical history, physical examination, and electrocardiographic data [abstract]. *J Am Coll Cardiol* 1996;27:101A.

(Simultaneous perfusion and first-pass function studies were acquired with stress technetium-99m sestamibi in 54 patients with severe, multivessel coronary disease. The composite perfusion and function evaluation improved prediction of the extent of coronary disease beyond history, electrocardiographic findings and even perfusion image information alone.)

197. Borges-Neto S, Shaw LK, Ravizinni GC, et al. Prediction of death and MI by perfusion and function assessment after revascularization: does perfusion imaging add prognostic information to ejection fraction [abstract]? *Circulation* 1999;100:I-584.

(Although the left ventricular ejection fraction was the best predictor of cardiac death after revascularization procedures, perfusion image findings were found to add to those of left ventricular function as a predictor of cardiac death or nonfatal infarction in 489 patients studied serially.)

198. Palmas W, Friedman JD, Diamond GA, et al. Incremental value of simultaneous assessment of myocardial function and perfusion with technetium-99m sestamibi for prediction of extent of coronary artery disease. *J Am Coll Cardiol* 1995;25:1024–1031.

(In this study of 70 consecutive patients, the addition of simultaneous SPECT perfusion imaging and first-pass evaluation of systolic left ventricular function to results of the treadmill exercise test added significantly to the ability to diagnose the presence and predict the extent of coronary disease. Receiver operating characteristic curve analysis demonstrated the relationship between risk in coronary disease and defect size. The relationship was made stronger when the effects of ejection fraction were included.)

199. Nicolson CS, Tatum JL, Jesse RL, et al. The value of gated tomographic Tc-99m sestamibi perfusion imaging in acute ischemic syndromes. *J Nucl Cardiol* 1995;2: S57–S62.

(Here abnormalities based in attenuation demonstrate normal wall motion, and regional reduction in systolic function is well seen. This permits the most specific identification of patients with acute ischemic syndromes presenting with ambiguous symptoms.

Nicolson et al. previously demonstrated the advantages of gated SPECT sestamibi for emergency department triage of patients presenting with chest pain. Compared with ungated studies, gated SPECT sestamibi improved specificity from 69% to 97% and increased the positive predictive value from 38% to 97% among 102 patients evaluated for possible acute myocardial infarction.)

200. Keng FYJ, Chandwaney RM, Mahmarian JJ, et al. Accuracy of gated SPECT imaging in diagnosing individual coronary artery stenosis: a comparison between ungated, gated end-systolic and gated end-diastolic images [abstract]. *J Am Coll Cardiol* 1999;33:409A.

(Gated stress myocardial perfusion scintigraphy was performed in 63 patients and compared with coronary angiography. Although added data regarding regional wall motion improved sensitivity, it reduced specificity and brought no change in overall accuracy.)

201. Sharir T, Lewin HC, Germano G, et al. Automatic quantitation of wall motion and thickening by gated SPECT: validation and application in identifying severe coronary artery disease [abstract]. *J Am Coll Cardiol* 1999;33:418A.

(In a group of coronary patients studied by gated SPECT, regional wall motion and thickening were more sensitive to severe coronary artery disease lesions than was the perfusion score. However, the perfusion score was more specific.)

202. Hachamovitch R, Berman D, Lewin H, et al. Incremental prognostic value of gated SPECT ejection fraction in patients undergoing dual-isotope exercise or adenosine stress SPECT [abstract]. *J Am Coll Cardiol* 1998;31:441A.

(Among 1032 consecutive patients studied by the dual-isotope protocol, those 130 with early revascularization were excluded. The remainder were followed for a mean of 1.7 yr. Gated SPECT added incremental prognostic value and permitted substratification of patients already well stratified on the basis of perfusion defects. Here, those with abnormal scans were stratified by left ventricular ejection fraction [LVEF] >50% to an event rate of 2.0%/yr and by LVEF <50% to an event rate of 5.8%/yr.)

203. Lewin HC, Thompson T, Shaw L, et al. The prognostic impact of ischemia as a function of ejection fraction on gated myocardial perfusion SPECT [abstract]. *J Am Coll Cardiol* 1999;33:469A.

(The authors studied outcomes among 2298 consecutive patients with poststress gated myocardial perfusion scintigraphy. Events included revascularization, and only stress defect score [SDS], not reversibility score or any viability index, was evaluated. With this analysis, event rate was uniformly high among those with left ventricular ejection fraction [LVEF] <35%, whereas events varied directly with SDS for those with LVEF >35%. Consideration of defect reversibility, the relative and cumulative size of fixed and reversible defects, as well as an index of viability, may better risk stratify patients with lower LVEF. This has already been done in some studies of viability, in which all patients studied had low LVEF [measured by another method] and were well risk stratified.)

204. Sharir T, Germano G, Kavanagh PB, et al. Incremental prognostic value of poststress ventricular volume by gated myocardial SPECT for the prediction of cardiac death [abstract]. *J Nucl Med* 1999;40:2P.

(The poststress end-systolic volume [ESV] had independent prognostic value and could substratify the risk related to perfusion image defects. An ESV <70 cc reduced the risk related to a markedly abnormal perfusion image, and an ESV >70 cc increased the risk related to mild-to-moderate defects.)

205. Nallamothu N, Araujo L, Russell J, et al. Prognostic value of simultaneous perfusion and function assessment using technetium-99m sestamibi. *Am J Cardiol* 1996;78: 562–564.

(The exercise perfusion pattern was a stronger predictor of outcomes, here primarily nonfatal infarction, than was the evaluation of left ventricular ejection fraction. Perhaps this related in part to the end point and the nature of the patient population.)

206. Sharir T, Germano G, Kavanagh PB, et al. Incremental prognostic value of post-stress left ventricular ejection fraction and volume by gated myocardial perfusion single photon emission computed tomography. *Circulation* 1999;100:1035–1042.

(A total of 1680 consecutive patients were studied with myocardial perfusion scintigraphy and the gated rest thallium-201 and stress technetium-99m sestamibi protocol and were followed for approximately 2 yr. Left ventricular ejection fraction [LVEF] <45%, end-systolic volume [ESV] >70 ml and end-diastolic volume >120 ml were established as optimal thresholds for the prediction of cardiac death. Death rates were related to these functional parameters and related perfusion defects. Patients with LVEF ≥45% or ESV <70 ml had mortality rates <1.2%/yr, even with severe perfusion defects, whereas those with LVEF <45% or ESV ≥70 ml had high mortality, even with mild-to-moderate defects. Multivariate Cox proportional hazards regression showed that perfusion defect characteristics and ESV were independent predictors of overall coronary events, whereas EDV and LVEF provided incremental prognostic value beyond perfusion data in predicting death or infarction.)

207. DePuey EG, Rozanski A. Using gated technetium-99m sestamibi single photon emission computed tomography (SPECT) to characterize fixed myocardial defects as infarct or artifact. *J Nucl Med* 1995;36:952–955.

(Gated sestamibi images and related regional systolic function were shown in these studies to be valuable for differentiating fixed defects related to infarction from those resulting from attenuation. Fixed image defects are most likely related to attenuation artifact rather than perfusion abnormalities. Application of this principle to a large group of clinical studies dramatically reduced the incidence of false-positive studies.)

208. Croon CD, Atsma DE, Dibbets P, et al. Gated SPECT myocardial imaging improves test accuracy in patients with persistent perfusion defects [abstract]. *J Nucl Med* 1999;40:163P.

(In 55 patients with documented prior infarction and 20 with none, wall motion and thickening on gated SPECT tetrofosmin myocardial perfusion scintigraphy permits the identification of regional viability in segments with severe fixed defects. Also, gated SPECT can detect ischemic or nonischemic cardiomyopathy by the finding of dysfunctional but perfused myocardium. Care must be applied, however, because regions of limited infarction may also show evidence of motion. The technique is best used as a tool to support the likelihood of attenuation integrated into the full analytic interpretive exercise.)

209. Smanio PE, Watson DD, Segalia DL, et al. Value of gating of technetium-99m sestamibi single photon emission computed tomographic imaging. *J Am Coll Cardiol* 1997;30:1687–1692.

(Electrocardiographic gating added to the diagnostic security of the interpretation of ungated SPECT images in 285 patients, generally moving toward normal studies in patients with low pretest likelihood and toward abnormal in patients with high pretest likelihood of coronary disease.)

210. Alderman EL, Bourassa MG, Cohen LS, et al. Ten-year follow-up of survival and myocardial infarction in the randomized Coronary Artery Surgery Study. *Circulation* 1990;82:1629–1646.

(Although studies generally indicate an advantage to surgical revascularization in the setting of multivessel [3-vessel] coronary involvement or a reduced left ventricular ejection fraction, the 7-yr follow-up of the Coronary Artery Surgery Study demonstrated an increased survival with surgical compared with medical treatment in patients with severe induced ischemia as indicated by >2 mm of horizontal ST depression, regardless of the baseline ejection fraction or the number of vessels involved. Again, the prognostic and therapeutic importance of induced ischemia is illustrated.)

211. Pollock SG, Abbott RD, Boucher CA, et al. Independent and incremental prognostic value of tests performed in hierarchical order to evaluate patients with suspected coronary artery disease. Validation of models based on these tests. *Circulation* 1992;85:237–248.

(The authors apply global χ^2 to analyze and demonstrate the independent prognostic value of image findings in thallium-201 [^{201}Tl] perfusion scintigraphy [excluding lung uptake], which were statistically and meaningfully superior to clinical variables, stress test variables and equal to that offered by coronary angiography. However, in this study, the prognostic values of perfusion imaging and angiographic variables were additive. Interesting was the further large incremental and independent prognostic value of lung uptake. Although perfusion-related variables appear to be preserved with technetium-99m [^{99m}Tc]-based agents, lung uptake seems to occur less frequently.

This study demonstrated the prognostic value of perfusion scintigraphy, and particularly the presence of lung uptake, among all clinical and stress test variables. The finding relates to a prolonged pulmonary transit of the radiotracer with increased extraction. With coronary disease, this finding suggests extensive severe disease. Lung uptake should not be confused with uptake in pectoral muscles and soft tissues of the chest wall. The latter increases in intensity in the rest or redistribution image; the former [true lung uptake] demonstrates vigorous washout on delayed imaging. Lung uptake is not as prominent with pharmacologic stress, nor as evident with ^{99m}Tc sestamibi imaging, as on imaging with ^{201}Tl.)

212. Weiss AT, Berman DS, Lew AS, et al. Transient ischemic dilation of the left ventricle on stress thallium-201 scintigraphy: a marker of severe and extensive coronary artery disease. *J Am Coll Cardiol* 1987;9:752–760.

213. Stolzenberg J. Dilation of the left ventricular cavity on stress thallium scan as an indicator of ischemic disease. *Clin Nucl Med* 1980;5:289–296.

(212,213: These authors examine the frequency and clinical implications of cavitary dilation with stress perfusion imaging. Although secondary dilation is generally a sign of widespread ischemia, dilation may be localized to regions of segmental ischemia. Sometimes, dilation may be more apparent than real, relating to the effects of reduced regional function or to imaging through overlying areas of reduced perfusion or on planar imaging. Similarly, cavitary photopenia may be induced with stress and relate to either overlying underperfused or dysfunctional myocardium [see reference 8].)

214. Iskandrian AS, Hakki AH, Segal BL. Assessment of jeopardized myocardium in patients with multivessel disease. *Am Heart J* 1983;106:1089–1096.

(The ability to identify the extent of vascular involvement and myocardium at ischemic risk is evaluated in this early article.)

215. Iskandrian AS, Chae SC, Heo J, et al. Independent and incremental prognostic value of exercise single-photon emission computed tomographic (SPECT) thallium imaging in coronary disease. *J Am Coll Cardiol* 1993;22:665–670.

(The authors followed 316 patients with angiographically documented coronary disease for a mean of 28 mo and demonstrated the incremental prognostic value of the perfusion scintigram beyond that of the angiogram! The size of the perfusion defect was the best prognostic indicator, and an abnormality ≥15% of the left ventricle was related to a poor outcome, compared with normal or even mildly abnormal scans.)

216. Mahmarian JJ, Pratt CM, Nishimura S, et al. Quantitative adenosine Tl-201 single-photon emission computed tomography for the early assessment of patients surviving acute myocardial infarction. *Circulation* 1993;87:1197–1210.

(Mahmarian et al. have suggested that adenosine thallium SPECT is as effective as exercise myocardial perfusion scintigraphy in stratifying patients in both the early period after myocardial infarction and in the long term. The size of the perfusion defect was highly predictive of mortality early after the event in this study applying SPECT thallium-201 to quantitate infarct size in 146 patients [approximately half with thrombolysis], 2–5 days after infarction. Here, infarct size >20% was related to a worse prognosis. More important, the left ventricular ejection fraction could be integrated with the size of related reversible defect to yield a strong graded index of risk. Enzyme values correlated poorly with image infarct size and prognosis.)

217. Miller TD, Christian TF, Hopfenspirger MR, et al. Infarct size after acute myocardial infarction measured by quantitative tomographic 99m-Tc sestamibi imaging predicts subsequent mortality. *Circulation* 1995;92:334–341.

(Studied with SPECT technetium-99m sestamibi at the time of admission and again at discharge were 274 patients with acute myocardial infarction who underwent reperfusion therapy. Mortality was directly related to the size of infarction, measured scintigraphically with sestamibi. Here, infarctions <12% of left ventricular size had a low related event rate, whereas infarct size >12% related to a 7% rate of death and nonfatal infarction over the first postinfarct year.

Each of these articles demonstrates the unpredictable difference between the amount of myocardium infarcted or at risk compared with the related coronary anatomy. This fact is probably a large part of the explanation for the excellent prognostic value of perfusion scintigraphic study and a good reason to support quantification of image parameters.)

218. Morise AP, Diamond GA, Detrano R, Bobbio M. Incremental value of exercise electrocardiography and thallium-201 testing in men and women for the presence and extent of coronary disease. *Am Heart J* 1995;130:267–276.

(Data from 1 center were used to develop incremental logic algorithms, which were then applied to 865 patients studied with stress perfusion scintigraphy and coronary angiography at 4 other centers. There was a significant increment in accuracy related to exercise testing and imaging for both the presence and extent of coronary disease, which were similar in men and women.)

219. Botvinick EH, O'Connell JW, Dae MW, et al. Analysis of thallium-201 "washout" from parametric color-coded images. *J Nucl Med* 1988;29:302–311.

(Botvinick et al. analyzed regional planar washout using parametric imaging to identify regional washout and, with it, gain insight into the meaning and content of the ventricular cavity and cavitary dilation. They developed software to superimpose postexercise and delayed thallium-201 [201Tl] images and calculate the regional washout. A functional image was generated with color-coded washout, pixel by pixel. It was noted that the region of the "cavity" shared normal washout rates with the parenchyma in normals, and cavitary washout was often divided into high and low values related to the characteristics of adjacent myocardial perfusion in regions subtended by the coronary vessels. This suggested that cavitary activity was related to that of the overlying myocardium and had broad implications for the interpretation of characteristics of the "cavity," including its origin, size and activity.

The presence of regional systolic dysfunction, with reduced systolic inward motion and thickening, can alone translate into apparent perfusion defects and cavitary photopenia on the basis of a partial volume effect and is likely the most common cause of such findings. In fact, the full effects of this factor on perfusion image findings, whether defects are perceived as fixed or reversible, and the subsequent impact on viability evaluation, have been little studied [see reference *246*].

Strauss et al. have evaluated the relationship between regional perfusion and 201Tl distribution [Strauss HW, Harrison K, Langan JK, et al. Relationship of thallium-201 to regional myocardial perfusion. *Circulation* 1975;51:641–650]. In an associated study, they demonstrated the effects of dilation and abnormal wall motion on apparent regional perfusion in an animal model. Here, aortic obstruction brought left ventricular dysfunction and dilation and the appearance of new perfusion defects related to ^{201}Tl, which had been injected before the intervention. Microspheres, injected after the aortic obstruction and sampled with ^{201}Tl after the animals were killed, demonstrated a continued homogeneous pattern of perfusion distribution, in spite of the apparent postobstruction ^{201}Tl image abnormalities.

Of course, in the presence of coronary disease, reduced perfusion accompanies reduced function. Here, as a result of severely reduced radioactivity or reduced motion with preserved activity, the involved myocardium overlying the cavity does little to obscure it and, instead, presents a window to it in specific planar projections or individual SPECT slices of the underlying myocardium. Thus, there is less "contamination" of the underlying planar and SPECT "cavity," presenting the appearance of dilation or photopenia.)

220. Maddahi J, Abdulla A, Garcia E, et al. Noninvasive identification of left main and triple-vessel coronary artery disease: improved accuracy using quantitative analysis of regional myocardial stress distribution and washout of Tl-201. *J Am Coll Cardiol* 1986;7:53–62.

(Here, the ability of the scintigraphic method is enhanced with quantitative analysis of uptake and washout.)

221. Pollock SG, Abbott RD, Boucher CA, et al. A model to predict multivessel coronary artery disease from the exercise thallium-201 stress test. *Am J Med* 1991;90: 345–352.

(Sixty-four percent of patients misclassified by visual analysis as having less extensive disease were correctly classified as having extensive disease by virtue of quantitative analysis of regional myocardial thallium-201 [^{201}Tl] washout. When the results of quantitative ^{201}Tl analysis were combined with those of blood pressure and electrocardiographic response to exercise, the sensitivity and specificity for identification of patients with left main and 3-main coronary disease were 86% and 76%, respectively, and the highest overall accuracy [82%] was obtained.)

222. Krishnan R, Lu J, Dae MW, Botvinick EH. Does myocardial perfusion scintigraphy demonstrate clinical utility in patients with markedly positive exercise tests? An assessment of the method in a high-risk subset. *Am Heart J* 1993;127:804–815.

(This article asked the question, "What value is stress perfusion scintigraphy in the setting of a 'markedly positive' exercise test?" For diagnostic purposes, in the presence of known disease or a high pretest likelihood, the image adds little and most such patients presenting with such stress tests go directly to angiography, without scintigraphy. However, if the pretest likelihood is not high, there is a spectrum of related disease from absent to high risk. Scintigraphy is applied usefully in such cases to risk stratify the group and base further evaluation on scintigraphic findings, which correlate well with the spectrum of anatomy in these cases.)

223. Kang X, Berman DS, Kimchi EY, et al. Prognostic value of a normal myocardial perfusion SPECT in patients undergoing coronary angiography. *J Am Coll Cardiol* 1998;31:409A.

(A unique and definitive study demonstrated the high predictive value of negative stress myocardial perfusion scintigraphy [MPS] in patients with and without coronary artery disease. It puts an end to the concern that a normal stress MPS may represent widespread and balanced ischemia.)

224. He ZX, Dakik HA, Vaduganathan P, et al. Clinical and angiographic significance of a normal thallium-201 tomographic study in patients with a strongly positive exercise electrocardiogram. *Am J Cardiol* 1996;78:638–641.

(Out of a total group of 23,059 patients undergoing exercise testing, the authors reviewed the available angiographic findings among all 817 [3.5%] patients with deep induced ST depressions on exercise electrocardiograph [ECG] and normal myocardial perfusion scintigraphy. Angiograms were performed in 52 patients with normal or near normal baseline ECGs. Only 32 had coronary artery disease, 16 [50%] with single-vessel disease, 56% with modest severity [<75% occlusion] and only 9% with subtotal or total occlusions.)

225.   Christian TF, Miller TD, Bailey KR, Gibbons RJ. The incremental value of exercise tomographic thallium-201 imaging for the detection of severe coronary artery disease in patients with normal electrocardiograms at rest. *Ann Int Med* 1994;121:825–832.

226.   Christian TF, Miller TD, Bailey KR, Gibbons RJ. Noninvasive identification of severe coronary artery disease using exercise tomographic thallium-201 imaging. *Am J Cardiol* 1992;70:14–20.

     (The ability of exercise thallium-201 [^{201}Tl] myocardial perfusion scintigraphy [MPS] to identify the presence of left main or 3-vessel coronary artery disease [CAD] was studied in 688 patients, 198 with extensive disease. Although many more were abnormal, roughly 30% of those with 3-vessel or left main CAD had involvement of these regions and could be identified as such on MPS analysis. This level of identification may relate in part to the presence of collaterals, the level of coronary flow demands and other factors. Clinical, stress test and image parameters related to left main or 3-vessel disease include: the magnitude of ST depression; the number of abnormal ^{201}Tl segments, diabetes and level of blood pressure augmentation. Clinical and exercise parameters and the presence of nonperfusion indicators will further aid identification of these anatomic subsets, as probably will the application of coronary dilator pharmacologic stress MPS. However, more important than the anatomic correlation is the relation of image findings to prognosis. The prognostic value of stress MPS is unmatched.

     225,226: The added diagnostic value of stress MPS for the identification of multivessel CAD is examined in these articles.)

227.   Patterson RE, Horowitz SF, Eng C, et al. Can noninvasive exercise test criteria identify patients with left main or 3-vessel coronary disease after a first myocardial infarction? *Am J Cardiol* 1983;51:361–370.

     (This is 1 of several analytic presentations by Patterson et al. Here, the authors analyze the ability of stress testing to identify high-risk coronary disease post-infarction. Cost-effectiveness issues are considered.)

228.   Sklar J, Kirch D, Johnson T, et al. Slow late myocardial clearance of thallium: a characteristic phenomenon in coronary artery disease. *Circulation* 1982;65:1504–1510.

     (Slow myocardial clearance is a finding that often indicates induced regional ischemia. However, factors related to the form and vigor of related stress strongly influence the findings. It has been most valuable when applied to exercise imaging and less so in association with pharmacologic stress.)

229.   Maddahi J, Van Train K, Don Michael TA, et al. Normal initial myocardial distribution and washout of Tl-201 at rest versus exercise. *Clin Nucl Med* 1985;10:11–18.

     (Washout values after a rest injection or with pharmacologic stress are relatively low compared with exercise-related values.)

230.   Bateman TM, Maddahi J, Gray RJ, et al. Diffuse slow washout of myocardial thallium-201: a new scintigraphic indicator of extensive coronary artery disease. *J Am Coll Cardiol* 1984;4:55–63.

     (The authors demonstrated that among 1265 consecutive patients with quantitatively analyzed planar stress–redistribution thallium-201 [^{201}Tl] scintigrams, 13 [1%] had the pattern of diffuse slow ^{201}Tl washout in the absence of a regional perfusion defect. Diffuse slow washout was defined as the presence of washout abnormalities in the distribution of all 3 major coronary arteries but not uniformly in all. Of these 13 patients, 9 [69%] were found to have left main or 3-vessel coronary disease. This incidence appears smaller yet with SPECT acquisition and relates to a very low negative predictive value. Diffuse slow washout was a rare indicator of extensive ischemia and related coronary disease in the absence of planar image defects. Because of the even greater infrequency of such findings, washout analysis is not recommended with ^{201}Tl SPECT. If one wishes to perform washout analysis, images acquired before reinjection must be analyzed.)

231. Teragawa H, Yamagata T, Kato M, et al. Assessment of the severity of coronary artery stenosis by the ratio of the regional washout rate determined by adenosine triphosphate stress Tl-201 SPECT. *J Nucl Cardiol* 1999;6:324–331.

(Teragawa et al. have demonstrated the value of regional thallium-201 washout on SPECT short-axis slices to determine the severity of coronary stenoses. In 31 patients with documented single-vessel coronary artery disease, the level of myocardial uptake on adenosine triphosphate pharmacologic stress testing was inversely related to the percentage of coronary artery stenosis.)

232. Williams KA, Schneider CM. Increased stress right ventricular activity on dual isotope perfusion SPECT. *J Am Coll Cardiol* 1999;34:420–427.

(A relative stress-induced increase in right ventricular perfusion [maximum right ventricular compared with maximum left ventricular activity] was found to be an accurate indicator of extensive coronary artery disease affecting the left ventricle. The authors do not indicate the incremental value of this sign [which must be computer analyzed] compared with better established methods, nor its relation to varying background.)

233. Bingham JB, McKusick KA, Strauss HW, et al. Influence of coronary artery disease on pulmonary uptake of Tl-201. *Am J Cardiol* 1980;46:821–828.

234. Gibson RS, Watson DD, Carabello BA, et al. Clinical implications of increased lung uptake of Tl-201 during exercise scintigraphy 2 weeks after myocardial infarction. *Am J Cardiol* 1982;49:1586–1593.

(233,234: Reviewed are the presumed etiology and clinical relevance of pulmonary uptake. These are also discussed in reference 8.)

235. Kushner FG, Okada RD, Kirschenbaum HD, et al. Lung Tl-201 uptake after stress testing in patients with coronary artery disease. *Circulation* 1981;63:341–348.

(Here, an attempt at standardization is made as pulmonary uptake in the left lung is related to the intensity of uptake in the adjacent anterior left ventricular wall in the anterior planar projection. This is still the method of choice, in cases in which the normal heart/lung ratio is ~<1.4. Of course, this depends on normal uptake in the anterior wall. Because all values are background corrected before calculation, background levels and background correction can bring variability and error. Pulmonary washout also can be assessed [see references 8 and 236]).

236. Levy R, Rozanski A, Berman DS, et al. Analysis of the degree of pulmonary thallium washout after exercise in patients with coronary artery disease. *J Am Coll Cardiol* 1983;2:719–726.

(Here, abnormal pulmonary thallium-201 washout was related to both the anatomic extent and functional severity of disease. Lung uptake was seen with greater frequency in patients with multivessel coronary disease and those with exercise-induced left ventricular dysfunction. Rapid washout is evident in abnormal pulmonary uptake but not in regions of normal thoracic uptake and serves to differentiate the 2.)

237. Marcassa C, Galli M, Baroffio C, Giannuzzi P. Prognostic value of resting thallium-201 lung uptake in patients with severe post-ischemic LV dysfunction [abstract]. *J Am Coll Cardiol* 1999;33:468A.

(In 74 consecutive patients with coronary artery disease and severe left ventricular dysfunction undergoing rest–redistribution thallium-201 myocardial perfusion scintigraphy, rest lung uptake was found to be a powerful predictor of adverse outcome.)

238. Krawczynska EG, Weintraub WS, Garcia EV, et al. Left ventricular dilatation and multivessel coronary artery disease on thallium-201 SPECT are important prognostic indicators in patients with large defects in the left anterior descending distribution. *Am J Cardiol* 1994;74:1233–1239.

(The title says it all. This clinical study identifies the image factors that lead one to the diagnosis of high-risk, proximal left anterior descending coronary artery [LAD] disease. Whether these are really defects in the distribution of 2 vascular regions or LAD involvement of distal inferior or anterolateral walls remains conjecture, but these areas may be appropriately involved in isolated LAD disease.)

239. McClellan JR, Travin MI, Herman SD, et al. Prognostic importance of scintigraphic left ventricular cavitary dilation during intravenous dipyridamole Tc-99m sestamibi myocardial tomographic imaging in predicting coronary events. *Am J Cardiol* 1997;79:600–605.

(In this study of 512 patients who had pharmacologic stress testing, transient cavitary dilation was related to a higher incidence of myocardial infarction, whereas fixed dilation related to a higher death rate and hospitalization for heart failure.)

240. Bulkley BH, Rouleau J, Strauss HW, et al. Idiopathic hypertrophic subaortic stenosis: detection by thallium-201 myocardial perfusion imaging. *N Engl J Med* 1979;293:1113–1118.

241. Cecil MP, Pilcher WC, Eisner RL, et al. Absence of defects in SPECT thallium-201 myocardial images in patients with systemic hypertension and left ventricular hypertrophy. *Am J Cardiol* 1994;74:43–46.

(240,241: The converse of a "dilated" cavity with thinned walls or similarly with ischemia, the small or vanishing "cavity" is seen with left ventricular hypertrophy. This again is more apparent than real and stems from the fact that the thick, radiointense overlying wall obscures vision of the underlying, radionuclide and counts-poor "cavity" in planar images. A similar phenomenon occurs when planar projection images are processed. Another way to look at the "cavity" is as an apparent rather than real scintigraphic structure, created by the counts difference between the left ventricular wall seen in tangent and that seen *en face*. In normals, the walls in tangent, presenting a much thicker cross section, are much thicker and radioactive than the walls viewed *en face*. This difference appears as a central clear area on planar images and the SPECT composite. As the wall *en face* approaches the thickness and intensity of the walls in tangent, as in hypertrophy, the "cavity disappears"! On SPECT imaging, wall thickness and thickening also have an effect that tends to reduce the apparent cavitary size. In the study by Cecil et al., hypertrophy obscured perfusion defects.)

242. Hansen CL, Sangrigoli R, Nkadi E, Kramer M. Comparison of pulmonary uptake with transient cavity dilation after exercise thallium-201 perfusion imaging. *J Am Coll Cardiol* 1999;33:1323–1327.

(Although pulmonary uptake and transient cavitary dilation have both been associated with advanced coronary artery disease, Hansen et al. report a weak correlation, suggesting the relationship with different pathophysiologic responses to exercise-induced ischemia. These findings support the hypothesis that transient cavitary dilation represents transient subendocardial ischemia rather than true physical ventricular dilation.)

243. Gewirtz H, Grotte GJ, Strauss HW, et al. The influence of left ventricular volume and wall motion on myocardial images. *Circulation* 1979;59:1172–1177.

244. Sinusas AJ, Shi QX, Vitols PJ, et al. Impact of regional ventricular function, geometry and dobutamine stress on quantitative ^{99m}Tc-sestamibi defect size. *Circulation* 1993;88:2224–2234.

(243,244: The findings on perfusion imaging are influenced by the related ventricular geometry and regional function, likely the result of a partial volume effect. The latter is the result of partial filling of a computer pixel or voxel. The unit will then be gray scale or color coded according to the mean pixel intensity, a lesser intensity than the peak value within the imaging unit.)

245. Dae M, Canhasi B, Olvera S, et al. The etiology and implications of dense cavitary "photopenia" on myocardial perfusion scintigraphy. *Invest Radiol* 1985;20:388–396.

   (When first noted, dense cavitary photopenia, presenting an area of deeply reduced radioactivity usually over a region near the cardiac apex, suggested the presence of a space occupying cavitary mass, displacing left ventricular cavitary radioactivity. However, brief reflection on the small amount of radiotracer [1%–2%] in the blood pool at the time of imaging suggests that this is not likely. Here, none of the patients with this finding had evidence of cavitary thrombus. Most, however, had evidence of an aneurysm and scar in the wall overlying the "cavitary photopenia." This phenomenon, then, is again more a reflection of the relationship between counts in the scarred wall, compared with those in the adjacent walls on planar and reconstructed SPECT projection images, than it is a reflection of any characteristic of the blood pool. The same findings may be induced transiently in relation to dense induced ischemia or simple perfusion heterogeneity in the absence of ischemia, as with vasodilator stress. The evident border between the photopenic and normal region sets the boundary for the ischemic or infarcted zone.)

246. Lette J, Lapointe J, Waters D, et al. Transient left ventricular cavitary dilation during dipyridamole-thallium imaging as an indicator of severe coronary artery disease. *Am J Cardiol* 1990;66:1163–1170.

   (The characteristic bullet- or cone-shaped left ventricle becomes permanently deformed, or remodeled, with infarction and may be transiently so with ischemia. The deformity, typically referred to as an aneurysm or severe segmental contraction abnormality, is evident in a bulging of the involved myocardium. Because such ischemia generally relates to the coronary distribution, such deformity is most common in the distal and apical regions. If imaged during a period of severe induced ischemia, this distal dilation may be seen to normalize on rest or redistribution imaging. The authors of this article discuss this configuration and its clinical importance in association with pharmacologic stress testing. Accompanying the dilation and its related reduced wall motion is a reduced influence of overlying myocardial activity on the apparent activity of the ventricular cavity, with the presence or dynamic development of "cavitary photopenia" [8,219,245].

247. Nishijima K, Miyahara Y, Furukawa K, et al. Simultaneous assessment of right ventricular function and hypertrophy by Tc-99m MIBI. *Clin Nucl Med* 1999;24:151–155.

   (The ratio of right ventricular [RV] uptake to left ventricular [LV] uptake correlated with pulmonary artery pressure in 23 patients with chronic pulmonary disease. First-pass blood pool evaluation was used in the same study to assess RV and LV function, gaining a full profile of pulmonary heart disease.)

248. Civelek AC, Shafique I, Brinker JA, et al. Reduced left ventricular cavity activity ("black hole sign") in thallium-201 SPECT perfusion images of anteroapical transmural myocardial infarction. *Am J Cardiol* 1991;68:1132–1137.

   (These phenomena of cavitary photopenia and dilation are evident on SPECT as well as planar imaging and with similar implications. They derive from the same mechanisms that produce them on planar imaging and are translated to the tomographic array via analysis of the planar projection data set. The authors of this article present the finding and discuss the cause and clinical implications of SPECT cavitary photopenia.)

249. Sciagraa R, Bisi G, Buonamici P, et al. Left ventricular cavity to myocardial count ratio in technetium-99m sestamibi SPECT in the detection of resting left ventricular dysfunction. *J Nucl Med* 1997;38:766–770.

   (There was a direct correlation between left ventricular dysfunction and the cavity-to-myocardial count ratio. Cavitary photopenia relates to reduced regional function or perfusion.)

250. Perrone-Filardi P, Pace L, Prastaro M, et al. Assessment of myocardial viability in patients with chronic coronary disease: rest-4 hour and 24 hour Tl-201 tomography versus dobutamine echocardiography. *Circulation* 1996;94:2712–2719.

(In this study, an almost linear relationship was found between the degree of myocardial thallium uptake and the likelihood that the related segment will improve functionally after revascularization. With the general consideration that relative myocardial uptake >50% suggested viability and functional improvement after revascularization, those segments with uptake between 50% and 60% related to an incidence of functional improvement after revascularization of only 56%, whereas 83% of segments improved among those that demonstrated regional thallium uptake >80%!)

251. Santana CA, Garcia EV, Vansant JP, et al. Three-dimensional color modulated display of myocardial SPECT perfusion distributions accurately assesses coronary artery disease [abstract]. *J Nucl Med* 1999;40:126P.

(The visual interpretation of the pattern on 3-dimensional displays of SPECT myocardial perfusion scintigraphy agreed well in 62 consecutive patient studies with visual interpretation of SPECT slices and may replace the visual slice assessment without loss of accuracy.)

252. Dunn RF, Kelly DT, Bailey IK, et al. Serial exercise thallium myocardial perfusion scanning and exercise electrocardiography in the diagnosis of coronary artery disease. *Aust NZ J Med* 1979;9:547–556.

(This article and reference *85* simply employed visual interpretation of image data to derive diagnostic accuracy.)

253. Berger BC, Watson DD, Taylor GJ, et al. Quantitative Tl-201 exercise scintigraphy for detection of coronary artery disease. *J Nucl Med* 1981;22:585–593.

254. Goris ML, Gordon E, Kim O. A stochastic interpretation of thallium myocardial perfusion scintigraphy. *Invest Radiol* 1985;20:253–262.

255. Kaul S, Boucher CA, Newell JB, et al. Determination of the quantitative thallium imaging variables that optimize detection of coronary artery disease. *J Am Coll Cardiol* 1986;7:527–536.

256. Massie B, Hollenberg M, Wisneski JA, et al. Scintigraphic quantitation of myocardial ischemia. A new approach. *Circulation* 1983;68:747–756.

(253–256: The authors of these articles, like others that commonly employ quantitative analysis of image data, applied objective criteria for detection of perfusion defects based on a comparison of image data with that of a normal database.)

257. Mishra J, Acio ER, Jaekyeong H, Iskandrian AE. Comparison of the polar maps methods and the summed stress score for predicting outcome in medically treated patients with coronary artery disease. *Am J Cardiol* 1999;83:258–260.

(SPECT scoring methods vary, but a summed 20-segment score seems quite popular and is well validated as an easily automated measure of coronary-related risk [*129*] that compares well with the polar map measure of defect size. The ability to risk stratify patients with coronary artery disease [CAD] was similar when polar maps or the summed stress score were used to develop the quantitative measure of defect size in 723 patients with chest pain studied by myocardial perfusion scintigraphy. Risks related to defects <15% were differentiated from those ≥15%, with similar risk differentiation when defect size was evaluated by both methods. Interesting was the fact that events did not relate to left ventricular ejection fraction or extent of CAD.)

258. Berman DS, Kang X, Van Train KF, et al. Comparative prognostic value of automated quantitative analysis versus semiquantitative visual analysis of exercise myocardial perfusion single-photon emission computed tomography. *J Am Coll Cardiol* 1998;32:1987–1995.

(Fully 1043 consecutive patients with dual-isotope rest thallium-201/stress technetium-99m sestamibi studies for known or suspected coronary artery disease were followed for more than 1 yr. Outcomes correlated very well with both quantitative polar map or visual segmental scores derived from SPECT data. This finding may be important, especially in labs where expert visual reading is not available. However, one must not simply accept computer-generated quantitation of defect scores until their origin is analyzed and found to be perfusion related.)

259. Thigpen KA, Ledges M, Munro SM, et al. Prognostic value of weighted quantitative analysis of coronary artery disease using rest Tl-201 and gated Tc-99m sestamibi imaging [abstract]. *J Nucl Med* 1999;40:42P.

(Defect size related to a volumetric analysis of left ventricular [LV] involvement also compared well with the 20-segment score. Stress myocardial perfusion scintigraphy defect size calculated by a score based on a 3-dimenstional volumetric estimate of LV involvement [3-D MSPECT; University of Michigan, Ann Arbor, MI], compared well with the 20-segment summed stress score, and the two methods predicted cardiac events equally well.)

260. Shanoudy H, Raggi P, Beller GA, et al. Comparison of technetium-99m tetrofosmin and thallium-201 single-photon emission computed tomographic imaging for detection of myocardial perfusion defects in patients with coronary artery disease. *J Am Coll Cardiol* 1998;31:331–337.

(Quantitative methods are applied to enhance the accuracy of tetrofosmin stress myocardial perfusion scintigraphy).

261. Kang X, Berman DS, Van Train KF, et al. Clinical validation of automatic quantitative defect size in rest technetium-99m sestamibi myocardial perfusion SPECT. *J Nucl Med* 1997;38:1441–1446.

(Kang et al. demonstrated the value of quantitative methods for measurement of defect size and severity [infarct size] and their correlation with left ventricular function, all generated from gated myocardial perfusion scintigraphy studies.)

262. Cohen Y, Acio E, Heo J, et al. Comparison of the prognostic value of qualitative versus quantitative stress tomographic perfusion imaging. *Am J Cardiol* 1999;83:945–948.

(The superiority of quantitative methods for risk stratification is demonstrated. Qualitative evaluation of exercise thallium-201 imaging was compared with quantitative measures in the prediction of outcome among 713 patients with a 78% prevalence of coronary artery disease on angiography. Although qualitative image evaluation contributed valuable prognostic information, it placed too many in an intermediate-risk subgroup, whereas the quantitative method correctly placed more patients in a low- or high-risk group and fewer in the intermediate-risk group.)

263. Atwood JE, Jensen D, Froelicher V, et al. Agreement in human interpretation of analog thallium myocardial perfusion images. *Circulation* 1981;64:601–609.

(This article presents early data regarding the reproducibility of myocardial perfusion scintigraphy. The values were excellent at the outset, but SPECT and objective markers of regional devices to identify artifact [prone imaging] and interpret perfusion with a deliberate analytic reading style and attention to technique have made them better. Attenuation correction promises to make them better yet.

When 4 experienced readers interpreted 100 analogue perfusion image sets on 2 occasions, there was agreement among 3 observers in 75% of abnormal and 68% of normal studies. There was wider disagreement in defect location. Posterior and lateral defects found lowest agreement. Agreement in defect intensity was high and in the range of 90%. These findings applied to analogue planar studies before SPECT, technetium-99m perfusion agents, high-resolution displays, polar maps and the analytic method of image interpretation.)

264. Okada RD, Boucher CA, Kirshenbaum HK, et al. Improved diagnostic accuracy of thallium-201 stress test using multiple observers and criteria derived from interobserver analysis of variance. *Am J Cardiol* 1980;46:619–624.

(Diagnostic accuracy was high among observers interpreting planar thallium-201 images. This article demonstrated an interobserver variability <10% and an intraobserver variability <5%.)

265. Segall GM, Stepp C, Kadkade PP, et al. Fast acquisition of myocardial SPECT images with Tc-99m sestamibi for the diagnosis of coronary artery disease. *J Nucl Cardiol* 1997;358–363.

(The study demonstrates that SPECT myocardial perfusion scintigraphy may be acquired in as little as 5–10 min with technetium-99m sestamibi and a 1-day rest/stress protocol and with preserved accuracy.)

266. Mahmarian JJ, Moye LA, Verani MS, et al. High reproducibility of myocardial perfusion defects in patients undergoing serial exercise thallium-201 tomography. *Am J Cardiol* 1995;75:1116–1119.

(This was an ancillary aspect of a double-blind, placebo-controlled study, testing the effects of transdermal nitroglycerin on myocardial perfusion scintigraphy [MPS] defect size [*281*]. This study reports no significant change in exercise MPS in that placebo group studied serially, 4–8 days apart. There was a 96% agreement in segmental abnormalities when studied serially, with serially measured mean defect size initially measured at 17.4 and subsequently measured at 16.6%. The upper limit of technical variability and reproducibility was demonstrated to be a defect change of 8%. Therefore, a change in SPECT defect size on serial study of 9% exceeds the 95% confidence interval and represents a real change beyond technical variability. Such quantitation with clear evaluation of reproducibility limits makes application of the method valuable for the assessment of the effects of treatment.)

267. Prigent F, Berman DS, Elashoff I, et al. Reproducibility of stress redistribution thallium-201 SPECT quantitative indexes of myocardium secondary to coronary artery disease. *Am J Cardiol* 1993;70:1255–1263.

(The reproducibility of quantitative indices of hypoperfusion were evaluated on serial thallium-201 SPECT images performed between 1 and 13 mo. Reproducibility was excellent, with measures of defect size ranging from 3.2%–4.5%. Mean absolute deviation for individual vascular areas ranged from 3.7%–9%. Both the accuracy and reproducibility of SPECT exceeded that for planar myocardial perfusion scintigraphy.)

268. MacDonald LA, Elliott MD, Leonard SM, et al. Variability of myocardial perfusion SPECT: contribution of repetitive processing, acquisition and testing [abstract]. *J Nucl Med* 1999;40:126P.

(Repeated acquisition and processing of 10 stress myocardial perfusion scintigraphy SPECT studies was performed in order to determine the variability related to serial study and processing. Repeat image processing related to a 1.87 standard error of the measurement [SEM] or about 40%–50% of the variability related to serial imaging in the same patient days apart [SEM 5.01 at rest and 4.04 at stress]. The remainder of the variability related to patient positioning and aspects of image acquisition, including variable motion and other factors.)

269. Germano G, Kavanagh JT, Wishner SH, et al. Repeatability of automatic left ventricular cavity volume measurements from myocardial perfusion SPECT. *J Nucl Cardiol* 1998;5:477–483.

(Left ventricular ejection fraction [LVEF] and volumes were calculated from serially acquired gated and ungated SPECT myocardial perfusion scintigraphy studies acquired in 926 patients. Reproducibility, as well as accuracy for LVEF and ventricular volumes, was well demonstrated.)

270. Iskandrian AS. Is quantification necessary in SPECT perfusion imaging [editorial]? *Am J Cardiol* 1995;75:1175–1176.

(This editorial concludes that, although quantitation is not absolutely necessary, prognostic if not diagnostic measures [as well as serial assessment to determine regression and progression and the benefits of related medical or interventional therapies] rely on the extent and depth of myocardial involvement. Quantitation is necessary for these purposes and is improved with technetium-based radiotracers.)

271. Hendel RC, Parker MA, Wackers FJTh, et al. Reduced variability of interpretation and improved image quality with a technetium-99m myocardial perfusion agent: comparison of thallium 201 and technetium 99m-labeled tetrofosmin. *J Nucl Cardiol* 1994;1:509–514.

(When technetium-99m [^{99m}Tc] tetrofosmin and thallium-201 stress imaging were performed in the same 216 patients within a 2-wk period, the ^{99m}Tc studies were of higher quality and demonstrated reduced interobserver variability.)

272. Golub RJ, Ahlberg AW, McClellan JR, et al. Interpretive reproducibility of stress Tc-99m sestamibi tomographic myocardial perfusion imaging. *J Nucl Cardiol* 1999; 6:257–269.

(Six readers, 3 less experienced [qualified in nuclear cardiology with 200 hr in radiation physics and at least 6 mo training in the field] and 3 well-experienced [similar training with years of clinical experience and >4000 images interpreted], interpreted 138 exercise and rest technetium-99m sestamibi studies in 101 patients with coronary artery disease [CAD] and in 37 patients with low CAD likelihood. Intraobserver agreement was high: 87%–94% for global evaluation, 82%–96% for left anterior descending coronary artery [LAD] and 88%–91% for non-LAD regions. Intraobserver agreement was similar among both experienced and less experienced readers. Overall, interobserver agreement was high: 73%–89% for global evaluation, 73%–93% for the LAD region and 76%–88% for non-LAD regions. Although higher for experienced [85%–87%, 89%–91%, 82%–86%] than less experienced [73%–84%, 73%–91%, 76%–86%] observers, interobserver agreement in global, LAD and non-LAD assessment was quite high for all. Reproducibility was good to excellent among readers over a range of experience.)

273. Haber HL, Beller GA, Watson DD, Gimple LW. Exercise thallium-201 scintigraphy after thrombolytic therapy with or without angioplasty for acute myocardial infarction. *Am J Cardiol* 1990;71:1257–1261.

(To evaluate exercise myocardial perfusion scintigraphy [MPS] after thrombolyisis, 88 patients were studied after thrombolytic therapy for acute infarction. MPS was more sensitive to induced ischemia and the identification of multivessel disease after thrombolysis than to stress ST changes. MPS redistribution and ST changes were complementary in their diagnostic abilities.)

274. Sutton JM, Topol EJ. Significance of a negative exercise thallium test in the presence of a critical residual stenosis after thrombolysis for acute myocardial infarction. *Circulation* 1991;83:1278–1286.

(The absence of reversible myocardial perfusion scintigraphy [MPS] defects in the presence of residual stenosis after thrombolytic therapy was found to relate to extensive myocardial necrosis and not inadequate exercise performance or MPS insensitivity.)

275. Wackers FJTh, Gibbons RJ, Verani MS, et al. Serial quantitative planar technetium-99m isonitrile imaging in acute myocardial infarction: efficacy for noninvasive assessment of thrombolytic therapy. *J Am Coll Cardiol* 1989;14: 861–873.

(Serial imaging of patients before and after thrombolytic therapy permitted measurement of myocardium at ischemic risk and final infarct size, where the difference was myocardium salvaged. The latter related to the success and timing of the intervention and the extent of myocardium at risk.)

276. Gibbons RJ, Verani MS, Behrenbeck T, et al. Feasibility of tomographic [99mTc]-hexakis-2-methoxy-2-methylpropyl-isonitrile imaging for the assessment of myocardial area at risk and the effect of treatment in acute myocardial infarction. *Circulation* 1980;80:1277–1286.

(SPECT sestamibi studies were performed in 11 patients before thrombolytic treatment with tissue-type plasminogen activator and within 4 hr of onset of acute myocardial infarction [AMI] marked by chest pain, as well as in 5 AMI patients who did not receive thrombolytic therapy. These studies were repeated 6–14 days later. Initial defect size ranged from 9%–68% of the left ventricle and was larger in anterior than inferior MI. Similar to studies performed in animals [442], the late defect size was smaller [0%–63% of the left ventricle] and correlated with late left ventricular ejection fraction and regional wall motion. Thrombolysis brought a significant reduction in defect size, not evident among those not so treated. SPECT imaging in patients undergoing thrombolytic treatment permits evaluation of myocardium at risk as well as the benefits of treatment.)

277. Gibson WS, Christian TF, Pellikka PA, et al. Serial tomographic imaging with technetium-99m sestamibi for the assessment of infarct-related arterial patency following reperfusion therapy. *J Nucl Med* 1992;33:2080–2085.

(273–277: Rest sestamibi images were acquired serially after acute myocardial infarction, on presentation and 18–48 hr later. Defect size was greater for anterior than inferior or lateral infarction. The change in defect size related to patency of the infarct-related artery.

Myocardial perfusion scintigraphy appears to maintain its accuracy and clinical value in the "post-thrombolytic" patient. The method has been well applied and of great value for the assessment of the benefit of thrombolysis in many blinded studies. However, at first glance diagnostic sensitivity, especially to multivessel disease, appears to be reduced. This may well be the result of different patient populations in the study after thrombolysis, compared with previous studies in which the incidence of nontransmural and prior infarction was greater, as was the incidence of multivessel disease. Nonetheless, perfusion scintigraphy has been very useful for evaluating the effects of thrombolysis [273,274]. Specifically, perfusion scintigraphy with technetium-99m sestamibi has been the research method employed to determine the value of thrombolysis and can do so in relatively small patient numbers. Here, a reduced image defect size on serial imaging, before and after thrombolysis, evident with great frequency in even small populations, provides the statistical validity needed to demonstrate the efficacy of the method, compared with the large numbers of patients needed to confirm improved survival [275,276]. Technetium-99m sestamibi has special advantages for evaluation of perfusion in relation to acute coronary syndromes and has been most widely applied [277]. All such evaluation depends on the reproducibility of the method. The validity of the findings, changes with therapy or the lack of changes must be related to the variability of the method with simple serial imaging without therapy. It is the small intra- and interobserver variability that permits the reliable detection of relatively modest therapy-induced changes.)

278. Williams DO, Braunwald E, Knatterud G, et al. One-year results of the thrombolysis in myocardial infarction investigation (TIMI) Phase II Trial. *Circulation* 1992;85:533–542.

279. Califf RM, White HD, Van de Werf F, et al. for the GUSTO Investigators. One-year results from the global utilization of streptokinase and TPA for occluded coronary arteries (GUSTO-I) trial. *Circulation* 1996;94:1233–1238.

(278,279: As a result of the low death rate experienced in patients enrolled in a variety of multicenter post-myocardial infarction thrombolytic trials in which highly selective, relatively young study populations without heart failure or hemodynamic instability were evaluated, many physicians believe that the death rate of patients hospitalized with acute myocardial infarction is in the range of 5%–10%. More realistically, this rate is in the range of 30%–40% among unselected populations.)

280. Aoki M, Sakai K, Koyanagi S, et al. Effects of nitroglycerin on coronary collateral function during exercise evaluated by quantitative analysis of thallium-201 single photon emission computed tomography. *Am Heart J* 1991;121:1361–1366.

281. Mahmarian JJ, Fenimore NL, Marks GF, et al. Transdermal nitroglycerin patch therapy reduces the extent of exercise-induced myocardial ischemia: results of a double-blind, placebo controlled trial using quantitative thallium-201 tomography. *J Am Coll Cardiol* 1994;24:25–32.

(280,281: It is the excellent reproducibility of the scintigraphic method which permits the serial evaluation of the effects of agents on coronary flow and their ability to effect ischemia.)

282. Frazier OH, March RJ, Horvath KA, et al. Transmyocardial revascularization with a carbon dioxide laser in patients with end-stage coronary artery disease. *N Engl J Med* 1999;341:1021–1028.

(In a prospective, controlled, multicenter trial, 91 coronary patients were randomly selected to receive laser transmyocardial revascularization and 101 to receive continued conventional medical therapy. After 12 mo, symptoms, measured quality of life and perfusion image defect score were significantly reduced only in the revascularization group.)

283. Hendel RC, Leonard SM, Toth B, et al. Improvement of myocardial perfusion following treatment with rhVEGF as evaluated by SPECT imaging [abstract]. *J Nucl Med* 1999;40:85P.

(Recombinant human vascular endothelial growth factor, rhVEGF, was infused in 15 patients with severe coronary artery disease and monitored by pre- and post-treatment SPECT myocardial perfusion scintigraphy. Those treated with a "high-dose" rhVEGF regimen demonstrated an improvement in the summed rest segmental scores after 30 days.)

284. Arora RR, Chou TM, Jain D, et al. The multicenter study of enhanced external counterpulsation (MUST-EECP): effect of EECP on exercise-induced myocardial ischemia and anginal episodes. *J Am Coll Cardiol* 1999;33:1833–1840.

(282–284: It is for reasons of reproducibility, objectivity and its quantifiable and prognostic nature that the perfusion imaging method was utilized in the earlier thrombolytic trials as a surrogate for hard outcomes. It permitted documentation of method value in only a limited patient numbers. It is for these reasons, too, that perfusion studies are used with regularity as the standard for documentation of the effects of new surgical methods to revascularize the myocardium [282] or of medications [283] or mechanical aids [284] to grow collaterals vessels.

It is the excellent reproducibility of the scintigraphic method that makes it an important part of the research protocol of several multicenter trials being conducted around the world, testing the effects of agents which, by different mechanisms, seek to provide medical coronary revascularization.)

285. Lewin HC, Sharir T, Germano G, et al. Reproducibility of dual isotope myocardial perfusion SPECT using a new quantitative perfusion SPECT (QPS) approach [abstract]. *J Am Coll Cardiol* 1999;33:483A.

(This 3-dimensional quantitative approach to image evaluation was demonstrated to be a highly stable and reproducible method, well able to reliably identify serial changes or changes ≥10% from baseline rest images.)

286. Hendel RC, Gibbons RJ, Bateman TM. Wintergreen panel summaries. Use of rotating (cine) planar projection images in the interpretation of a tomographic myocardial perfusion study. *J Nucl Cardiol* 1999;6:234–240.

(The importance of evaluation of the rotating planar projection images must be a part of the interpretation of every SPECT study. Planar images help to confirm SPECT findings but also help to assess patient motion, attenuation artifact, presence and severity of extracardiac activity and the presence of gating artifact, as well as providing important quality control measures.)

287. Kiat H, Van Train KF, Friedman JD, et al. Quantitative stress-redistribution thallium-201 SPECT prone imaging: methodologic development and validation. *J Nucl Med* 1992;33:1509–1515.

(The benefit of prone imaging for resolving the cause of inferior defects, motion artifacts and others is now well established but still not fully appreciated or applied.)

288. Starksen NF, O'Connell JW, Dae MW, et al. Basal interventricular septal thallium-201 defects: real or artifact? *Clin Nucl Med* 1993;18:291–297.

(The authors report a case in which an image documented reversible perfusion defect at the base of the interventricular septum. In fact, such defects are too often more apparent than real, resulting from mismatching of short-axis slices or inconsistencies of axial processing.)

289. Garcia EV, Cooke CD, Folks RD, et al. Expert system (PERFEX) interpretation of myocardial perfusion tomograms: validation using 655 prospective patients [abstract]. *J Nucl Med* 1999;40:126P.

(This computerized expert system method, the most advanced available, applied 253 heuristic rules in 461 patient myocardial perfusion scintigraphy studies with angiographic documentation of coronary anatomy and compared its accuracy with visual interpretation, where polar map defects compared with the normal database were identified as abnormal. Although it increased sensitivity from 87% to 93%, specificity was poor with visual analysis and fell with application of the expert system. Of course, simple visual image analysis is not the best interpretive method that can be applied by expert readers. A fully integrated evaluation of all image data, using polar map findings as a reading guide but without automatic acceptance of polar map findings, would likely do better yet.)

290. William KA, Schneider CM, Bryant TA, Rajoub H. Prediction of long-term outcome with simultaneous stress Tc-99m-sestamibi SPECT and first-pass radionuclide angiography [abstract]. *J Am Coll Cardiol* 1999;33:469A.

(Outcomes over 4 yr were related to clinical and image findings as well as to exercise first-pass evaluation of left ventricular ejection fraction and wall motion in 324 patients undergoing exercise SPECT sestamibi myocardial perfusion scintigraphy [MPS] for clinical indications. Much of the prognostic data was in the rest and stress first-pass blood pool images. When combined with the clinical and exercise data, stress MPS was comparable only with the combination of clinical data plus rest radionuclide angiography.)

291. Ficaro EP, Fessler JA, Shreve PD, et al. Simultaneous transmission/emission myocardial perfusion tomography. Diagnostic accuracy of attenuation-corrected ^{99m}Tc-sestamibi single-photon emission computed tomography. *Circulation* 1996;93:463–473.

(With a 3-head detector SPECT system equipped with an americium-241 transmission line source, simultaneous transmission–emission tomography was performed on 60 patients with coronary artery disease [CAD] and 59 patients with a low likelihood of CAD. Attenuation corrected [AC] and non-AC images were blindly compared in each set with a qualitative approach and applying specific polar maps based in an AC [or not] normal population. For the low likelihood group, visual and quantitative analysis normalcy rates increased from 0.88 and 0.76 to 0.98 and 0.95, respectively, for AC. For the CAD group, sensitivity and specificity increased with AC, from 0.78 and 0.46 to 0.84 and 0.82, respectively, with qualitative visual analysis and from 0.84 and 0.46 to 0.88 and 0.82, respectively, with quantitative analysis. Defect localization also improved with AC. The authors contend that clinical application of this AC method should be carefully considered. Although such AC systems are being sold, supportive studies like this are not the rule. Results of the application of AC in clinical practice have been spotty at best and have not yet demonstrated reliability and clinical value.)

292. Lim T, Lee DS, Cheon GJ, et al. Additive diagnostic efficacy of scatter and attenuation-corrected myocardial SPECT in the diagnosis of coronary artery disease [abstract]. *J Nucl Med* 1999;40:89P.

(Among 45 studies interpreted by less experienced readers, attenuation-corrected images increased diagnostic sensitivity from 78% to 88% but did not affect the accuracy of interpretation for experienced readers.)

293. Pretrius PH, Narayanan MV, Dahlberg ST, et al. Review of physiological and anatomical factors impacting count uniformity in attenuation and scatter corrected Tc-99m sestamibi SPECT slices [abstract]. *J Nucl Med* 1999;40:113P.

(The study demonstrated that reduced apical activity, commonly seen in normal myocardial perfusion scintigraphy, is likely a true anatomic finding but, like reduced anterior and inferior activity, is also likely affected by respiratory motion. The latter may also be responsible for the overlap of inferior left ventricular wall activity with subdiaphragmatic extracardiac activity.)

294. Gibbons RJ. Myocardial perfusion imaging for detection of CAD. Extracting all the information. Presented at: Annual meeting of the American Society of Nuclear Cardiology; June 1998; Toronto, Canada.

(The factors that determine the extent of added value related to test performance are detailed.)

295. Zhu YY, Lee W, Botvinick EH, et al. The clinical and pathophysiologic implications of pain, ST abnormalities, and scintigraphic changes induced during dipyridamole infusion: their relationships to the peripheral hemodynamic response. *Am Heart J* 1988;116:1071.

(This was the first study demonstrating the dissociation between the central and peripheral hemodynamic effect of dipyridamole. Sensitivity of dipyridamole pharmacologic stress was well maintained, even in the absence of a hemodynamic response.)

296. Cerqueira M, Mahmarian JJ, Borer JS, et al. Wintergreen panel summaries. Monitoring aggressive therapy for CAD. *J Nucl Cardiol* 1999;6:148–155.

(This is an excellent status report of the application of myocardial perfusion scintigraphy for the serial evaluation of anti-ischemic therapies. It also plots a direction for future development.)

297. Chouraqui P, Maddahi J, Ostrzega E, et al. Quantitative exercise thallium-201 rotational tomography for evaluation of patients with prior myocardial infarction. *Am J Cardiol* 1990;2:151–157.

(The accuracy for detection of patients with multivessel coronary disease, measurement of infarct size and assessment of regional viability by quantitative thallium-201 [201Tl] SPECT was excellent and superior to that of planar methods in 66 patients studied with stress 201Tl SPECT and coronary angiography.)

298. Mahmarian J, Femmore NL, Marks GE, et al. Transdermal nitroglycerin patch therapy reduces the extent of exercise-induced myocardial ischemia: results of a double-blind, placebo-controlled trial using quantitative thallium-201 tomography. *J Am Coll Cardiol* 1994;24:25–32.

(In this double-blind, placebo-controlled trial, 40 patients with stress perfusion defects who were weaned from antianginal drugs were randomized to receive intermittent nitroglycerin patch therapy or placebo. Repeat exercise myocardial perfusion scintigraphy, about 4–8 days later, revealed a significant reduction in defect size only in the nitroglycerin-treated group, greatest in those with the largest baseline defects. This was without change in double product, indicating a true augmentation of perfusion.)

299. Shehata A, Gilliam LD, Mascitelli VA, et al. Impact of acute propanolol administration on dobutamine-induced myocardial ischemia as evaluated by myocardial perfusion imaging and echocardiography. *Am J Cardiol* 1997;80:268–272.

(Seventeen patients with known reversible perfusion defects were studied with dobutamine stress electrocardiography, myocardial perfusion scintigraphy and echocardiography stress testing, on or off beta blockers. There was a lower heart rate and double product on beta blockers with smaller perfusion defects and fewer induced wall motion abnormalities, even with a higher dobutamine dose. Defects in 4 of 17 patients were seen only during the control phase, with reduced sensitivity of all methods on beta blockers.)

300. Mahmarian J, Moye LA, Nasser GA, et al. Nicotine patch therapy in smoking cessation reduces the extent of exercise-induced myocardial ischemia. *J Am Coll Cardiol* 1997;30:125–130.

(When used to promote smoking cessation, nicotine patches significantly reduced the size of exercise-induced perfusion defects and related myocardial ischemia.)

301. Dakik H, Kleiman NS, Farmer JA, et al. Intensive medical therapy versus coronary angioplasty for suppressing myocardial ischemia in survivors of acute myocardial infarction: a prospective randomized pilot study. *Circulation* 1998;98:2017–2023.

(To determine the benefit of percutaneous transluminal coronary angioplasty [PTCA] revascularization over medical therapy in stable survivors of acute myocardial infarction [MI] with large stress myocardial perfusion scintigraphy [MPS] defects [>20% of the left ventricle] and large reversible components [>10%], the authors performed this prospective study in 44 stable post-MI patients with such defects at baseline adenosine MPS, performed 2–8 days after the event. As if taking advantage of the effect described in references *593–596*, Dakik et al. studied adenosine MPS performed in patients who had been off of antianginal therapy for a mean of 4.5 ± 2.9 days, in comparison with the results of adenosine MPS performed later, after optimization of maximal medical therapy or revascularization procedure, 43 ± 2.3 days in a select population of post-MI patients, all with large total defect size, >20% of the left ventricular mass and induced ischemia >10% of the left ventricle! Both medical and revascularization therapy brought a comparable benefit with a similar reduction in total and reversible defect size. When stress MPS was repeated 20–60 days later, the reduction in stress defect size and the size of the reversible defect were similar in the medical and PTCA groups. The larger the reduction in the size of the reversible defect, the less likely was death or any event in follow-up. Cardiac events were evident in 7 of 44 [16%] patients followed over a period of 12 ± 5 mo. Those without events had greater reductions in induced reversible defect size [$-13\% \pm 9\%$ versus $-5\% \pm 7\%$; $P = 0.02$], and event-free survival was significantly better [96%] in the 24 patients with a reduction in reversible defect size $\geq 9\%$ than in those without such change [$P = 0.009$]. This result was independent of and unrelated to the form of treatment given.

The authors concluded that the adenosine defect size and its response to medical therapy provide an important prognostic index and guide to therapy. Both medical and revascularization therapy were better able to provide a reduced risk and improved outcome based on normalization of the stress image with reduced reversible defect size. It should be noted that in this study, the 9% value was set by the reproducibility and variability of the method. A change of 9% or more was a statistically significant change and beyond the variability of the method. This was not the first study to demonstrate the prognostic significance of stress MPS on therapy or the excellent prognosis of an improved stress MPS on any therapy [see reference *303*]. The Angioplasty Compared to Medicine study reviewed similar findings.)

302. Sharir T, Rabinowitz B, Livschitz S, et al. Underestimation of extent and severity of coronary artery disease by dipyridamole stress Tl-201 single photon emission computed tomographic myocardial perfusion imaging in patients taking antianginal drugs. *J Am Coll Cardiol* 1998;31:1540–1546.

(Contrary to prior and apparently established belief, continued use of antianginal drugs before dipyridamole [and low-level exercise] thallium-201 SPECT may reduce defect extent and severity of defects, potentially underestimating coronary artery disease and the extent of myocardium at ischemic risk.)

303. Parisi AS, Hartigan PM, Folland SD, et al. Evaluation of exercise thallium scintigraphy versus exercise electrocardiography in predicting survival outcomes and morbid cardiac events in patients with single and double-vessel disease: findings from the Angioplasty Compared to Medicine (ACME) Study. *J Am Coll Cardiol* 1997;3:1256–1263.

(Here, survival was improved with the reduction of induced ischemic ST changes on Holter recording. In the Angioplasty Compared to Medicine [ACME] study, 270 patients with coronary artery disease were randomized to medical or revascularization therapy. Thallium-201 stress planar myocardial perfusion scintigraphy [MPS] was performed at baseline and after 6 mo of treatment. Outcome was significantly better among those whose defect normalized with either therapy than among those with persistent image evidence of ischemia [.92 versus .82; $P < 0.02$]. This study indicates that MPS can be used to both assess initial risk and track its amelioration with treatment.)

304. Rahimtoola SA. The hibernating myocardium. *Am Heart J* 1989;117:211–221.

(This classic article presents all known at the time about the condition of "resting ischemia" or viable but dysfunctional myocardium. Unlike "stunned" myocardium, it is not a clearly postischemic condition. However, it may represent repetitive stunning.)

305. Heller GV, Brown KA. Prognosis of acute and chronic coronary artery disease by myocardial perfusion imaging. *Symp Cardiol Clin* 1994;12:271–287.

306. Gibbons RJ. Role of nuclear cardiology for determining management of patients with stable coronary disease. *J Nucl Cardiol* 1994;1:S118–S130.

(305,306: Presented are excellent reviews of the prognostic value of myocardial perfusion scintigraphy in acute and chronic coronary disease, as well as a clinical evaluation that demonstrates the prognostic value of the method in coronary disease.)

307. Pancholy SB, Fattah AA, Kamal AM, et al. Independent and incremental prognostic value of exercise thallium single-photon emission computed tomographic imaging in women. *J Nucl Cardiol* 1995;2:110–116.

(In addition to anterior breast attenuation, the relatively smaller size of the female heart and end-systolic volume <20 cc have been reported to represent a particular problem reducing test sensitivity. In addition, because of the limited resolution of the method, end-systolic volume may be underestimated and left ventricular ejection fraction exaggerated. Nonetheless, this study demonstrated the independent and added prognostic value of SPECT thallium-201 perfusion imaging in 212 women undergoing coronary angiography. Multivariate survival analysis demonstrated that a large perfusion abnormality and age were the only independent predictors of events and that women with large perfusion abnormalities [>15% of the left ventricular myocardium] had significantly worse event-free survival than women with no or small defects [<15%; $P = 0.0001$]. In this same study, myocardial perfusion scintigraphy demonstrated added prognostic value beyond coronary angiography.)

308. Rozanski A. Myocardial perfusion SPECT in conjunction with exercise and pharmacologic stress: prognostic applications in the clinical management of patients with coronary artery disease. In: DePuey EG, Berman DS, Garcia EV, eds. *Cardiac SPECT Imaging*. New York, NY: Raven Press, Ltd.; 1995:201–236.

(A thorough review of the use of myocardial perfusion scintigraphy for prognosis.)

309. Stratmann HG, Williams GA, Wittry MD, et al. Exercise technetium-99m sestamibi tomography for cardiac risk stratification of patients with stable chest pain. *Circulation* 1994;89:615–622.

(Here, workers studied 521 patients for more than 1 yr after rest–stress technetium-99m sestamibi SPECT study and found that both exercise-related and reversible perfusion defects had independent predictive values for hard cardiac events. Over the course of follow-up, a normal scan related to a 0.5% event rate, whereas an abnormal scan related to a 7% event rate!)

310. Kotler TS, Maddahi J, Kiat H, et al. Benefit from surgery in patients with triple vessel coronary disease may be predicted by evidence of ischemia on exercise-redistribution Tl-201 scintigraphy [abstract]. *Clin Nucl Med* 1987;12:P14.

311. Kotler TS, Maddahi J, Berman DS, Diamond GA. Is thallium scintigraphy better than coronary angiography for prognosis? *Circulation* 1986;74:2042–2051.
    (310,311: These 2 articles demonstrate the impressive prognostic advantage of perfusion scintigraphic data and its superiority even over anatomy. Here, scintigraphic findings were better able to substratify prognosis and the benefits of surgical management among otherwise apparently uniform anatomic groups of coronary patients. Kotler et al. [*310*] have shown that a subgroup of patients with 3-vessel coronary disease with an average 1-yr event rate of 17% could be further classified prognostically into risk subgroups ranging from 6.3% to 57.1%, based on the extent and severity of reversible and nonreversible thallium-201 [^{201}Tl] defects. In the other study by Kotler et al. [*311*], it was further demonstrated in a nonrandomized population of patients that surgically treated patients had a similar coronary event rate compared with those who received medical therapy, when the number of reversible ^{201}Tl defects was no more than 1. Only in a subgroup of patients with 2 or more reversible segments was bypass surgery shown to be superior to medical therapy with respect to 1-yr event rate [11% versus 4%, respectively].)

312. Gill JB, Ruddy TD, Newell JB, et al. Prognostic importance of thallium uptake by the lungs during exercise in coronary artery disease. *N Engl J Med* 1987;317:1485–1489.
    (The authors demonstrate the important prognostic value of pulmonary uptake.)

313. Kaul S, Finkelstein DM, Homma S, et al. Superiority of quantitative exercise thallium-201 variables in determining long-term prognosis in ambulatory patients with chest pain: a comparison with cardiac catheterization. *J Am Coll Cardiol* 1988;12:25–34.
    (The prognostic importance of pulmonary thallium-201 [^{201}Tl] uptake has been further confirmed by Kaul et al., who found that a quantitative index of pulmonary uptake of ^{201}Tl, the heart-to-lung ratio of ^{201}Tl, was the single most powerful variable for prognosis in symptomatic, ambulatory patients undergoing catheterization.)

314. Wilson RF, Marcus ML, White CW. Prediction of the physiologic significance of coronary arterial lesions by quantitative lesion geometry in patients with limited coronary artery disease. *Circulation* 1987;75:723–732.
    (Many studies demonstrating the inability of quantitative angiography to predict the physiologic significance of a coronary stenosis were conducted in patients with widespread coronary artery disease or used methods that could not measure the maximal flow reserve. These authors demonstrated that the percentage of stenosis evident in the anatomic lesion at coronary angiography relates poorly to the local coronary flow reserve. It is this critical parameter that myocardial perfusion scintigraphy quantifies best. In this study, coronary flow reserve measured in patients with discrete, limited lesions, correlated well with luminal stenosis measured by quantitative angiography.)

315. Vogel RA. The radiographic assessment of coronary blood flow parameters. *Circulation* 1985;72:460–465.
    (Coronary flow reserve, measured noninvasively in patients with digital angiographic methods, correlated extremely well with the findings on stress perfusion and stress blood pool scintigraphy but relatively poorly with those of coronary angiography.)

groups on the basis of image findings. Scintigraphic prognosis was much better defined and prognostic subgroups better separated in females, in whom scintigraphic abnormalities acquired in relation to the same ischemic stress were weighted more heavily toward a poor prognosis and a higher event rate. Therefore, and contrary to popular belief, perfusion scintigraphy better stratifies coronary risk in females, where the same scintigraphic abnormality appears to relate to a worse prognosis than in males. This had no relation to the selection process, in which the likelihood of coronary angiography was related to the same defect size and related provocation in both sexes.)

338. Iskander S, Iskandrian A. Risk assessment using single photon emission computed tomographic technetium-99m sestamibi imaging. *J Am Coll Cardiol* 1998;32:57–62.

(Analyzed were the published reports of the relationships between findings on technetium-99m sestamibi myocardial perfusion scintigraphy and coronary-related events and included data from more than 12,000 patients. Patients with normal images presented a 0.6% annual hard event rate, whereas an abnormal scan related to a 7.4% rate, 12-fold higher! Quantitation of defects increased the ability to risk stratify.)

339. Veilleux M, Lette J, Mansur A, et al. Prognostic implications of transient left ventricular cavity dilation during exercise and dipyridamole-thallium imaging. *Can J Cardiol* 1994;10:259–262.

(Patients with perfusion scintigraphic cavitary dilation induced with dipyridamole were at greater risk of events [50%] than when it was induced with exercise [9%].)

340. Shaw LJ, Miller DD, Romeis JC, et al. Prognostic value of noninvasive risk stratification and coronary revascularization in nonelderly and elderly patients referred for evaluation of clinically suspected coronary artery disease. *J Am Geriatr Soc* 1996;44:1190–1197.

(Shaw et al. evaluated test utilization and predictors of outcome as a function of age and gender in 1,345 patients, 505 of whom were older than 65, who underwent stress testing or stress myocardial perfusion scintigraphy. They found both significant age- and gender-based differences in test utilization, cost of testing and subsequent outcomes, with outcomes better related to image findings in the elderly with a lower cost per event identified.)

341. Berman DS, Hachamovitch R, Shaw L, et al. Prognostic risk stratification with SPECT imaging: results from a 20,340 patient multicenter registry [abstract]. *J Am Coll Cardiol* 1998;31:410A.

(This large number of patients without known coronary disease undergoing dynamic or pharmacologic stress SPECT perfusion scintigraphy by a variety of protocols at 3 institutions were prospectively analyzed with a follow-up of 1.8 ± 1 yr. The summed stress image score stratified patients well according to the risk of cardiac death or nonfatal infarction.)

342. Hachamovitch R, Berman DS, Kiat H, et al. What is the warranty period for a normal scan? Temporal changes in risk in patients with normal exercise sestamibi SPECT [abstract]. *Circulation* 1995;92:I-522.

(After telling a patient that his or her image was normal, how many times have we been asked, "OK, so I have a normal image. How long does the guarantee last?" Here, the duration of that "warranty" of a benign future and low event rate related to a normal or probably normal SPECT perfusion scintigram was evaluated. Here, the event rate was determined serially over a 3-yr period in a large number of patients undergoing myocardial perfusion scintigraphy [MPS] with normal or probably normal findings, with and without known coronary artery disease [CAD], in order to determine if there was a specific period after which the event rate escalated. Patients with CAD were noted to have a mild but significant bump in their event rate in their second yr of follow-up, whereas those without known CAD were noted to have a mild bump in event rate after 2–3 yr. The latter, increasing from 0.9 in yr 1 to 2.8 and 3.8 in the second and third follow-up yr was related well to age, with those older than 65 yr demonstrating a 4% event rate in the second poststudy year and those younger than 65 yr continuing to demonstrate a low event rate. This suggests, as well, the approximate necessary interval between MPS evaluations in patients thought to be at continued potential coronary risk.)

343. Brown KA, Rowen M. Prognostic value of a normal exercise myocardial perfusion imaging study in patients with angiographically significant coronary artery disease. *Am J Cardiol* 1993;71:865–867.

    (Among many studies involving more than 3500 patients spanning a variety of methods and including patients with known coronary artery disease, a normal stress myocardial perfusion scintigraphy carries an event rate <1%.)

344. Abdel-Farrah A, Kamal AM, Pancholy SS, et al. Prognostic implications of normal exercise tomographic thallium images in patients with angiographic evidence of significant coronary artery disease. *Am J Cardiol* 1994;74:769–771.

    (The article demonstrates that medically treated patients, even in the presence of coronary artery disease, have a benign prognosis in the presence of a normal myocardial perfusion scintigraphy. The event rate related to a normal stress echocardiogram far exceeds the hard event rate in patients with a negative stress perfusion scintigram, even in the presence of known coronary artery disease [*844*].)

345. Pavin D, Deloca J, Siegenthaler N, et al. Long-term (10-year) prognostic value of a normal thallium-201 myocardial exercise scintigram in patients with coronary artery disease documented by angiography. *Eur Heart J* 1997;18:69–77.

    (This article sought to assess the prognostic significance of a normal exercise thallium-201 myocardial perfusion scintigraphy [MPS] in patients with coronary artery disease [CAD]. Here, the incidence of cardiac death or infarction was studied in 69 symptomatic patients [group I] with normal exercise MPS without Q-wave infarction and with documented CAD, 136 patients [group II] with reversible defects on MPS and CAD and 102 patients [group III] with a normal exercise MPS and normal coronaries. Patients in group I had a higher incidence of single-vessel disease compared with those in group II [83% and 35%, respectively; $P < 0.0001$] and with more distal disease [55% and 23%, respectively; $P < 0.0001$]. Most patients in group I with normal images with CAD were treated medically [65%] with a low event rate [1 fatal and 8 nonfatal infarcts during 8.6 yr] and showed no difference in event rate between patients in group III and patients with normal images and no CAD. Patients with normal images in the presence of CAD generally have mild CAD and a good prognosis. Another study [*313*] demonstrates the infrequency of angiography among those with normal stress SPECT MPS and the low event rate associated with negative tests among those with or without angiography.)

346. Nallamothu N, Johnson JH, Bagheri B, et al. Utility of stress single-photon emission computed tomography (SPECT) perfusion imaging in predicting outcome after coronary artery bypass grafting. *Am J Cardiol* 1997;80:1517–1521.

    (Studied were the predictors of outcome in 255 patients with coronary artery disease, at a mean of 5 yr after coronary artery bypass graft [CABG]. SPECT variables of multivessel perfusion defects, defect size and lung uptake were predictors of death and all events by uni- and multivariate analysis. Stress SPECT myocardial perfusion scintigraphy was useful in stratifying patients after CABG.)

347. Soman P, Parsons A, Lahiri N, et al. The prognostic value of a normal Tc-99m sestamibi SPECT study in suspected coronary artery disease. *J Nucl Cardiol* 1999;6:252–256.

    (The investigators evaluated rates of death or nonfatal infarction over a 3-yr period among 473 patients with normal stress technetium-99m sestamibi SPECT myocardial perfusion scintigraphy. The population included 201 women, 89% with symptoms suggestive of coronary artery disease and 65% with abnormal stress tests. The annualized mortality rate was 0.2%, with no infarctions.)

348. Jain D, Joska T, Hamida A, et al. Prognostic significance of normal exercise myocardial perfusion imaging in conjunction with suboptimal workload [abstract]. *J Am Coll Cardiol* 1999;33:469A.

(Among 457 patients with a suboptimal stress test, normal exercise myocardial perfusion scintigraphy [MPS] and <85% of maximal predicted rate for age, those 188 with known coronary artery disease [CAD] had a higher hard cardiac event rate [3%/yr] and revascularization rate [7%/yr], than those 289 without documented CAD [1% and 1.1%/yr]. Those with normal MPS despite a suboptimal rate response had a low, 1.8% event rate. However, those with known CAD had a 3-fold greater event rate and a 7-fold greater revascularization rate than those without definite evidence of CAD. Further, in those with known CAD, but not in those without CAD documentation, event rates rose as achieved rate fell below the 85% level. Vasodilator pharmacologic stress MPS should be preferred in those with a suboptimal heart rate response and normal MPS, especially those with known CAD. Of course, those with image abnormalities or even typical symptoms and diagnostic electrocardiographic changes may provide satisfactory stress tests, even at a low achieved rate. What does this data say about the thesis of Mahmarian et al. [*464,671*] that negative tests on antianginal therapy, even at low achieved double product, are diagnostic of a good outcome? What does it say about the validity of pharmacologic stress testing with a beta blocker?)

349. Chatziioannou SN, Moore WH, Ford PV, et al. Prognostic value of myocardial perfusion imaging in patients with high exercise tolerance. *Circulation* 1999;99:867–872.

(Among 388 patients who reached stage IV of the Bruce protocol, 231 [59.5%] had normal and 157 [40.5%] had abnormal related myocardial perfusion scintigraphy [MPS] findings. In follow-up over 18 ± 2.7 mo, 19 had early revascularization related to the MPS findings and/or the patent condition and were not included in the analysis. Among 21 others with adverse events [late revascularization, myocardial infarction or death], 17 had abnormal MPS, which was shown by Cox proportional hazards regression analysis to be an excellent predictor of cardiac events in patients with high exercise tolerance. The addition of the Duke Treadmill Score did not improve the predictive power, and the addition of the stress electrocardiogram had no better predictive power than the MPS findings alone. Although high exercise tolerance makes events less likely, risk can be stratified well among appropriate members of this group with application of MPS.)

350. Applegate RJ, Dell'Italia LJ, Crawford MH. Usefulness of two-dimensional echocardiography during low-level exercise testing early after uncomplicated acute myocardial infarction. *Am J Cardiol* 1987;60:10–14.

(Postexercise left ventricular ejection fraction [LVEF] and decremental wall motion were prognostic parameters on exercise echocardiography performed in 17 patients after infarction. However, they could predict no more than 44%–63% of events, whereas negative findings presented an event rate of 13%–20%. Yet, wall motion is subjective and poorly reproducible and LVEF is never measured on stress echocardiography, because of studies demonstrating its inaccuracy and poor reproducibility. Unlike the early studies of MPS that served as a basis for subsequent developments, much of the early echocardiographic literature presents findings based on poorly reproducible data or methods since abandoned.)

351. Krivokapich J, Child JS, Gerber RS, et al. Prognostic usefulness of positive or negative exercise stress echocardiography for predicting events in ensuing twelve months. *Am J Cardiol* 1993;71:646–651.

(Although a positive stress echocardiogram presented a 3-fold higher event rate compared with a normal stress test, there was a 34% event rate with a positive test and a 10% event rate with a negative test. Although stress echocardiography has a high predictive value of a positive test, in some studies this is incredibly high, suggesting a selection process in which the positive echocardiographic response is nearly always related to an event. Conversely, too many studies demonstrate the high event rate of a normal stress echocardiographic response.)

352. Ryan T, Armstrong WF, O'Donnell JA, Feigenbaum H. Risk stratification after acute myocardial infarction by means of exercise two-dimensional echocardiography. *Am Heart J* 1987;114:1305–1311.

(Exercise echocardiography is more sensitive and specific than exercise electro-cardiography. Qualitative, induced wall motion abnormalities in the presence of rest abnormalities after infarction were diagnostic of events in 40 patients studied by exercise echocardiography. Even if we accept such data without questioning its objectivity and reproducibility, there was and remains no data permitting a graded risk stratification. Rather, the method simply claims to divide the postinfarct population into those with normal stress images without events and those with induced wall motion abnormalities who will have events. Such perfection in risk stratification has not stood up, and end points were soft. Desirable would be objective, quantifiable parameters that relate to hard end points in a continuous fashion.)

353. Picano E, Landi P, Bolognese L, et al. for the EPIC study group. Prognostic value of dipyridamole echocardiography early after acute myocardial infarction: a large scale, multicenter trial. *Am J Med* 1993;95:608–618.

(Picano et al. published the results of a large, prospective multicenter trial examining the efficacy of stress echocardiography after myocardial infarction. A total of 923 patients were considered in this analysis based upon recruitment from 11 different laboratories. Although new stress-induced wall motion abnormalities were the most powerful predictor of cardiac death, the rate of cardiac death in patients with normal scans was still 2%–3%. Thus, as in the other studies discussed, stress echocardiography failed to identify a patient cohort defined as low risk by the Agency for Health Care Policy Research Guidelines and who could be successfully managed without further testing [31]. The authors claim that dipyridamole echocardiography was an excellent prognostic method in patients after acute myocardial infarction. Others have been unable to demonstrate even the diagnostic value of the method.)

354. Miller DD, Heller G, Travin M, et al. Economic study of noninvasive economics group: a multicenter study of 2,737 patients examining the multivariate prognostic value of stress single photon emission computed tomography (SPECT) myocardial perfusion scintigraphy [abstract]. *J Am Coll Cardiol* 1996;27:286A.

(This is a comprehensive evaluation of the economic impact of the prognostic impact of stress myocardial perfusion scintigraphy.)

355. Maddahi J, Kiat H, Resser K, et al. Prediction of coronary events by Tl-201 quantitation of jeopardized myocardium and clinical and exercise variables. *J Nucl Med* 1988;29:770–778.

(The size of the quantitative planar perfusion defect was the most important predictor of events.)

356. Machecourt J, Longaere P, Fagret D, et al. Prognostic value of thallium-201 single photon emission computed tomographic myocardial perfusion imaging according to extent of myocardial defect. Study in 1926 patients with follow-up at 33 months. *J Am Coll Cardiol* 1994;23:1096–1102.

(Among this large number of patients with stable angina, a normal stress thallium-201 SPECT myocardial perfusion scintigraphy indicated a low-risk patient, and the extent of induced defect is an important prognostic predictive factor.)

357. Brown KA. Prognostic value of myocardial perfusion imaging: state of the art and new directions. *J Nucl Cardiol* 1996;3:516–537.

(Exercise testing alone appeared to be unsatisfactory for risk stratification after infarction, with a 25% sensitivity to events among 10 studies reviewed here, in which ST changes were themselves nonpredictive of events.)

358. Miller TD, Christian TF, Hodge DO, et al. Prognostic value of exercise Tl-201 perfusion imaging in a community population: overall mortality. *Am Heart J* 1998;135:663–670.
(Established as a prognostic tool in a tertiary care, referral setting, this study was performed to establish the prognostic value of exercise perfusion imaging among 446 residents of Olmstead, MN. Age, infarction history, lung uptake and the number of abnormal image segments were variables that contained the most independent information. Among those older than the mean population age [60 yr], the 5-yr survival in those with abnormal images was 84% compared with 97% among those with normal scans.)

359. Miller DD, Gersh BJ. Risk sensitive therapeutic strategies for coronary artery disease: toward testing-driven therapy in stable angina patients with low to intermediate risk cardiac imaging results. *J Nucl Cardiol* 1997;4:409–417.
(Presented is an analysis of the diagnostic and risk stratification strategies to identify patients with stable angina who are at lower risk for events but who would benefit greatly from aggressive medical management. Evidence presented makes a strong case for the cost-effective application of noninvasive stress perfusion imaging.)

360. Cohen MC, Curran PJ, L'Italien GJ, et al. Long-term prognostic value of preoperative dipyridamole thallium imaging and clinical indexes in patients with diabetes mellitus undergoing peripheral vascular surgery. *Am J Cardiol* 1999;83:1038–1042.
(Age, the presence of resting electrocardiographic abnormalities and an abnormal thallium scan were independent predictors of late death. Combined clinical and scan variables may identify a population in whom intensive medical or surgical interventions may be warranted to reduce both perioperative and late cardiac events.)

361. Shaw LJ, Hachamovitch R, Cohen M, et al. Cost implications of selective preoperative risk screening in the care of candidates for peripheral vascular operations. *Am J Managed Care* 1997;3:1817–1827.
(The authors developed a decision model based on the available literature. They found that the application of [pharmacologic] stress myocardial perfusion scintigraphy was cost effective, with much cost savings, for patients aged 60–80 yr and with intermediate pretest likelihood, with cost per quality-adjusted life year ranging from $33,338–$21,790, all well within acceptable values for practical clinical application, with increasing likelihood of coronary artery disease.)

362. Mathews T, Wongsuwan S, VanDecker W, et al. Outcome of patients with vasodilator-induced ST depression and normal SPECT perfusion imaging [abstract]. *J Am Coll Cardiol* 1999;33:448A.
(Among 2772 consecutive patients studied by adenosine or dipyridamole stress myocardial perfusion scintigraphy, 40 [1.4%], including 33 women, had induced ST depression and normal images. After a mean follow-up period of 22 mo, there were no "hard" events, but 3 patients went to revascularization. Although uncommon, normal images relate to a low hard event rate, even in association with vasodilator-induced ST changes.)

363. Narula J, Amanulla A, Petrov A, et al. Fate of negative adenosine SPECT perfusion images [abstract]. *J Am Coll Cardiol* 1999;33:479A.
(The authors studied 89 selected patients who had an initial normal adenosine stress SPECT myocardial perfusion scintigraphy and a second such study for clinical indications a mean of 21 ± 15 mo later. Thirty percent of studies became abnormal on the second evaluation. Image conversions were most likely to occur in association with typical symptoms or abnormal electrocardiography. Although the study is highly biased by patient selection, the "warranty period" may vary depending on disease likelihood.)

364. Fuster V, Badimon L, Badimon JJ, et al. The pathogenesis of coronary artery disease and the acute coronary syndromes. *N Engl J Med* 1992;326:242–250;310–318.
(This excellent review of the pathogenesis of coronary disease considers the variety of factors that relate to the development of atheromata and subsequent

occlusion. The latter relate to factors currently under investigation. Lesion stability or instability is probably as important prognostically as the degree of coronary stenosis. However, only the latter is addressed by stress testing methods.)

365. Wilson RF, Holiday MD, White CW. Quantitative angiographic morphology of coronary stenoses leading to myocardial infarction or unstable angina. *Circulation* 1986;73:286–294.

(This article excited many readers when it analyzed a group of patients who had serial coronary angiography for clinical indications before and after an infarction. Noted was the fact that there was a poor relationship between the initial distribution of stenoses and the vessel that will likely occlude with the subsequent event. In fact, quantitative coronary angiography supports the greater likelihood of significantly and severely stenotic vessels to occlude. However, within the methods of the study, many occlusions appeared to occur in normal or less than significantly stenotic vessels. In spite of the omission of many patients who were revascularized and the variable and often lengthy time between examinations, the article does support the fact that events are determined by more than the simple measurement of stenosis severity. The latter is among several factors determining events. Stress perfusion imaging is probably prognostic by virtue of its relationship to the total mass of atheromata, the ischemic burden, which in some indirect manner relates to the likelihood of occlusion.)

366. Farb AF, Tang AL, Burke AP, et al. Sudden cardiac death: frequency of active coronary lesions, inactive coronary lesions and myocardial infarction. *Circulation* 1995;95:1701–1709.

(Active lesions, determined morphologically, were seen in relation to 89% of acute infarctions but were seen in only 46% of those with healed infarction and in 50% of those with coronary disease but no prior infarction. The likelihood of coronary events, especially acute infarction, relates to dynamic coronary disease as well as to the total extent and severity of disease, the ischemic burden.)

367. Little WC, Constantinescu M, Applegate RJ, et al. Can coronary angiography predict the site of a subsequent myocardial infarction in patients with mild to moderate coronary artery disease? *Circulation* 1988;78:1157–1166.

(The coronary angiograms of 42 consecutive patients who underwent angiography both before and after an acute myocardial infarction were reviewed in an effort to determine whether anatomic lesions and angiographic stenosis can predict the site of subsequent coronary occlusion. Twenty-nine patients had a newly occluded vessel, 25 with at least 1 artery >50% stenotic. However, 19 of 29 [66%] arteries that subsequently occluded had <50% stenosis, and in 28 of 29 [97%] the initial stenosis was <70%. There was always some abnormality at the site of subsequent occlusion, and 10 of 29 [34%] vessels involved the most severe stenosis. There was no relationship between the severity of initial stenosis and the time of occlusion. This data suggests that the severity of coronary stenosis may be inadequate to predict the time or location of subsequent occlusion. However, patients with severe instrumented stenoses were excluded, and these retrospective studies included serial angiograms performed years apart.)

368. Ambrose JA, Fuster V. Can we predict future acute coronary events in patients with stable coronary artery disease? *JAMA* 1997;277:343–437.

(This is a thorough review of the science behind the relationship between stenosis severity and the likelihood of occlusion.)

369. Bateman TM. Impact of myocardial perfusion imaging on patient management implications for cost-effectiveness. *Perspect Nucl Cardiol* 1997;3:3–6.

(The cost-effective nature of stress myocardial perfusion scintigraphy is considered.)

370. Giroud D, Li JM, Urban P, et al. Relation of the site of acute myocardial infarction to the most severe coronary arterial stenosis at prior angiography. *Am J Cardiol* 1992;69:729–732.

(Serial coronary angiograms were performed in 92 patients soon after and at a variable time [1–144 mo] preceding an acute myocardial infarction. On the second angiogram, the site of occlusion was related to the previously most stenotic vessel in only 29 [32%] patients and 72 [78%] of responsible vessels had less than significant stenosis. All those with revascularization between the 2 angiograms were excluded.)

371. Alderman EL, Corley SD, Fisher LD, et al. Five-year angiographic follow-up of factors associated with progression of coronary artery disease in the Coronary Artery Surgery Study (CASS). *J Am Coll Cardiol* 1993;22:1141–1154.

(The original CASS randomized 780 patients to medical or surgical therapy. It demonstrated the benefits of surgery when ventricular dysfunction with left ventricular ejection fraction [LVEF] <50%. Unlike other studies, there was no benefit of revascularization with advanced left main or 3-vessel disease and preserved LV function. These findings were later confirmed on 10-yr follow-up. Five participating institutions performed serial angiography on >50% of their randomized subjects, seeking factors that might indicate likely disease and stenosis progression.

Lesion severity was 1 factor, with lesion morphology, that correlated with subsequent occlusion. When analyzed quantitatively, on a vessel-by-vessel basis, and because of the inverse relationship between lesion severity and the percentage incidence of such vessels, the likelihood of an event precipitated by occlusion of a tightly stenotic vessel far exceeds that related to occlusion of any insignificantly stenotic vessel, even when most events occur in less stenotic vessels.)

372. Nagakomi A, Celermajer DS, Lumley T, et al. Angiographic coronary narrowing is a surrogate marker for the extent of coronary atherosclerosis. *Am J Cardiol* 1996;78:516–519.

(The authors sought to determine the relationship between the severity of coronary artery disease and the extent of coronary atherosclerosis in 350 consecutive patients referred for elective angiography. There was a strong linear relationship between coronary disease severity and the extent of coronary involvement [atherosclerosis]. This may explain the relationship between the number of vessels with obstructive lesions and subsequent coronary events, although many such events occur at sites of minor plaque and stenosis.)

373. Frais M, Botvinick EH, Shosa D, O'Connell W. Are regions of ischemia detected on stress perfusion scintigraphy predictive of sites of subsequent myocardial infarction? *Br Heart J* 1982;47:357–364.

374. Morris S, Mascitelli VA, Lawrence DS, et al. Acute Tc-99m SPECT myocardial perfusion imaging during spontaneous angina and stress imaging: the same defect, same location [abstract]? *Circulation* 1995;92:I-677.

(373,374: Contrary to the demonstrated lack of correlation between lesion severity and subsequent infarction, these works demonstrate the excellent relationship between the location of new infarction and the area of prior exercise-induced scintigraphic defect. Reference *373* correlates the location of infarction to that of prior stress-induced ischemia, and *374* relates regions of stress-induced malperfusion to the defect noted on the subsequent acute presentation with chest pain.)

375. Miller GL, Herman SD, Heller GV, et al. Relation between perfusion defects on stress Tc-99m sestamibi SPECT scintigraphy and the location of a subsequent acute myocardial infarction. *Am J Cardiol* 1996;78:26–30.

(In this study, most infarctions occurred in regions with defects on prior imaging study and previously demonstrated myocardium at ischemic risk among 25 patients who had an acute infarction some time after perfusion scintigraphy. The location of new infarction related well to the area of prior exercise-induced scintigraphic defect when infarction occurred spontaneously, and the area at risk accurately paralleled the area subsequently lost.)

376. Galvin JM, Brown KA. The site of acute myocardial infarction is related to the coronary territory of transient defects on prior myocardial perfusion imaging. *J Nucl Cardiol* 1996;3:382–388.

(Records of 34 patients with transient defects on myocardial perfusion scintigraphy [MPS] performed before an acute infarction were reviewed. Among those 14 with infarction <2 yr after the scan, 11 had infarction in the region of induced ischemia but only 5 of 20 studied during 2 yr before infarction had infarction in the ischemic zone. There was a strong correlation between regional ischemia and the sight of subsequent infarction when MPS was performed in relatively close temporal relation to the subsequent event.)

377. Klausner S, Botvinick E, Shames D, et al. The application of radionuclide infarct scintigraphy to diagnose perioperative myocardial infarction following revascularization. *Circulation* 1977;56:173–178.

378. Klausner S, Botvinick E, Shames D, et al. Scintigraphic distribution of acute myocardial infarction after cardiac surgery. *Herz* 1977;2:171–177.

    (377,378: In this study [377] and the summary report [378], infarction again appeared to occur in relation to the most severe stenosis. An exception related to infarcts occurring perioperatively after bypass surgery, in which the relationship was more variable, as may be expected, because intraoperative events and surgical technique strongly influence natural pathophysiology.)

379. Hoeg JM. Evaluating coronary heart disease risk. Tiles in the mosaic. *JAMA* 1997;277:1387–1390.

    (The "ischemic burden" appears to be generally well correlated with the coronary flow reserve. The findings on stress perfusion imaging provide the best available correlation with the the coronary flow reserve and "ischemic burden.")

380. Miller DD, Shaw LJ, Travin MI, Heller GV. Downstream economic impact of failing to document myocardial ischemia before coronary angiography in stable angina patients. *Circulation* 1994;94:160–168.

    (Once the risk of cardiac events is established, aggressive or conservative management can be appropriately applied. The lack of adequate prognostication results in the failure to deliver adequate treatment and the subsequent clinical and ecomomic costs.)

381. Udelson JE, Bonow RO, Allman KC, Dilzisian V, et al. Wintergreen panel summaries. Assessing myocardial viability in left ventricular dysfunction and heart failure. *J Nucl Cardiol* 1999;6:156–172.

    (This is a review and summary statement from a large panel of researchers on scintigraphic methods for viability assessment. Also presented is a statement of the needs and yet unachieved goals in this area and suggestions regarding the most desirable direction of future investigation.)

382. Shaw LJ, Kesler KL, Marwick TH, et al. Development of a stress myocardial perfusion imaging model to predict cardiac death [abstract]. *Circulation* 1996;94:I-20.
    (The high-risk perfuson scan is considered.)

383. Iskandrian AS, Johnson J, Le TT, et al. Comparison of the treadmill score and single-photon emission computed tomographic thallium imaging in risk assessment. *J Nucl Cardiol* 1995;1:144–149.

    (In this study of 503 patients, the prognostic information of stress thallium-201 SPECT was additive to that supplied by the stress test itself and clinical data.)

384. National Cooperative Study Group: Unstable Angina. National Cooperative Study group to compare surgical and medical therapy. II: In-hospital experience and initial follow-up results in patients with one, two and three vessel disease. *Am J Cardiol* 1978;42:839–848.

    (This is 1 of several clinical trials in patients with unstable angina that has demonstrated the lack of significant differences in the rate of death or nonfatal infarction among those with unstable angina treated medically or with revascularization. However, in the Veterans Affairs Study [385], those with reduced left ventricular ejection fraction treated medically did worse than those treated with coronary artery bypass graft.)

385. Scott SM, Deupree RH, Sharma GVRK, Luchi RJ. VA study of unstable angina: 10 year results show duration of surgical advantage for patients with impaired ejection fraction. *Circulation* 1994;90(suppl):120–123.

(The surgical survival advantage over medical therapy among patients with unstable angina and reduced left ventricular ejection fraction was maintained for 5 yr but diminished at 10 yr after onset.)

386. Luchi RJ, Scott SM, Deupree RH. Comparison of medical and surgical treatment for unstable angina. *N Engl J Med* 1987;316:977–984.

(This prospective study of 468 men with unstable angina divided into medical and surgical groups found no difference in outcome unless there was a reduced left ventricular ejection fraction [LVEF]. The curves relating survival to LVEF were different for the groups and demonstrated a benefit of coronary artery bypass graft when LVEF is reduced.)

387. The TIMI IIIB Investigators. Effects of tissue plasminogen activator and a comparison of early invasive and conservative strategies in unstable angina and non-Q-wave myocardial infarction. *Circulation* 1994;89:1545–1556.

(The study evaluated 1473 patients with unstable angina or non-Q myocardial infarction seeking the benefit of thrombolysis versus medical therapy and also an early revascularization therapy with medical therapy. Overall mortality was low [2.4%], as was infarction or reinfarction [6.3%] at 6 wk. This was true employing an early aggressive or conservative approach. The former reduced hospital days and use of antianginal drugs. Thrombolysis was not beneficial and was potentially harmful.)

388. Anderson HV, Cannon CP, Stone PH, et al. One year results of the thrombolysis in myocardial infarction TIMI Phase IIIB clinical trial. A randomized comparison of tissue type plasminogen activator versus placebo and early invasive versus early conservative strategies in unstable anginal and non-Q wave myocardial infarction. *J Am Coll Cardiol* 1995;26:1643–1650.

(The TIMI IIIB Trial randomized 1473 patients with unstable angina or a non-Q infarction to an invasive approach with angiography within 48 hr or conservative management with angiography only for refractory angina or evidence of ischemia on stress electrocardiography or perfusion image. The overall mortality and infarction rate was 6% and did not differ between management groups.)

389. Theroux P, Waters D, Qiu S, et al. Aspirin versus heparin to prevent myocardial infarction during the acute phase of unstable angina. *Circulation* 1993;88:2045–2048.

(This article presents data demonstrating that heparin prevents myocardial infarction better than aspirin during the acute phase of unstable angina.)

390. Grambow DW, Topol EJ. Effect of maximal medical therapy on refractoriness of unstable angina patients who respond to medical treatment. *Am J Cardiol* 1992;70:557–581.

(A group of 125 patients with unstable angina were studied over a 5-yr period to define the incidence of refractory unstable angina in this time of advanced drug therapy. Refractory chest pain was noted in 8.8% of those treated with maximal aggressive medical therapy. The rate of acute myocardial infarction or death among those managed medically was 3%. In-hospital strategies included continued medical management [32%], percutaneous transluminal coronary angioplasty [40%] and coronary artery bypass graft [27%].)

391. Wilcox I, Freedman SB, Allman KC, et al. Prognostic significance of a predischarge exercise test in patients with suspected unstable coronary artery disease. *Am J Cardiol* 1991;18:677–683.

(The exercise test performed at predischarge provided independent prognostic information to clinical and electrocardiographic data in medically treated patients with unstable angina. Of course, stress myocardial perfusion scintigraphy provides better risk stratification.)

392. Butman SM, Olsen HG, Gardin JM, et al. Submaximal exercise testing after stabilization of unstable angina pectoris. *J Am Coll Cardiol* 1984;4:667–673.

(In stabilized patients with unstable angina, submaximal exercise testing demonstrated an ability to predict the outcome in the first year after hospital discharge. Those with a positive test should be considered for further diagnostic studies.)

393. Swahn E, Magnus A, Berglund U, et al. Predictive importance of clinical findings and a predischarge exercise test in patients with suspected unstable coronary artery disease. *Am J Cardiol* 1987;59:208–214.

(In a study of 13,500 patients, induced ST depression did identify a higher-risk group, yet even "low risk" was substantial, and 26% of these patients had a previous non-Q infarction.

A variety of studies present evidence that myocardial perfusion imaging and specifically reversible defects may provide prognostic data that could assess risk in patients with unstable angina and so help guide medical therapy.)

394. Brown KA. Prognostic value of thallium-201 myocardial perfusion imaging in patients with unstable angina who respond to medical treatment. *J Am Coll Cardiol* 1991;17:1053–1057.

(Among 52 unstable angina patients studied with exercise myocardial perfusion scintigraphy by Brown, the only significant predictor of hard events among all clinical and exercise variables was the presence of a reversible defect. Those with reversible defects had a hard event rate of 26%, whereas those with none had a 3% rate over the 39 mo of the study [<1%/year]. The stress electrocardiograph had no prognostic value in these patients.)

395. Stratmann HG, Younis LT, Wittry MD, et al. Exercise technetium-99m myocardial tomography for the risk stratification of men with medically treated unstable angina pectoris. *Am J Cardiol* 1995;76:236–240.

(The prognostic value of predischarge maximal exercise SPECT sestamibi myocardial perfusion scintigraphy [MPS] was evaluated in 126 consecutive men hospitalized and stabilized medically with unstable angina. There were 35 events, including cardiac death [5], nonfatal infarction [6] and rehospitalization for unstable angina [24] over a 1-yr follow-up. Any event occurred in 12% with normal images, 39% with abnormal images and 60% with reversible defects. There was a 2% hard event rate with normal scans, compared with 14% with abnormal scans and 29% with reversible defects. Stress MPS is an excellent way to risk stratify patients with unstable angina.)

396. Madsen JK, Stubgaard M, Utne HE, et al. Prognosis and thallium-201 scintigraphy in patients admitted with chest pain without confirmed acute myocardial infarction. *Br Heart J* 1998;59:184–189.

(Madsen et al. found that 21% of those with [compared to only 3% of those without] a reversible defect on symptom-limited stress myocardial perfusion scintigraphy, performed after admission for a noninfarction chest pain syndrome, suffered a nonfatal infarction or death over a mean 14-mo follow-up period.)

397. Brown KA. Management of unstable angina: the role of noninvasive risk stratification. In: Maddahi J, Iskandrian A, eds. Nuclear cardiology and managed care: from challenge to opportunity. *J Nucl Cardiol* 1997;4(suppl):S164–S168.

(The value of stress *MPS* in the diagnosis and risk stratification of unstable angina is examined.)

398. Hillert MC, Narahara KA, Smitherman TC, et al. Thallium-201 perfusion imaging after the treatment of unstable angina pectoris: relationship to clinical outcome. *West J Med* 1996;145:335–340.

(Hillert et al. found that 15 of 19 patients with reversible thallium-201 defects suffered infarction or recurrent unstable angina compared with 2 of 18 [$P < 0.001$] without evidence of redistribution on 12-wk follow-up.)

399. Marmur JD, Freeman MR, Langer A, Armstrong PW. Prognosis in medically stabilized unstable angina: early Holter ST monitoring compared with predischarge exercise thallium tomography. *Ann Int Med* 1990;113:575–581.

(Marmur et al. evaluated the predictive value of a positive stress electrocardiogram, stress myocardial perfusion scintigraphy, Holter and coronary angiogram in 54 patients presenting with unstable angina and found that the only predictor of events was the presence of reversible defects.)

400. Christian TF, Clements IP, Gibbons RJ. Noninvasive identification of myocardium at risk in patients with acute myocardial infarction and nondiagnostic electrocardiograms with technetium-99m sestamibi. *Circulation* 1991;83:1615–1620.

(Here, 14 patients with typical symptoms of acute infarction but without diagnostic electrocardiographic [ECG] changes were studied with rest perfusion scintigraphy. Twelve had gross image defects, and 11 of these had occluded related coronary arteries. Perfusion scintigrams in the acute presenting stage of infarction may identify a subgroup who could benefit from thrombolysis, even though they did not demonstrate classic ECG changes. The area of myocardium at risk was not insignificant, averaging 21% of the left ventricle.)

401. Zhu YY, Botvinick EH, Dae MW, et al. Dipyridamole perfusion scintigraphy: the experience with its application in 170 patients with known or suspected unstable angina. *Am Heart J* 1991;121:33–40.

(Presented are the safety, accuracy and potential clinical utility of dipyridamole perfusion scintigraphy with thallium-201 in 170 consecutive patients, 78 with suspected and 92 with known unstable angina. The method was safe and diagnostically accurate even in the sickest patients, including some on nitroglycerin drips and 1 with an intra-aortic balloon pump. Those studied with suspected unstable angina were among those tested, for diagnostic reasons, in the setting of atypical rest chest pain. Those studied with known unstable angina were generally so evaluated to assess the extent and location of myocardium at ischemic risk, often with the thought of performing a "culprit" angioplasty.)

402. Wackers FJTh, Lie KI, Liem KL, et al. Potential value of thallium-201 scintigraphy as a means of selecting patients for the coronary care unit. *Br Heart J* 1979;41:111–117.

(An apparent strong advantage of the scintigraphic method in the emergency department is its ability to identify abnormalities in the setting of unstable angina, even hours after pain resolution, as documented here. The findings in this classic report have been reproduced in many studies applied more recently to similar populations and noted above.)

403. Stratmann HG, Tamesis BR, Younis LT, et al. Prognostic value of predischarge dipyridamole technetium-99m sestamibi myocardial tomography in medically treated patients with unstable angina. *Am Heart J* 1995;130:734–740.

(Stratmann et al. performed myocardial perfusion scintigraphy before discharge in 128 medically treated patients with unstable angina who were at intermediate pretest clinical risk. They were then followed for 16 ± 11 mo. Events, both "hard" and "soft," were noted in 10% with normal studies and 69% with defects [$P < 0.01$], and the scan findings were the only independent predictors of outcome. It appears that a noninvasive strategy of risk stratification based in stress perfusion imaging can separate well high- from low-risk subgroups and serve as a basis for selecting those most likely to benefit from aggressive management.)

404. Nyman I, Larsson H, Areskog M. The predictive value of silent ischemia at an exercise test before discharge after an initial episode of unstable coronary artery disease. RISC study group. *Am Heart J* 1992;123:324–331.

405. Madsen JK, Thomsen BI, Mellemgaard K. Independent prognostic risk factors for patients referred because of suspected acute myocardial infarction without

confirmed diagnosis. Prognosis after discharge in relation to medical history and non-invasive investigations. *Br Heart J* 1988;9:611–618.

(404,405: The perfusion scintigraphic method is particularly applicable in patients who have minimal risk factors or in patients with clear-cut unstable angina who respond quickly to medical therapy. In these medically stabilized patients, either exercise or pharmacological stress testing with perfusion imaging can effectively stratify patients into low- and high-risk subsets.)

406. Lin SS, Lauer MS, Marwick TH. Risk stratification of patients with medically treated unstable angina using exercise echocardiography. *Am J Cardiol* 1998;82:720–724.

(The "incremental prognostic value" of exercise echocardiography was evaluated in 226 consecutive patients studied with medically treated unstable angina. Clinical risk was low in 108, intermediate in 116 and high in 2 by the Unstable Angina Guidelines [31]. Ischemia was identified by stress electrocardiography [ECG] in 33 patients and by stress echocardiography in 55 patients. Overall, 38 patients had early revascularization and 28 suffered cardiac death, nonfatal infarction or late revascularization. Although an ischemic echocardiographic finding at stress was associated with a 9% overall 1-yr event rate, a negative study had a 3% event rate, figures that were not clinically different from the 8% and 3.5% rates of stress ECG! A negative echocardiogram had an unacceptably high level of related events.)

407. Lee TH, Rouan GW, Weisberg MC, et al. Clinical characteristics and natural history of patients with acute myocardial infarction sent home from the emergency room. *Am J Cardiol* 1987;60:219–224.

(Discharge from the emergency department with an acute myocardial infarction is associated with a poor outcome, and a missed acute myocardial infarction is the leading cause of medical malpractice litigation. For these reasons, most physicians treat presenting patients conservatively and admit too many patients to the hospital with what eventually prove to be noncardiac chest pains. Because of this practice, acute infarctions amount to <30% of critical care unit admissions. Although the group with ruled-out myocardial infarctions have excellent short-term prognoses, they absorb most of the costs.)

408. Gaspoz J-M, Lee TH, Weinstein MC, et al. Cost-effectiveness of a new short-stay unit to "rule-out" acute myocardial infarction in low risk patients. *J Am Coll Cardiol* 1994;24:1249–1259.

(Alternatives to the coronary care unit for patients with low-to-moderate likelihood [risk] are being developed and applied. Coronary observation units are being developed in order to reduce the length of stay and the intensity of nursing care after admission of patients with a low likelihood of myocardial infarction. This is an early analysis.)

409. Goldman L, Cook EF, Brand DA, et al. A computer protocol to predict myocardial infarction in emergency department patients with chest pain. *N Engl J Med* 1988;318:797–803.

(Based on population studies relating the rest electrocardiogram and available clinical parameters to the likelihood of infarction, the application of clinical algorithms is the simplest approach to estimate the risk of acute myocardial infarction in patients presenting to the emergency department with possible acute infarction.)

410. Lee TH, Jarez G, Cook EF, et al. Ruling out acute myocardial infarction. A prospective multicenter validation of a 12-hour strategy for patients at low risk. *N Engl J Med* 1991;324:1239–1246.

(In 2684 patients, Lee et al. prospectively validated an algorithm predicting the risk of acute myocardial infarction based on both clinical and electrocardiographic [ECG] data acquired in the emergency department. Overall, 331 [35%] of those patients assigned to the low-risk group with normal or nondiagnostic ECG had a final diagnosis of either acute myocardial infarction or unstable angina.)

411. Goldman L, Cook EF, Johnson PA, et al. Prediction of the need for intensive care in patients who present to emergency departments with acute chest pain. *N Engl J Med* 1996;334:1498–1504.

(When separating out the very high- and very low-risk patients, many in the intermediate category are left in limbo without diagnosis or an approach to management.)

412. Adams JE, Bodor GS, Davila Roman VG, et al. Cardiac troponin I. A marker with high specificity for cardiac injury. *Circulation* 1993;88:101–106.

(Cardiac enzymes, including creatinine kinase isoforms, troponins T and I, and myoglobin, offer considerable promise for speeding the diagnosis of acute myocardial infarction and increasing the specificity of this diagnosis.)

413. Duca M, Giri S, Wu AHB, et al. Comparison of acute rest perfusion imaging and serum markers of myocardial injury in patients with chest pain syndromes. *J Nucl Med* 1999;6:570–576.

(When Duca et al. studied the appearance of image abnormalities and elevation of troponin I and T among 75 patients admitted to the emergency department with chest pain and a nondiagnostic electrocardiogram, acute rest sestamibi/tetrofosmin was more sensitive for acute myocardial infarction diagnosis than serum enzymes, with preserved specificity.)

414. Lewis WR, Amsterdam EA. Utility and safety of immediate exercise testing of low-risk patients admitted to the hospital for suspected acute myocardial infarction. *Am J Cardiol* 1994;74:987–990.

(Stress testing alone appeared adequate to triage chest pain patients in this early study. But did test results contribute to patient management in this very low-likelihood population?)

415. Kirp JD, Turnispseed S, Lewis WR, Amsterdam EA. Evaluation of chest pain in low-risk patients presenting to the emergency department: the role of the immediate exercise testing. *Ann Emerg Med* 1998;32:1–7.

(Twenty-eight [13%] patients had positive exercise electrocardiograms. Of these patients, 23 had further evaluation that revealed evidence of coronary artery disease in 13 [57%]. Negative exercise test results were recorded in 125 [59%] patients, and 59 [28%] had nondiagnostic tests. All patients with negative stress tests and 93% with nondiagnostic exercise tests were discharged directly from the emergency department. Thirty-day follow-up was done in 201 [95%] patients and revealed no myocardial infarction or death in any patient. One patient with positive exercise test presented within 30 days with mild congestive heart failure.)

416. Stomel R, Grant R, Eagle KA. Lessons learned from a community hospital chest pain center. *Am J Cardiol* 1999;83:1033–1037.

(Stomel et al. reported on the effects of the establishment of a chest pain center, with the implementation of stress-testing screening in patients presenting with chest pain syndromes with intermediate risk. Hospital admissions fell 21%, and referral to the center increased 1726%. Among 333 patients with an intermediate risk, there were no deaths and only 1 non-Q infarction. However, stress testing was normal in 11 who were subsequently proven to have coronary artery disease, 4 with revascularization. Nine false positives were recorded among 13 patients with positive stress tests!)

417. Stein JH, Neumann A, Preston LM, et al. Admission echocardiography predicts in-hospital cardiac events in patients with unstable angina [abstract]. *J Am Coll Cardiol* 1996;27:377A.

(The authors studied 63 patients with unstable angina with an echocardiogram at admission and demonstrated a high sensitivity and poor specificity for outcome events in patients with unstable angina.)

418. Gibler WB, Runyon JP, Levy RC, et al. A rapid diagnostic and treatment center for patients with chest pain in the emergency department. *Ann Emerg Med* 1995;25:1–8.

(Here, the sensitivity of wall motion abnormalities was reduced in the absence of chest pain, and echocardiography was of little value when performed late, ~5 hr after presentation.)

419. Sabia P, Afrookteh A, Touchstone DA, et al. Value of regional wall motion abnormality in the emergency room diagnosis of acute myocardial infarction: a prospective study using two-dimensional echocardiography. *Circulation* 1991;84(suppl I):I-85–I-92.

(The authors applied 2-dimensional echocardiography in 180 high-risk patients presenting to the emergency department. There was a finite failure rate. Diagnostic criteria included segmental wall motion abnormalities in a coronary distribution. However, diffuse wall motion abnormalities were taken as noncoronary in origin. Among 30 patients with acute myocardial infarction [AMI], 27 [90%] had segmental wall motion abnormalities, only 9 with diagnostic electrocardiographic changes. However, 60 others without AMI also had segmental abnormalities! Diffuse wall motion abnormalities were seen in 22 [13%], none with AMI. If diffuse abnormalities were excluded, sensitivity of segmental abnormalities was 93% with a specificity 49%, a predictive value of a negative test of 100% and a predictive value of a positive test of only 31%. However, in other studies, diffuse wall motion abnormalities, taken as evidence of ischemic disease and compatible with AMI, were associated with AMI and added to test sensitivity.)

420. Jesse RL, Kontos MC. Evaluation of chest pain in the emergency department. *Curr Prob Cardiol* 1997;22:149–236.

(The authors demonstrated a high [100%] sensitivity in 89 patients with transmural myocardial infarction [MI] and a modest [86%] sensitivity in 79 patients with a non-Q MI, using rest echocardiography. Overall there was difficulty recognizing wall motion abnormalities with small transmural or non-Q MI, and diffuse wall motion abnormalities were nonspecific for coronary artery disease.)

421. Kontos MC, Arrowood JA, Paulson WH, et al. Ability of echocardiography in the emergency department to detect myocardial ischemia in patients presenting with chest pain [abstract]. *J Am Soc Echocardiol* 1995;8:346A.

(The authors studied 140 patients with possible acute coronary syndromes by rest echocardiography. The sensitivity for identification of an acute coronary syndrome was 84% with a negative predictive value of 82%.)

422. Trippi JA, Kopp G, Lee KS, et al. The feasibility of dobutamine stress echocardiography in the emergency department with telemedicine interpretation. *J Am Soc Echocardiol* 1996;9:113–118.

(Dobutamine stress echocardiography was performed by the on-call ultrasonographer and emergency department staff. The study was then transmitted to the on-call cardiologist, who read the study on a lap-top computer. The discharge of 41 patients after a normal dobutamine stress echocardiogram brought a decrease in costs without adverse events at 30 days.)

423. Wackers FJTh, Lie KI, Liem KL, et al. Thallium-201 scintigraphy in unstable angina pectoris. *Circulation* 1978;57:738–742.

(Wackers et al. imaged 98 patients with chest pain after acute myocardial infarction was "ruled out." They found 57% of images studied within 6 hr of chest pain resolution were positive, but only 8% were abnormal if imaged >12 hr after pain resolution. An abnormal scan with an abnormal, albeit nonspecific, electrocardiogram predicted a poor outcome, with a 94% sensitivity.)

424. Wackers FJTh, Lie KI, Liem KL, et al. Potential value of thallium-201 scintigraphy as a means of selecting patients for the coronary care unit. *Br Heart J* 1979;41:111–117.

(Wackers et al. imaged 203 patients with atypical histories and nondiagnostic electrocardiography within weeks of their last chest pain episode. All 34 with infarction and 27 [58%] of those with unstable angina were positive, but none were abnormal among 98 patients with stable angina or noncardiac chest pain.)

425. Van der Wieken LR, Kan G, Belfer AJ, et al. Thallium-201 scanning to decide CCU admission in patients with non-diagnostic electrocardiograms. *Int J Cardiol* 1983;4:285–295.

(The authors imaged 149 patients admitted to rule out acute myocardial infarction [AMI] without prior histories and with normal or nondiagnostic electrocardiography a mean of 5 hr from the last chest pain. They found 39 of 57 abnormal scans among those with MI, a 90% sensitivity and 80% specificity for AMI, with a positive predictive value of 61% and a negative predictive value of 96%. If 13 equivocal scans were called abnormal, the sensitivity was 97% with a negative predictive value of 99%.)

426. Wackers FJTh, Busemann-Sokole E, Samson G, et al. Value and limitations of thallium-201 scintigraphy in the acute phase of myocardial infarction. *N Engl J Med* 1976;295:1–5.

(Wackers et al. imaged 200 myocardial infarction patients with planar thallium-201 within 10 days of symptom onset. Images were abnormal in 83%, including all those studied within 6 hr.)

427. Bilodeau L, Theroux P, Gregoire J, et al. Technetium-99m sestamibi tomography in patients with spontaneous chest pain: correlations with clinical, electrocardiographic and angiographic findings. *J Am Coll Cardiol* 1991;18:1684–1691.

(Patients with spontaneous chest pain were studied with rest perfusion imaging. Bilodeau et al. imaged 45 patients who were admitted for unstable angina without prior infarction. There was a 96% sensitivity and 79% specificity for the diagnosis of cardiac pain when patients were imaged during active chest pain. However, the electrocardiogram acquired during active chest pain demonstrated a sensitivity of 65%.

The method was able to visualize the regional abnormalities and subsequent resolution well and was more sensitive and specific than the rest electrocardiogram. The image defects correlated well with angiography and provided important diagnostic and localizing information that impacts management.

Myocardial perfusion scintigraphy is of great potential clinical value in patients with spontaneous chest pain and thrombolytic therapy. Here, the lack of redistribution of the technetium-99m–based agent sestamibi provides the needed logistics for appropriate application. The agent may be injected at the time of presentation, with imaging hours after instrumentation and when stable. This image reflects the presenting perfusion deficit and can then be compared with a subsequent rest study performed after reperfusion to assess myocardium salvaged.)

428. Gregoire J, Theroux P. Detection and assessment of unstable angina using myocardial perfusion imaging: comparison between technetium-99m sestamibi SPECT and 12-lead electrocardiogram. *Am J Cardiol* 190;66:42E–46E.

(Myocardial perfusion scintigraphy has been applied as well to the diagnostic and prognostic evaluation of patients with unstable angina, the implications and distribution of acute myocardial infarction, the effects of thrombolysis and acute percutaneous transluminal coronary angioplasty.)

429. Varetto T, Cantalupe D, Altieri A, Orlandi C. Emergency room technetium-99m sestamibi imaging to rule out acute myocardial ischemic events in patients with nondiagnostic electrocardiograms. *J Am Coll Cardiol* 1993;22:1804–1808.

(The authors studied 64 patients in an effort to determine the value of rest SPECT technetium-99m sestamibi myocardial perfusion scintigraphy in the emergency department. There were image abnormalities in 30 patients; 13 with acute infarction and 14 others with proven coronary artery disease [CAD]. None of the 34 with normal images was shown to have CAD. All 6 events occurred in those with image abnormalities.)

430. Hilton TC, Thompson RC, Williams HJ, et al. Technetium-99m sestamibi myocardial perfusion imaging in the emergency room for evaluation of chest pain. *J Am Coll Cardiol* 1994;23:1016–1022.

(This article rekindled interest in the application of rest technetium-99m [^{99m}Tc] myocardial perfusion scintigraphy [MPS] for the triage of patients presenting to the emergency department with chest pain and a normal or nondiagnostic electrocardiogram [ECG]. Here, 102 patients with ongoing typical chest pain and a normal or nondiagnostic ECG were studied with rest SPECT ^{99m}Tc sestamibi MPS. Multivariate analysis identified scan abnormalities as the only independent predictor of adverse cardiac events [$P = 0.009$]. Only 1 of 70 [1.4%] with a normal scan had a subsequent event, whereas 2 of 15 [13%] with equivocal scans and 12 of 17 [71%] abnormal scans had events [$P = 0.004$]. The method was highly accurate in an otherwise ambiguous population.)

431. Hilton TC, Fulmer H, Abuan T, et al. Ninety-day follow-up of patients in the emergency department with chest pain who undergo initial single-photon emission computed tomographic perfusion scintigraphy with technetium 99m labeled sestamibi. *J Nucl Cardiol* 1997;4:174–177.

(Here, 150 patients with typical chest pain and a normal or nondiagnostic electrocardiogram were studied with rest SPECT technetium-99m sestamibi myocardial perfusion scintigraphy [MPS] and followed for >90 days. The results duplicated those in the authors' earlier study [442] demonstrating that the previously observed excellent prognostic ability of the rest MPS method extends over at least 90 days.

Both 434 and 435 were studies in patients injected during ongoing chest pain. Clearly, sensitivity would be expected to fall with time after pain resolution.)

432. Stowers SA. Myocardial perfusion scintigraphy for assessment of acute ischemia syndromes: can we seize the moment? *J Nucl Cardiol* 1995;2:274–277.

433. Wackers FJTh, Heller GV, Stowers SA, et al. Normal rest tetrofosmin SPECT imaging in patients with chest pain and normal or nondiagnostic ECG in the emergency department is associated with lower need for subsequent cardiac catheterization and revascularization [abstract]. *J Am Coll Cardiol* 1997;29:196A.

(Wackers et al. demonstrated the benefits of a normal rest SPECT perfusion image performed with tetrofosmin in patients presenting to the emergency department with chest pain and normal or nondiagnostic electrocardiography.)

434. Tatum JL, Ornato JP, Jesse RL, et al. A diagnostic strategy using Tc-99m sestamibi for evaluation of patients with chest pain in the emergency room [abstract]. *Circulation* 1994;90:I-367.

(Tatum et al. studied 135 patients presenting to the emergency department with chest pain with rest SPECT sestamibi imaging. There were 27 with abnormal images, 18 among 19 [95%] with coronary artery disease [CAD] and acute myocardial infarction or unstable angina. Among 88 with normal images, coronary disease was documented in only 1, an overall specificity of 88% [87/96], with a positive and negative predictive values of 67% and 98%, respectively. There were wall motion abnormalities in 8 patients who did not have CAD.)

435. Radensky PW, Hilton TC, Fulmer H, et al. Potential cost effectiveness of initial myocardial perfusion imaging for assessment of emergency department patients with chest pain. *Am J Cardiol* 1997:79:595–599.

(Radensky et al. studied the potential cost effectiveness of initial myocardial perfusion imaging for the triage of patients presenting to the emergency department [ED] with chest pain. In the "scan strategy," those with abnormal images were admitted, whereas those with normal scans were sent home. The "no scan strategy" employed clinical and electrocardiographic variables to triage patients. Those with >3 risk factors or abnormalities were admitted, whereas all others were sent home. The costs were lowest among patients discharged from the ED [$715 per patient].

Overall, the scan strategy cost $5,019 per patient, and the no scan strategy cost $6,051 per patient.)

436. Tatum JL, Jesse RL, Kontos MC, et al. Comprehensive strategy for evaluation of the patient presenting to the emergency department with chest pain. *Ann Emerg Med* 1997;29:116–123.

(In their largest population reported, Tatum et al. applied rest sestamibi images to risk stratify 1187 consecutive patients with acute chest pain. The image sensitivity for acute infarction diagnosis was 100%, and specificity was 78%. Here, 32% of patients with abnormal scans and only 3% with normal scans had revascularization. Over a 1-yr follow-up, there was not a single death or infarction in any patient with a normal scan, but a 19% "hard event" rate was noted among those with abnormal scans.)

437. Kontos MC, Jesse RL, Anderson FP, et al. Comparison of myocardial perfusion imaging and cardiac troponin I in patients admitted to the emergency department with chest pain. *Circulation* 1999;99:2073–2078.

(Studied were 620 patients presenting to the emergency department with acute chest pain syndromes. Early rest perfusion imaging and serial troponin I had similar sensitivity for identification of acute myocardial infarction [AMI]. Although specificity for AMI was less than that of troponin I, imaging had a greater ability to predict significant coronary artery disease in patients without AMI.)

438. Kontos MC, Alimard R, Krishnaswami A, et al. Use of acute emergency department perfusion imaging results in more appropriate use of coronary angiography [abstract]. *Circulation* 1999;100:I-584.

(These authors compared the use of rest sestamibi in screening low-risk patients presenting to the emergency department with a similar group not so evaluated. Those evaluated by myocardial perfusion scintigraphy had a lower rate of referral to catheterization [18.7% versus 13.1%] but with a greater proportion of significant disease [6.8% versus 5.7%] and with no greater risk.)

439. Udelson J. The emergency room assessment of sestamibi for the evaluation of chest pain clinical trial-in data analysis and preparation. Paper presented at: Annual meeting of the American Hospital Association, November 1999.

(This large prospective randomized trial was conducted at 7 clinical centers in the northeast United States, in 2456 patients [50% women, 50% men] with a low likelihood of presenting with acute myocardial infarction [AMI] to the ED to rule out AMI. There was a 20% reduction in hospital admissions without loss of sensitivity for AMI or unstable angina diagnosis. But the sestamibi study, when available in half the studies, was not used in management decisions. How great would be the clinical and economic benefit if the scan were integrated into clinical decision making?)

440. Christian TF, Gibbons RJ, Clements IP, et al. Estimates of myocardium at risk and collateral flow in acute myocardial infarction using electrocardiographic indexes with comparison to radionuclide and angiographic measures. *J Am Coll Cardiol* 1995;26:388–393.

(The method has demonstrated its ability to identify the extent of myocardium at ischemic risk in acute myocardial infarction but is thought to be at some disadvantage in the presence of a prior infarction [image defect]. This can be turned to advantage, and impressive comparisons can be made with this reproducible, quantifiable method in the presence of a readily accessible prior study.)

441. Sciammarella MG, Wolfe CL, Lizotte P, et al. Cost-effectiveness with preservation of diagnostic accuracy among patients presenting to the emergency department with chest pain [abstract]. *J Invest Med* 1998;46:155A.

(In this small study of 30 patients admitted with ambiguous presentations to rule out myocardial infarction, 7 had image abnormalities, each with an acute coronary syndrome. Only 1 of the remainder was seen to have ischemia on subsequent stress imaging, the symptoms of which were subsequently demonstrated to have a non-cardiac cause. Even in this small study, if patients with normal gated sestamibi studies were sent home, $33,640 would be saved and no events would be lost. This has now been extended to nearly 100 patients with similar results.)

442. Misbach G, Botvinick E, Tyberg J, Parmley W. Functional infarct size. In: Heiss HW, ed. *Advances in Clinical Cardiology.* New York, NY: Witzstrock Pub House Inc.; 1980:115–126.

(Early animal studies demonstrated an ability of the method to identify regional infarction as small as 1 cm^2 in area and 5–10 gm in weight. This work also demonstrated the relationship between regional infarction, global and regional wall motion and serial functional changes.)

443. Medrano R, Weilbaecher D, Young JB, et al. Assessment of myocardial viability with technetium 99m-sestamibi in patients undergoing cardiac transplantation: a scintigraphic-pathologic study. *Circulation* 1996;94:1010–1017.

(Fifteen patients were injected with sestamibi and imaged before heart transplantation. SPECT image infarct size, measured on slices, correlated linearly and well [$r = 0.88$; $P < 0.001$] with the pathologic infarct size measured after surgery.)

444. Maes AF, Borgers M, Flameng W, et al. Assessment of myocardial viability in chronic coronary artery disease using technetium-99m sestamibi SPECT. *J Am Coll Cardiol* 1997;29:62–68.

(Technetium-99m sestamibi uptake was significantly higher in viable areas confirmed by PET and in areas with improved contractility 3 mo after byass graft surgery. Fifteen patients were injected with sestamibi and imaged before heart transplantation. SPECT image infarct size, measured on slices, correlated linearly and well [$r = 0.88$; $P < 0.001$] with the pathologic infarct size measured after surgery. There was a linear relationship between percent fibrosis and sestamibi uptake, with an optimal threshold of 50% for prediction of functional recovery, with positive and negative predictive values of 82% and 78%, respectively. This data strongly support the ability of the method to quantitate infarct size and suggests that sestamibi uptake is comparable to that of thallium-201 for viability evaluation, with the same levels of regional uptake.)

445. DeCoster PM, Wijns W, Cauwe F. Area at risk determination by technetium-99m hexakis-2-methoxy-isobutyl-isonitrile in experimental reperfused myocardial infarction. *Circulation* 1990;82:2151–2162.

(Technetium-99m sestamibi was able to delineate well the regional myocardium subtended by a coronary occlusion.)

446. Udelson JE, Coleman PS, Metherall J, et al. Predicting recovery of severe regional dysfunction: comparison of resting scintigraphy with 201-Tl and 99m-Tc-sestamibi. *Circulation* 1994;89:2552–2561.

(Comparisons were made between rest and redistribution thallium-201 [^{201}Tl] activity and sestamibi activity 1 hr after rest injection in 31 patients with coronary disease and left ventricular dysfunction. There was a 90% concordance of regional activity between the 2 studies. Quantitative ^{201}Tl and sestamibi regional activities were no different among those with reversible and irreversible left ventricular dysfunction. Sestamibi uptake parallels that of ^{201}Tl in patients with coronary disease and left ventricular dysfunction. Quantitative analysis of regional activity of ^{201}Tl and sestamibi after rest injection each differentiated viable myocardium from scar with similar abilities to predict reversibility of dysfunctional myocardium. Sestamibi appeared able to identify viable myocardium well, in spite of the absence of redistribution.)

447. Sinusas AJ, Trautman KA, Bergin JD, et al. Quantification of "area at risk" during coronary occlusion and degree of myocardial salvage after reperfusion with technetium-99m-methoxyisobutyl-isonitrile. *Circulation* 1990;82:1424–1437.

(When technetium-99m sestamibi was administered to animals with myocardial infarction and the postmortem infarction was compared with the distribution of the radionuclide on autoradiography, excellent linear correlation was noted.)

448. Chareonthaitawee P, Christian TF, Hirose K, et al. The relationship of infarct size with the extent of left ventricular remodeling following myocardial infarction. *J Am Coll Cardiol* 1995;25:567–573.

449. Christian TF, Behrenbeck T, Gersh BJ, Gibbons RJ. Relation of left ventricular volume and function over one year after acute myocardial infarction to infarct size determined by technetium-99m sestamibi. *Am J Cardiol* 1991;68:21–26.

(448,449: These authors related the extent of ventricular remodeling, an important mechanical factor bearing on prognosis, to scintigraphic infarct size.)

450. Prigent FM, Maddahi J, Van Train KF, et al. Comparison of thallium-201 SPECT and planar imaging methods for quantification of experimental myocardial infarct size. *Am Heart J* 1991;122:972–979.

(Although planar and SPECT infarct image sizes both correlated well with pathology, SPECT, without overlapping walls and with full interrogation of the myocardium, has been shown to have clear superiority for such anatomic resolution.)

451. Christian TF, Gibbons RL. Myocardial perfusion imaging in myocardial infarction and unstable angina. In: Verani MS, ed. *Cardiology Clinics.* Philadelphia, PA: W.B. Saunders; 1994:247–261.

(The authors of this chapter review the data demonstrating that the area at ischemic risk correlates well with the final infarct size in animal studies of occlusion and occlusion followed by reperfusion.)

452. Christian TF, Schwartz RS, Gibbons RJ. Determinants of infarct size in reperfusion therapy for acute myocardial infarction. *Circulation* 1992;86:81–90.

(Myocardium at ischemic risk was evaluated in 89 patients with first infarction who underwent successful reperfusion therapy. Myocardium at risk, collateral presence and grade were each associated with final infarct size. These, but *not* time to reperfusion, were among factors judged, by a multivariate analysis using a noninvasive approach, to significantly influence infarct size. With an invasive approach, time to reperfusion gains significance. Each of these factors is important in the preservation of myocardial viability. The extent of collaterals can be determined by assessment of the risk region with radionuclide administration during occlusion [453–455]. This method may be applied clinically and so provide information regarding the final infarct size [445,447].)

453. Christian TF, O'Connor MK, Schwartz RS, et al. A noninvasive Tc-99m sestamibi-based method to assess coronary collateral flow during acute myocardial infarction: evaluation in closed chest animal models of coronary artery occlusion with reperfusion. *J Nucl Med* 1997;38:1840–1846.

454. Shen MYH, Shi QZ, Dione DP, et al. Quantitative SPECT Tc-99m sestamibi provides an accurate assessment of infarct zone collateral flow; experimental validation [abstract]. *J Am Coll Cardiol* 1994;23:422A.

(453,454: The extent of coronary collateral supply can be estimated from the severity of the perfusion defect when the radionuclide is administered during coronary occlusion. Such an evaluation provides an estimate of the size of the potential infarction, including risk area, should the vessel be lost.)

455. Wahr DW, Ports TA, Botvinick EH, et al. The effects of coronary angioplasty and reperfusion on distribution of myocardial flow. *Circulation* 1985;72:334–343.

(To assess the effects of percutaneous transluminal coronary angioplasty [PTCA] and intracoronary streptokinase on regional coronary perfusion, radioactive albumin particles [technetium-99m macroaggregated albumin; MAA] were injected into the uninvolved coronary artery before successful PTCA [n = 33] or successful thrombolysis [n = 8]. After treatment, indium-111 MAA was administered into the same contralateral vessel, except in 10 patients, in whom it was placed in the instrumented vessel. Dual-isotope images, acquired in registry, were color coded for each radionuclide and compared with angiography. Control studies agreed with anatomy but showed no serial change. When MAA was injected into the uninvolved vessel, the region of distribution retracted but expanded after the procedure, when injected in the treated vessel, indicating withdrawal of collateral support, not always evident angiographically, where vessels <100 μ are not well visualized. After the successful procedure, angiographic collaterals vanished on the immediate postprocedure angiogram. Although the procedure did not necessarily result in perfusion of unperfused regions, it did result in perfusion of underperfused regions, generally collateralized and with the result that the fuller region was restored to perfusion by the primary, rather than the collateral, vessel. Not only is perfusion optimized, but perfusion is no longer collateral dependent, and a safety net is provided for subsequent events with renewed availability of a collateral network.)

456. Pellikka PA, Behrenbeck T, Verani MS, et al. Serial changes in myocardial perfusion using tomographic technetium-99m-hexakis-2-methooxy-2-methylpropyl-isonitrile imaging following reperfusion therapy of myocardial infarction. *J Nucl Med* 1990;31:1269–1275.

457. Galli M, Mariassa C, Bolli R, et al. Spontaneous delayed recovery of perfusion and contraction after the first five weeks after anterior infarction. *Circulation* 1994;90:1386–1397.

(456,457: Infarct size appears to improve slowly over time, possibly in relation to growing collaterals or the resolution of "stunned myocardium." Although serial imaging can document arterial patency, imaging early [<48 hr] may overestimate infarct size [*458*].

458. Misbach GA, Botvinick EH, Tyberg JV, et al. The functional implications of scintigraphic measures of ischemia and infarction. *Am Heart J* 1983;106:996–1002.

(Functional infarct size [the left ventricular ejection fraction and percent akinetic segment] appeared to diminish with time. Percent akinetic segment late [1–2 wk] after infarction correlated best with pathologic infarct size, suggesting the source of additional ventricular dysfunction early after infarction in "stunning."

Evaluated scintigraphically in this dog study, infarct size may shrink progressively for weeks after the event, and, with it, there may be improved left ventricular function, likely evidence of improved perfusion and resolving ischemia or stunning after the event. Care must be taken in assessing defect size in all settings, as it is enhanced by the partial volume effect related to regional dysfunction.)

459. Sinusas AJ, Watson DD, Cannon JR Jr, Beller GA. Effect of ischemia and post-ischemia dysfunction on myocardial uptake of technetium-99m labeled methoxy-isobutyl isonitrile and thallium-201. *J Am Coll Cardiol* 1989;14:1785–1793.

(There appears to be an incongruity, in that "stunned" myocardium may appear to relate to a resolving fixed defect or to reversible defects with stress. Improved function, as with resolution of stunned myocardium, may appear to demonstrate myocardial salvage, when, in fact, stunning should not relate to a perfusion defect.)

460. Vera P, Nobili F, Copello F, et al. Thallium gated SPECT in patients with major myocardial infarction: effect of filtering and zooming in comparison with equilibrium radionuclide imaging and left ventriculography. *J Nucl Med* 1999;40:513–521.

(Accurate left ventricular ejection fraction [LVEF] calculation may be performed with SPECT gated thallium-201 myocardial perfusion scintigraphy, even in patients with a large myocardial infarction. However, this article reveals that filtering and zooming appear to greatly influence the calculation of LVEF, as well as ventricular volumes that may be increasingly overestimated as infarct size increases.)

461. Perez-Gonzalez J, Botvinick E, Dunn R, et al. The late prognostic value of acute scintigraphic measurement of myocardial infarction size. *Circulation* 1982;66: 960–967.

(Perez-Gonzalez et al. demonstrated the prognostic value of perfusion defect size, scintigraphic infarct size and left ventricular ejection fraction in uncomplicated patients after infarction.)

462. Becker LC, Silverman KJ, Bulkley BH, et al. Comparison of early thallium-201 scintigraphy and gated blood pool imaging for predicting mortality in patients with acute myocardial infarction. *Circulation* 1983;67:1272–1282.

(Shown here is the interaction of function, as left ventricular ejection fraction [LVEF], and perfusion, as defect size, in the determination of prognosis after infarction. The 2 interact so that a given perfusion defect, here grossly measured, representing scar and myocardium at ischemic risk, influences prognosis more in the setting of a lower LVEF.)

463. American Heart Association. *Heart and Stroke Statistical Update.* Chicago, IL: American Heart Association; 1997:10.

(In the United States, about 1,500,000 people suffer an acute myocardial infarction each year and one-third of these die.)

464. Mahmarian JJ, Mahmarian AC, Marks GF, et al. Role of adenosine thallium-201 tomography for defining long-term risk in patients after acute myocardial infarction. *J Am Coll Cardiol* 1995;25:1333–1340.

(This is 1 of many studies showing the prognostic value of residual scintigraphic ischemia early after acute infarction. Those with residual ischemia have a higher event rate after myocardial infarction, and the risk increases with the extent of myocardium at ischemic risk. Here, as in reference *216*, Mahmarian et al. demonstrated the prognostic importance of infarct and related ischemia size. The total ischemic defect size interacted with the left ventricular ejection fraction [LVEF] to determine prognosis, with death and recurrent infarction more frequent among those with large defects, a risk that was compounded by a low LVEF. Conversely, the prognosis related to any defect was worsened by a low LVEF, and the prognosis related to any LVEF was progressively worsened by the presence of increasing defect size.)

465. Dakik HA, Mahmarian JJ, Kimball KT, et al. Prognostic value of exercise Tl-201 tomography in patients treated with thrombolytic therapy during acute myocardial infarction. *Circulation* 1996;94:2735–2742.

(Dakik et al. demonstrated the importance of infarct size with an infarct >20% related to a poor prognosis, compared with infarct size <20%. The authors demonstrated the interaction of quantitative exercise thallium-201 [^{201}Tl] SPECT imaging parameters, including image defect size, with left ventricular ejection fraction [LVEF] to provide important independent and incremental, long-term prognostic information in 71 patients with acute infarction studied after thrombolysis and before discharge. Quantitative exercise ^{201}Tl SPECT imaging parameters, including image defect size, interact with the LVEF to provide important independent and incremental, long-term prognostic information in patients studied after thrombolysis. Most important was that SPECT provided incremental prognostic information compared with clinical data, but coronary angiography provided no further advantage to risk stratification compared with that provided by the perfusion scan in combination with clinical data and the LVEF.)

466. Zaret BL, Wackers FJTh, Terrin ML, et al. for The TIMI Study Group. Value of radionuclide rest and exercise left ventricular ejection fraction in assessing survival of patients after thrombolytic therapy for acute myocardial infarction: results of thrombolysis in myocardial infarction (TIMI) Phase II Study. *J Am Coll Cardiol* 1995;26:72–79.

(Rest left ventricular ejection fraction [LVEF], but not exercise EF or their difference, was an important prognostic index after thrombolytic therapy. At any level of LVEF, mortality was lower than in patients in the prethrombolytic phase not so treated.)

467. Travin Ml, Dessouki AMR, Cameron T, Heller GV. Use of exercise technetium-99m sestamibi SPECT imaging to detect residual ischemia and for risk stratification after acute myocardial infarction. *Am J Cardiol* 1995;75:665–669.

(Events were determined over a 15-mo period in 134 postinfarction patients studied within 10 days after the event with exercise myocardial perfusion scintigraphy. Induced ischemia or defects in multiple vascular areas identified 12 of 13 patients with events, including all deaths. Defect extent remained a strong prognostic factor in those 54 patients having thrombolytic therapy, better than clinical and electrocardiographic parameters. A normal study was again associated with a low event rate.)

468. Gibbons RJ, Holmes DR, Reeder GS, et al. Immediate angioplasty compared with the administration of a thrombolytic agent followed by conservative treatment for myocardial infarction. The Mayo Coronary Care Unit and Catheterization Laboratory Groups. *N Engl J Med* 1993;328:685–691.

(Among 103 patients randomized, based on pre- and postintervention evaluation and myocardial perfusion scintigraphy, there was no evident difference in myocardial salvage resulting from immediate percutaneous transluminal coronary angioplasty [PTCA] or thrombolytic therapy. Time to balloon inflation was greater than time to thrombolytic agent infusion onset. However, in daily practice, it is unusual to find a normal image after thrombolysis, but this is seen frequently after immediate PTCA. Perhaps time to revascularization is the critical factor rather than the method applied.)

469. Silverman KJ, Becker LC, Bulkey BH, et al. Value of early thallium-201 scintigraphy for predicting mortality in patients with acute myocardial infarction. *Circulation* 1980;61:996–1003.

(Rest thallium-201 imaging is highly prognostic after myocardial infarction, with additional incremental prognostic information contributed by evidence of redistribution, the presence of induced chest pain, ST changes [with exercise or dipyridamole] and other findings at exercise testing.)

470. Gioia G, Milan E, Giubbini R, et al. Prognostic value of tomographic rest-redistribution thallium-201 imaging in medically treated patients with coronary artery disease and left ventricular dysfunction. *J Nucl Cardiol* 1996;3:150–156.

(Gioia et al. studied 81 patients with rest–redistribution imaging and demonstrated a 26% cardiac death rate over 31 mo among those with fixed defects, compared with 58% in those with reversible defects. These relationships have been related as well to the size of the defect and likely relate as well to the state of left ventricular function.)

471. Klarich KW, Christian TF, Higano ST, Gibbons RJ. Variability of myocardium at risk for acute myocardial infarction. *Am J Cardiol* 1999;83:1191–1195.

(When 193 patients with acute myocardial infarction and ST elevation were injected with technetium-99m sestamibi before reperfusion, the great variability of myocardium at ischemic risk [MIR] was identified. Although MIR was greatest for left anterior descending coronary artery [LAD] occlusions, the measure increased with proximal location in both LAD and left circumflex coronary artery beds. Overall, the extent of MIR varied greatly with the grade of sestamibi flow, the specific artery involved and the proximal nature of the lesion. Risk likely relates better to the extent of MIR, a physiologic parameter, than to the vessel or number of vessels involved, each anatomic measures of coronary artery disease.)

472. Gibbons RJ, Miller TD, Christian TF. Infarct size measured by single photon emission computed tomographic imaging with Tc-99m sestamibi. Measure of the efficacy of therapy in acute myocardial infarction. *Circulation* 2000;101:101–108.

(Gibbons et al. [486] presented a review of 7 randomized trial and 6 multicenter trials that demonstrate the prognostic value of infarct size. Recommended is the application of the method as an end point in early pilot studies to evaluate efficacy, in dose-ranging studies and as a surrogate end point to evaluate advantages of new therapies.)

473. Sanz KA, Castaner A, Betriu A, et al. Determinants of prognosis in survivors of myocardial infarction: a prospective clinical angiographic study. *N Engl J Med* 1992;306:1065–1070.

(Several studies have long demonstrated that coronary angiography generally offers no further prognostic information beyond myocardial perfusion scintigraphy in uncomplicated patients with acute infarction.)

474. Gibson RS, Watson DD, Craddock GB, et al. Prediction of cardiac events after uncomplicated myocardial infarction: a prospective study comparing pre-discharge exercise thallium-201 scintigraphy and coronary angiography. *Circulation* 1983;68: 321–336.

(Gibson et al. studied a group of 140 patients with documented acute myocardial infarction [AMI] comparing the results of submaximal treadmill testing, submaximal exercise thallium-201 scintigraphy and coronary arteriography. They demonstrated that low-level exercise testing, performed in conjunction with planar thallium imaging performed before discharge after AMI, more effectively stratified patients into low- and high-risk groups than did clinical variables, exercise electrocardiography [ECG] or the findings on coronary angiography. Thallium-201 defects involving 2 vascular territories, the presence of reversible defects and the presence of abnormal lung uptake were highly predictive of subsequent cardiac events, more so than the coronary angiogram. Patients in this study who did not manifest exercise-induced angina or ST segment depression nonetheless had a moderate subsequent rate of cardiac events on follow-up, as did patients who were found to have single-vessel disease at the time of cardiac catheterization. Patients with normal or low-risk thallium scans in this study, however, had a very low risk for subsequent events, lower than those with a normal stress ECG and even lower than those with "normal" coronary angiograms.

This was an early and important prethrombolytic study demonstrating the important prognostic value of stress perfusion scintigraphy and its superiority to the coronary anatomy after infarction. Stress perfusion scintigraphy was a better prognostic indicator after infarction than the results of stress testing and even coronary angiography. Such improved risk stratification, often with advantageous identification of a low-risk subgroup, is a primary benefit of the perfusion scintigraphic method.)

475. Brown KA, Weiss RM, Clements JP, et al. Usefulness of residual ischemic myocardium within prior infarct zone for identifying patients at high risk late after acute myocardial infarction. *Am J Cardiol* 1987;60:15–19.

476. Gibson RS, Beller GA, Gheorghiade M, et al. The prevalence and clinical significance of residual myocardial ischemia 2 weeks after uncomplicated non-Q-wave myocardial infarction: a prospective natural history study. *Circulation* 1986;73: 1186–1198.

477. Wilson WW, Gibson RS, Nygaard TW, et al. Acute myocardial infarction associated with single-vessel coronary artery disease: an analysis of clinical outcome and the prognostic importance of vessel patency and residual ischemic myocardium. *J Am Coll Cardiol* 1988;11:223–234.

(475–477: These articles demonstrate the prognostic value of stress myocardial perfusion scintigraphy after infarction.)

478. Shaw LJ, Peterson ED, Kesler K, et al. A meta-analysis of predischarge risk stratification after acute myocardial infarction with stress electrocardiographic, myocardial perfusion and ventricular function imaging. *Am J Cardiol* 1996;78:1327–1337.

(Abnormal discharge test results were correlated with outcome in studies of patients after infarction. Reports of 54 studies included 19,874 patients and were mostly retrospective and small. One-year mortality ranged from 2.55 for dobuta-mine echocardiography to 9.3% for exercise radionuclide angiography. Dipyri-damole myocardial scintigraphy perfusion [MPS] was related to more subsequent events than was exercise evaluation. Positive predictive values for most noninvasive tests were low, <.10 for death and <.20 for death or acute myocardial infarction [AMI]. The authors suggest that more rigorous studies be performed to establish relative test values.

Shaw et al. applied exercise MPS to risk stratify 1910 patients after infarction. Reversible defects in multiple segments in a multivessel distribution related to a death rate of 8% with an AMI rate of 18%, whereas absence of such extensive defects related to 2% death or infarction event rate.)

479. Leppo JA, O'Brien J, Rothendler JA, et al. Dipyridamole-thallium-201 scintigraphy in the prediction of future cardiac events after acute myocardial infarction. *N Engl J Med* 1984;310:1014–1018.

(Leppo et al. evaluated dipyridamole thallium-201 [201Tl] testing before discharge in order to predict death or recurrent myocardial infarction in patients with prior myo-cardial infarction. Among all other variables tested, only the presence of redistribution on dipyridamole 201Tl study was a significant predictor of a subsequent cardiac event.)

480. Brown KA, O'Meara J, Chambers CE, et al. Ability of dipyridamole-thallium-201 imaging one to four days after acute myocardial infarction to predict in-hospital and late recurrent myocardial ischemic events. *Am J Cardiol* 1990;65:160–167.

481. Gimple LW, Hutter AM, Guiney TE, et al. Prognostic utility of predischarge dipyri-damole-thallium imaging compared to predischarge submaximal exercise electro-cardiography and maximal exercise thallium imaging after uncomplicated acute myocardial infarction. *Am J Cardiol* 1989;64:1243–1248.

(480,481: Early postinfarction dipyridamole evaluation is both safe and effective for risk stratification.)

482. Younis LT, Byers S, Shaw L, et al. Prognostic value of intravenous dipyridamole thallium scintigraphy after an acute myocardial ischemic event. *Am J Cardiol* 1989;64:161–166.

(Shaw et al. applied exercise myocardial perfusion scintigraphy to risk stratify 1910 patients after infarction. Reversible defects in multiple segments in a multi-vessel distribution related to a death rate of 8% with an AMI rate of 18%, whereas absence of such extensive defects related to 2% death or infarction event rate.)

483. Wolfe CL, Lee W, Botvinick EH, et al. The utility of dipyridamole thallium scintig-raphy in predicting ischemic events after myocardial infarction. *Circulation* 1988;78 (suppl II):II-431–II-437.

(480–483: In these articles, the dipyridamole thallium-201 study was demon-strated to be significantly more predictive of subsequent myocardial events than the exercise electrocardiogram.)

484. Daou D, Le Guludec D, Faraggi M, et al. Nonlimited exercise test combined with high-dose dipyridamole for thallium-201 myocardial single-photon emission com-puted tomography in coronary artery disease. *Am J Cardiol* 1995;76:753–758.

(Although dipyridamole stress was more sensitive than submaximal exercise testing, the authors found that high-dose dipyridamole combined with "nonlim-ited" exercise testing presented superior results than dipyridamole stress alone, results that were comparable with those with maximum exercise testing.)

485. Yao S, Quereshi E, Bornstein A, et al. Impact of early predischarge dipyridamole myocardial perfusion SPECT on cost-effective utilization following acute myocar-dial infarction [abstract]. *J Nucl Med* 1999;40:43P.

(Assessed was the 1-yr outcome, days hospitalized and cost, based on the tim-ing of performance of dipyridamole myocardial perfusion scintigraphy [MPS] among 432 patients with uncomplicated acute infarction. The performance of early [≤4 days] MPS in 244 patients was accompanied by a shortened length of hospital stay without increase in adverse events, compared with that in 188 patients studied later. Early dipyridamole MPS is a safe and effective method for reducing hospital stay after acute myocardial infarction.)

486. Brown KA, Heller GV, Landin RS, et al. Early dipyridamole Tc-99m sestamibi single photon emission computed tomographic imaging 2–4 days after acute myocardial infarction predicts in-hospital and postdischarge cardiac events. Comparison with submaximal exercise imaging. *Circulation* 1999;100:2060–2066.

   (Here, the prognostic value of dipyridamole stress myocardial perfusion scintigraphy [MPS] early after an initial acute myocardial infarction and the superiority of MPS to submaximal exercise testing was established in 451 randomized patients. Dipyridamole MPS predicted early and late cardiac events well and was a far better predictor of postinfarct events than the submaximal exercise MPS. The method was safe and permits management decisions to be made earlier after infarction.)

487. Wackers FJTh, Zaret BL. Risk stratification soon after acute infarction [editorial]. *Circulation* 1999;100:2040–2042.

   (The conclusions and implications of reference *499* are strongly supported in this accompanying editorial. This data should make changes in guidelines for patients after infarction.)

488. Bodenheimer MM, Wackers FJTh, Schwartz RG, et al. Prognostic significance of a fixed defect 1 to 6 months after onset of acute myocardial infarction or unstable angina. *Am J Cardiol* 1994;74:1196–1200.

   (Bodenheimer et al. demonstrated the risk of fixed defects in patients with known coronary artery disease to be similar to that in patients with reversible defects of the same magnitude and much worse than those with normal scans. Yet, evidence of redistribution, [myocardium at ischemic risk] adds to the risk related to extensive fixed defects.)

489. Moss AJ, Goldstein RE, Hall WJ, et al. Detection and significance of myocardial ischemia in stable patients after recovery from an acute coronary event. *JAMA* 1993;269:2379–2385.

   (Moss et al. found no benefit to noninvasive testing in patients studied after acute myocardial infarction or unstable angina. Because evaluation was limited to patients with normal rest electrocardiograms and a large number of patients who presented were revascularized and excluded from the study, the apparent lack of noninvasive test utility here is likely related to the selective population studied, with a large number of excluded patients and the very low risk in those studied. This work does not refute the value of the method but rather demonstrates the reduced contribution of noninvasive testing in patients who have already been risk stratified and are at relatively low risk.)

490. Clements IP, Christian TF, Higano ST, et al. Residual flow to the infarct zone as a determinant of infarct size after direct angioplasty. *Circulation* 1993;88:1527–1533.

   (Technetium-99m sestamibi administration on presentation and subsequent imaging after thrombolysis or acute percutaneous transluminal coronary angioplasty present evidence of the initial perfusion defect and the results of intervention. The extent of myocardium salvaged can be gained, as demonstrated in this article.)

491. Miller DG, Donohue TJ, Caracciolo EA, et al. "False positive" stress myocardial perfusion tomographic studies are significantly reduced by comparison to physiologic post-stenotic coronary flow reserve, not anatomic quantitative stenosis severity [abstract]. *J Am Coll Cardiol* 1994;23:256A.

   (Intracoronary ultrasound and Doppler measurements were made at rest and with coronary dilation in vessels subtending reversible defects on prior stress myocardial perfusion scintigraphy but without apparent angiographic stenoses.

The overwhelming number of such vessels evaluated revealed unsuspected stenoses or abnormalities in the ability to augment flow in response to a dilator. Surprisingly, the anatomy often revealed lengthy but even atheromatous deposits, presenting a smooth and presumably normal contour to angiographic evaluation. Here, intra-coronary Doppler measurement of flow augmentation with a direct coronary dilator correlates better with the findings on pharmacologic stress perfusion scintigraphy than does the qualitative assessment of the coronary anatomy. Again, coronary anatomy is found wanting when compared with perfusion scintigraphy and other physiologic markers of perfusion.)

492. Donohue TJ, Miller DD, Bach RG, et al. Correlation of post-stenotic hyperemic coronary flow velocity and pressure with abnormal stress myocardial perfusion imaging in coronary artery disease. *Am J Cardiol* 1996;77:948–954.

(The functional significance of a coronary lesion is often determined by stress myocardial perfusion scintigraphy [MPS]. In this study, poststenotic flow velocity and pressure were related to the findings on stress MPS in 50 patients undergoing coronary angiography within 1 wk of exercise [29 patients] or dipyridamole [21 patients] MPS. Distal coronary flow velocity reserve [CFRV] was abnormal in 22 of 25 with a reversible defect on MPS but normal in 25 with none. Thirteen of 25 with defects had high trans-stenotic gradients, whereas 20 of 25 without defects had no or a minor gradient. CFRV was better correlated with image findings than with translesion gradients, and quantitative angiographic measures of stenosis did not differentiate between those with normal or abnormal MPS. Stress MPS defects are correlated well with CFRV.)

493. Uren NG, Crake T, Lefroy DC, et al. Delayed recovery of coronary resistance vessel function after coronary angioplasty. *J Am Coll Cardiol* 1993;21:612–621.

(491–493: Intracoronary Doppler measurement of flow augmentation with a direct coronary dilator correlates better with the findings on pharmacologic stress perfusion scintigraphy than does the qualitative assessment of the coronary anatomy [*491*]. Regardless of the apparent anatomic effect on the epicardial vessels, percutaneous transluminal coronary angioplasty [PTCA] does not immediately restore normal coronary flow hemodynamics. However, these do improve serially with time, likely an aspect of the healing process.

There does indeed appear to be a healing process after PTCA. The coronary flow is not always immediately restored to normal after restoring the epicardial lumen. Although sometimes a stress-related perfusion defect is noted early after even "successful" angioplasty, the authors of reference *492* demonstrate that such defects are, in fact, generally related to true persistent, hemodynamic abnormalities. Although this is not a common finding days to weeks after revascularization, it can, at times, mislead the physician to believe that the epicardial vessel has restenosed. For this reason, imaging is best applied to symptomatic patients early after PTCA. Others have shown that the persistence of image evidence of a blunted coronary flow relates to an increased risk of subsequent occlusion [*493*].)

494. Christian TF, Behrenbeck T, Pellikka PA, et al. Mismatch of left ventricular function and infarct size demonstrated by technetium-99m isonitrile imaging after reperfusion therapy for acute myocardial infarction: identification of myocardial stunning and hyperkinesia. *J Am Coll Cardiol* 1990;16:1632–1638.

(It is now clear that patients after thrombolysis or primary [acute] angioplasty have varied prognoses. They are evaluated well after the acute intervention and at serial times remote from the intervention to assess the state of coronary perfusion and prognosis and to determine the value of acute revascularization, in terms of salvaged myocardium. In these studies, the postintervention defect size was predictive of ejection fraction late, after resolution of stunning. Perfusion imaging has been applied to gain an important objective end point, short of death or infarction, to determine the efficacy of the thrombolytic method. This permits identification of a benefit while sampling fewer patient numbers.)

495. Miller TD, Gersh BJ, Christian TF, et al. Limited prognostic value of thallium-201 exercise treadmill testing early after myocardial infarction in patients treated with thrombolysis. *Am Heart J* 1995;130:259–266.

   (A group of 210 patients treated with thrombolysis alone [n = 131] or with associated angioplasty [n = 79], who underwent stress perfusion SPECT scintigraphy a mean of 9 days after infarction, were followed and analyzed retrospectively. Unlike the findings in postinfarction patients studied in the "prethrombolytic era," no single exercise or perfusion image variable, including those associated with a poor outcome in nonthrombolytic patients, could predict the outcome. Articles such as this have led to the supposition that such stress imaging parameters are of no use in the "post-thrombolytic era." Certainly the anatomy and pathophysiology are changed, and these may affect the course of lesion progression and its predictability. There was only a single death and 11 nonfatal infarctions over a 2-yr follow-up period. Careful analysis and subsequent use, however, suggests that the utility of these methods persist. Reviews and editorials presented here support this fact.)

496. Beller GA. Noninvasive assessment of prognosis after acute myocardial infarction in the thrombolytic era and age of interventional cardiology [editorial]. *J Nucl Cardiol* 1995;2:159–162.

   (The perfusion method appears to have a reduced sensitivity to the detection of multivessel coronary disease after thrombolysis. Explanations include: the lower incidence of patients with prior infarction in those studied post-thrombolysis; a lower incidence of multivessel disease in patients treated with thrombolysis; restoration of flow post-thrombolysis reduces the visibility of related perfusion defects; and a low incidence of non-Q infarctions and their related high incidence of induced perfusion defects. The text also notes the limited, low-risk [only 1.2% mortality] nature of the 939 included patients [31% post-thrombolysis, 39% postangioplasty and 67% postangiography] who were analyzed to yield the results of the Multicenter Study of Myocardial Ischemia [MSMI], which demonstrated no prognostic advantage to stress testing with or without imaging! Excluded were 1839 patients who underwent bypass surgery after the index event, 955 who were on digoxin or other drugs that were believed to influence the stress test, 947 patients with bundle branch block, rest ST abnormalities or atrial fibrillation and all who could not perform adequate treadmill testing! Further, most MSMI patients were signed up late after the index event, after the expected period when most subsequent events would occur. This agrees with the editorial statement made by Dr. K Brown in reference to this same MSMI study, where he noted, "The applicability of the results of this study to other patient groups, especially those that have not yet undergone risk stratification, is nil.")

497. Nishimura T. Assessment of acute thrombolysis with newly developed single-photon emission computed tomographic techniques [editorial]. *J Nucl Cardiol* 1995;2:163–166.

   (The author evaluates "freeze" and "memory" or technetium-99m [^{99m}Tc] sestamibi and "hot-spot," ^{99m}Tc pyrophosphate, antimyosin or metabolic fatty acid imaging, in the evaluation of patients undergoing thrombolytic therapy. Freeze imaging permits simultaneous evaluation of the area at ischemic risk as well as salvaged myocardium, and memory imaging aids evaluation of necrosis or viability in the area related to the event and can aid clinical assessment with measures not directly related to perfusion.)

498. Beller GA. Determining prognosis after acute myocardial infarction in the thrombolytic era [editorial]. *Clin Res* 1997;315:761–762.

   (Beller assesses the methods for risk stratification after infarction in the thrombolytic era and, specifically, the value of perfusion scintigraphy.)

499. Santoro GM, Bisi G, Sciagra R, et al. Single photon emission computed tomography with technetium-99m-hexakis-2-methoxyisobutyl isonitrile in acute myocardial

infarction before and after thrombolytic treatment: assessment of salvaged myocardium and prediction of late functional recovery. *J Am Coll Cardiol* 1990;12:301–314.

(Comparing prethrombolytic with post-thrombolytic "infarct size" acquired at least 18 hr after thrombolytic therapy, technetium-99m sestamibi myocardial perfusion scintigraphy has been used as well to determine the extent of myocardium salvaged by thrombolysis compared with conservative treatment [275,276].)

500. Christian TF, Gibbons RJ, Gersh BJ, et al. Effect of infarct location on myocardial salvage assessed by technetium-99m isonitrile. *J Am Coll Cardiol* 1991;17:1303–1308.

(Although anterior infarcts were larger as a result of the extent of the perfusion zone of the affected vessel and demonstrated a greater reduction in defect size after revascularization, both anterior and inferior infarcts showed a significant reduction in defect size after reperfusion therapy [$P < 0.001$ for both].)

501. Behrenbeck T, Pellikka PA, Huber KC, et al. Primary angioplasty in myocardial infarction: assessment of improved myocardial perfusion with technetium-99m-isonitrile. *J Am Coll Cardiol* 1991;17:365–372.

(The beneficial effects of acute angioplasty were documented in pre- and postintervention images by Behrenbeck et al. Here, reports suggest little intrinsic difference between thrombolytic therapy and acute percutaneous transluminal coronary angioplasty [PTCA], if each is delivered early and with early establishment of vessel patency. Although acute PTCA requires mobilization and utilization of increased resources, it more generally assures early patency, in which stability is increased with stenting.)

502. Reimer KA, Jennings RB, Cobb FR, et al. Animal models for protecting ischemic myocardium: results of the NHLBI cooperative study. Comparison of unconscious and conscious dog models. *Circ Res* 1985;56:651–665.

(Animal experiments were performed with coronary occlusion and release to measure the extent of myocardium at risk and to determine that the region of risk was modulated by the extent of collateral flow, the duration of occlusion and the severity of myocardial oxygen demands.)

503. Austin GE, Ratliff NB, Hollman J, et al. Intimal proliferation of smooth muscle cells as an explanation for recurrent coronary artery stenosis after percutaneous transluminal coronary angioplasty. *J Am Coll Cardiol* 1985;6:369–375.

(Technetium-99m sestamibi may be injected on presentation and subsequent stress perfusion scintigraphy applied to assess the amount of myocardium at ischemic risk and to aid in prognosis. Of course, much like in the initiation of coronary occlusion with acute infarction, lesion stability after instrumentation plays a larger role, along with lesion severity, in the likelihood of subsequent occlusion or restenosis as discussed in this article. Unlike atherosclerosis, a fibrocellular growth process has been noted to develop after percutaneous transluminal coronary angiography.)

504. Beller GA. Radionuclide imaging in acute myocardial infarction. In: Beller GA, ed. *Clinical Nuclear Cardiology*. Philadelphia, PA: W.B. Saunders Co.; 1995:193–235.

(Beller presents a complete review of the subject, including the importance of perfusion imaging in the evaluation of the post-thrombolytic patient [273,277, 467,474].)

505. Baron H, Sciammerella M, Lenihan K, et al. Repeated administration of adenosine and heparin reduces myocardial ischemia in patients with chronic stable angina [abstract]. *Circulation* 1997;96(suppl I):I-342.

(In 21 patients and 7 controls, it appeared that the daily infusion of adenosine and heparin for 2 wk brought reduced exercise-induced defect size, unexplained by exercise time or any reduction in the achieved double product. The mechanism is unclear but may relate to collateral growth.)

530. Hecht HS, Shaw RE, Chin HL, et al. Silent ischemia after coronary angioplasty: evaluation of restenosis and extent of ischemia in asymptomatic patients by tomographic thallium-201 exercise imaging and comparison with asymptomatic patients. *J Am Coll Cardiol* 1991;17:670–677.

(529,530: Listed are some of the numerous studies that have evaluated the role of myocardial perfusion scintigraphy in the assessment of patients after percutaneous transluminal coronary angioplasty.)

531. Gibbons RJ, Balady GJ, Beaseley JW, et al. ACC/AHA guidelines for exercise testing: executive summary. Report of the ACC/AHA Task Force on Practical Guidelines. *Circulation* 1997;96:345–354.

(Although guidelines suggest the application of myocardial perfusion scintigraphy only in the setting of renewed symptoms anytime after an intervention, the imaging method is of great value in targeting those patients needing invasive re-evaluation and in other settings. These include asymptomatic patients after a complicated or incomplete angioplasty or coronary artery bypass graft [CABG], those having percutaneous transluminal coronary angioplasty [PTCA] of a potentially life-threatening lesion 5 yr after PTCA and 19 yr after CABG, as well as patients with atypical symptoms or ambiguous presentations.)

532. Reed DC, Beller GA, Nygaard TW, et al. The clinical efficacy and scintigraphic evaluation of post-coronary bypass patients undergoing percutaneous transluminal coronary angioplasty for recurrent angina pectoris. *Am Heart J* 1989;117:60–71.

(This article demonstrates the accuracy and clinical value of the scintigraphic method in evaluating the results of percutaneous transluminal coronary angioplasty and postintervention treatment applied to stenosis in postsurgical bypass grafts.)

533. Klein LW, Avula SB, Uretz E, et al. Utility of various clinical, noninvasive, and invasive procedures for determining the causes of recurrence of myocardial ischemia or infarction more than 1 year after percutaneous transluminal coronary angioplasty. *Am J Cardiol* 1995;75:1003–1006.

(In 76 consecutive patients who presented with recurrent symptoms >1 yr after successful coronary angioplasty, only coronary angiography could differentiate between restenosis, disease progression and quiescence. Performed in only 40 patients, stress perfusion imaging had a modest sensitivity of 77% but a low specificity in these patients who all underwent angiography.)

534. Hecht, HS. Radionuclide techniques in the selection of patients for PTCA and in post-PTCA evaluation. *Symp Nucl Cardiol* 1994;12:373–383.

535. Beller, GA. Radionuclide evaluation of coronary bypass surgery and percutaneous transluminal coronary angioplasty. In: Beller GA, ed. *Clinical Nuclear Cardiology.* Philadelphia, PA: W.B. Saunders; 1995:337–353.

(This chapter reviews the results of perfusion scintigraphy, immediately, early [within 4 wk] and later after percutaneous transluminal coronary angioplasty [PTCA]. Evaluation in the minutes after revascularization could demonstrate the postreperfusion hyperemic response. In an important minority of subjects, in the early weeks after reperfusion the image may reveal a persistent defect as a result of altered flow reserve, in spite of successful restoration of epicardial vessel patency. Progressive improvement in flow reserve results in a normal image weeks after a successful intervention hyperemia. The method is appropriately applied to evaluate renewed symptoms anytime after PTCA or to electively assess the results of the procedure, if desired, 3–4 wk and more after revascularization.

534,535: The method of perfusion scintigraphy appears to retain its diagnostic and prognostic accuracy after revascularization. It is a valuable tool to apply for the evaluation of symptoms and retained vessel or graft patency after coronary bypass graft surgery or PTCA.)

536. Lakkis NM, Mahmarian JJ, Verani MS. Exercise thallium-201 single photon emission computed tomography for evaluation of coronary artery bypass graft patency. *Am J Cardiol* 1995;76:107–111.

(There was an 84% sensitivity of stress thallium-201 SPECT for diagnosing graft stenosis in 50 patients with typical or atypical symptoms, studied a mean of 52 mo after coronary bypass surgery.)

537. Breisblatt WM, Barnes JV, Weiland F, Spaccavento LJ. Incomplete revascularization in multivessel percutaneous transluminal coronary angioplasty. The role for stress thallium-201 imaging. *J Am Coll Cardiol* 1988;11:1183–1190.

(This article highlights the localizing ability of perfusion scintigraphy and its ability to identify the most severely stenotic lesion in pathophysiologic terms. This "culprit lesion" may then be approached to relieve symptoms and possibly risk in patients with multivessel disease who are too ill or who refuse to undergo full revascularization. Other applications include the assessment of the significance of a questionably stenotic lesion or to determine whether a vessel that might be anatomically amenable to angioplasty is the cause of ischemic symptoms in a patient with several other unapproachable vessels. Although postrevascularization scintigraphy generally reveals further evidence of ischemia or ischemic potential in another vascular bed, many patients successfully and comfortably passed the 1-yr follow-up period.)

538. Wharton TP Jr, Neill WA, Oxendine JM, Painter LN. Effect of duration of regional myocardial ischemia and degree of reactive hyperemia on the magnitude of the initial thallium-201 defect. *Circulation* 1980;62:516–521.

(This article demonstrates that the intensity of a given defect varies as a function of the severity and duration of imposed ischemia and on the extent of postischemic hyperemia.)

539. Kronenberg MW, Pobertson RM, Born ML, et al. Thallium-201 uptake in variant angina: probable demonstration of myocardial reactive hyperemia in man. *Circulation* 1982;66:1332–1338.

(The presence of a perfusion defect in the presence of coronary spasm depends on the state of the vasculature at the time of radionuclide administration. If injected at the cessation of spasm, a "hot spot" may result and correspond to the region of postischemic hyperemia.)

540. Hecht HS. Radionuclide techniques in the selection of patients for PTCA and post PTCA evaluation. *Symp Nucl Cardiol*. 1994;12:373–382.

(The prognostic value of perfusion scintigraphic findings after percutaneous transluminal coronary angioplasty are determined and discussed in this review article.)

541. Wijns W, Serruys PW, Simoons ML, et al. Predictive value of early maximal exercise test and thallium scintigraphy after successful percutaneous transluminal coronary angioplasty. *Br Heart J* 1985;53:194–200.

(To determine the value of stress myocardial perfusion scintigraphy [MPS] for predicting restenosis after percutaneous transluminal coronary angioplasty [PTCA] and recurrence of angina, exercise MPS was performed in 91 asymptomatic patients a median of 5 wk after a technically successful PTCA. The presence or absence of defects on MPS was highly predictive of restenosis and subsequent infarction, but the results of the stress electrocardiogram were not.)

542. Manyari DE, Knudtson M, Kloiber R, et al. Sequential thallium-201 myocardial perfusion studies after successful percutaneous transluminal coronary artery angioplasty: delayed resolution of exercise induced scintigraphic abnormalities. *Circulation* 1988;77:86–95.

(541,542: Wijns et al. and Manyari et al. demonstrated that a normal scan after percutaneous transluminal coronary angioplasty [PTCA] related to a good early prognosis, whereas an abnormal scan early indicated a poor prognosis and high likelihood for restenosis. Although post-PTCA defects may be seen in the presence of an apparently successfully dilated epicardial vessel, these generally resolve with time, as flow reserve normalizes, and have been related to an increased incidence of closure in such vessels [523,526–528].)

543. Milan E, Zoccarato O, Terzi A, et al. Technetium-99m sestamibi SPECT to detect restenosis after successful percutaneous coronary angioplasty. *J Nucl Med* 1996;37: 1300–1305.

(Milan et al. demonstrated the superiority of perfusion imaging over stress testing for the diagnosis and prediction of restenosis after percutaneous transluminal coronary angioplasty.)

544. Kiat H, Ansari A, Berman DS, et al. Abnormal myocardial perfusion single photon emission computed tomography and normal coronary angiogram: the role of intracoronary vascular ultrasound in providing diagnostic confirmation. *Am Heart J* 1995;130:182–186.

(A case is reported with apparently normal angiographic coronary anatomy in the presence of an apparent stress-induced perfusion defect. Intracoronary ultrasound demonstrated the presence of severe disease, unrecognized angiographically. This study and works like it support the presence of hemodynamically significant disease in the presence of apparent false-positive perfusion scintigrams. Others have shown similar scintigraphic corroboration based on Doppler measurements of coronary flow reserve. Clearly, the anatomic "gold standard" often leaves something to be desired, as judged by the pathophysiologic perfusion marker.)

545. Nkoma VT, Hodge DO, Gibbons RJ, et al. The impact of time from coronary angioplasty on the detection of restenosis by exercise perfusion imaging: an incremental analysis [abstract]. *J Am Coll Cardiol* 1999;33:482A.

(A group of 390 patients who had successful percutaneous transluminal coronary angioplasty, exercise thallium-201 myocardial perfusion scintigraphy within the subsequent year and repeat coronary angiography were evaluated for the ability to predict restenosis. Restenosis, evident in 329 patients [84%], was supported by clinical [age, sex, symptoms] and exercise test [heart rate, ST changes] variables. However, beyond these, the extent of MPS redistribution added 26% in correct classification.)

546. Krawszynska EG, Alazraki NP, Kosinski AS, et al. Quantitative thallium SPECT (QTl-S) at one year post revascularization helps to predict outcome in diabetic patients [abstract]. *J Am Coll Cardiol* 1999;33:470A.

(Among 336 diabetic patients with multivessel coronary artery disease studied at 1 yr after revascularization, stress myocardial perfusion scintigraphy was well able to risk stratify event-free survival from 100%, without evidence of reversible defect, to 86% with mild-to-moderate defect reversibility score, to 58% with severe reversible defects.)

547. Schricke U, Kastrati A, Neverve J, et al. Prognostic value of scintigraphically assessed myocardial salvage for functional outcome in patients with acute myocardial infarction 6 months after stent supported primary angioplasty [abstract]. *J Nucl Med* 1999;40:7P.

(The extent of myocardial salvage measured on myocardial perfusion scintigraphy as the difference in defect size pre- and postintervention is a predictor of functional outcome after infarction. Functional improvement occurred in proportion to the serial decrement [improvement] in defect size after stenting, with continued improvement over 6 mo.

548. Nakamura S, Hamada S, Suigiura T, et al. Quantitative estimation of myocardial salvage after primary coronary angioplasty in patients with angiographic no reflow [abstract]. *J Am Coll Cardiol* 1999;33:39A.

(Epicardial flow grade [TIMI flow grade] after primary angioplasty serves as an angiographic marker of the "no reflow phenomenon." When angiographic and scintigraphic patterns of flow were evaluated before and after primary percutaneous transluminal coronary angioplasty [PTCA], 2 patient groups were identified: 1 with few changes in defect size after primary PTCA [n = 40] and those with significant improvement compared with the pre-PTCA study [n = 42]. Although angiographic evidence of "no reflow" was highly specific for scintigraphic "no reflow" and little evidence of defect improvement with revascularization, angiography was insensitive to scintigraphic evidence of improvement post-PTCA! Many with apparent no reflow angiographically, improved on myocardial perfusion scintigraphy after revascularization.)

549. Mishra IP, Iskandrian AE. Stress myocardial perfusion after coronary angioplasty. *Am J Cardiol* 1998;81:766–769.

(This is an in-depth editorial on the subject. It concludes that stress myocardial perfusion scintigraphy is valuable after percutaneous transluminal coronary angioplasty with reversible abnormalities indicating residual, downstream, sidebranch, remote or restenosis.)

550. Lauer MS, Lytle B, Pashkow F, et al. Prediction of death and myocardial infarction by screening with exercise thallium testing after coronary artery bypass grafting. *Lancet* 1998;351:615–622.

(In a group of 873 symptom-free patients studied with exercise perfusion scintigraphy after coronary artery bypass graft, thallium-201 defects and exercise capacity were strong and independent predictors of subsequent death and nonfatal infarction.)

551. Desideri A, Candelpergher G, Zanco P, et al. Exercise technetium-99m sestamibi single-photon emission computed tomography late after coronary artery bypass surgery: long-term follow-up. *Clin Cardiol* 1997;20:779–784.

(Desideri et al. demonstrated a greater predictive value and a significantly higher χ^2 for stress myocardial perfusion scintigraphy than the clinical history, symptoms or results of exercise testing.)

552. Lai S, Berman DS, Kang X, et al. Prognostic value of stress myocardial perfusion SPECT in patients with history of coronary artery bypass grafting [abstract]. *J Nucl Med* 1999;40:6P.

(Among 1758 patients who had stress [35% adenosine, 65% exercise] myocardial perfusion scintigraphy 6.9 ± 5.2 yr after coronary artery bypass graft [CABG], patient age, time after CABG and summed stress score were independently associated with cardiac death. After adjusting for age and elapsed time after CABG, stress defects with scores ≥9 related to increased mortality, and this risk increased proportionately to defect size.)

553. Zellweger MJ, Dubois EA, Lai S, et al. Risk of late death in patients early and late after CABG using stress myocardial perfusion SPECT: implications for appropriate clinical strategies [abstract]. *J Nucl Med* 1999;40:7P.

(Studied with stress myocardial perfusion scintigraphy [MPS] were 1707 patients, 80% males, with exercise in 1111 and pharmacologic stress in 596, who were separated into those who had coronary artery bypass graft [CABG] <5 or >5 yr earlier. The cardiac death rate was low in asymptomatic patients studied within 5 yr of CABG. However, the cardiac death rate was intermediate in those studied after 5 yr and are well risk stratified by stress MPS.)

554. Batemen TM. Selection of patients following cardiac interventions (CABG/PTCA) who will benefit from myocardial perfusion/function imaging. Part of symposium: Patient Selection for Nuclear Cardiology Procedures: Meeting the Demands of the Cardiologist. Annual meeting of the American Society of Nuclear Cardiology; March 1998; Atlanta, GA.

(According to guidelines, the routine image evaluation of asymptomatic patients after revascularization is inappropriate. Published American College of Cardiology/American Heart Association guidelines [161,531] support stress testing or stress imaging evaluation after revascularization for patients presenting with renewed symptoms or in selected asymptomatic patients with electrocardiographic [ECG] changes or an ischemic stress ECG response. Further, the study is appropriate to quantitate left ventricular function and may be appropriately applied in the setting of incomplete revascularization, baseline multivessel disease, after a perioperative infarction or with new or worsening heart failure.)

555. Palmas W, Bingham S, Diamond GA, et al. Incremental prognostic value of exercise thallium-201 myocardial single photon emission computed tomography late after coronary artery bypass surgery. *J Am Coll Cardiol* 1995;25:403–409.

(After evaluation of treadmill exercise data in this study, thallium-201 myocardial perfusion SPECT provided incremental prognostic information in patients studied late [>90 days] after coronary artery bypass graft.)

556. Miller TD, Christian TF, Hodge DO, et al. Prognostic value of exercise thallium-201 imaging performed within 2 yr of coronary artery bypass graft surgery. *J Am Coll Cardiol* 1998;31:848–854.

(In this study, the exercise and thallium-201 exercise image variables were evaluated prospectively for their prognostic value among 411 patients who underwent exercise imaging and were followed for a median duration of 5.8 yr. The number of reversible defects was the only variable in multivariate analysis to demonstrate a significant association with early and late infarctions and cardiac death. The 5-yr, event-free survival rate for patients without angina and a normal image was 93%, but 71% for those with angina and a medium or large defect. Exercise perfusion imaging performed within 2 yr of coronary artery bypass graft could stratify patients well into low- and high-risk subgroups.)

557. Shaw L, Chaitman B, Hilton TC, et al. Prognostic value of dipyridamole thallium-201 imaging in elderly patients. *J Am Coll Cardiol* 1992;19:1390–1398.

(Dipyridamole SPECT was successfully able to risk stratify patients aged 65 and older, including those studied after coronary artery bypass graft. Here, patients with normal scans had <1% event rate over the first year of follow-up. In addition, the perfusion scan added incremental prognostic information over nonimaging variables. Similar stratification was achieved by others [607,608].)

558. The BARI Investigators. Comparison of coronary bypass surgery with angioplasty in patients with multivessel disease. The Bypass Angioplasty Revascularization Investigation (BARI). *N Engl J Med* 1996;335:217–225.

(This was a randomized multicenter study comparing the 2 initial approaches to revascularization. Compared with coronary artery bypass graft [CABG], an initial percutaneous transluminal coronary artery [PTCA] strategy did not reduce survival in patients with multivessel disease, although subsequent revascularization was more frequent. For diabetics, survival was better after CABG than PTCA.)

559. Greenberg BH, Hart R, Botvinick EH, et al. Thallium-201 myocardial perfusion scintigraphy to evaluate patients after coronary bypass surgery. *Am J Cardiol* 1978;42:167–176.

(This is 1 of many articles that document the accuracy of perfusion scintigraphy for the evaluation of regional perfusion and graft patency after bypass graft surgery.)

560. Verani MS, Marcus ML, Spoto G, et al. Thallium-201 myocardial perfusion scintigrams in the evaluation of aorto-coronary saphenous bypass surgery. *J Nucl Med* 1978;19:765–772.

(558,560: These are 2 of many articles that document the accuracy of perfusion scintigraphy for the evaluation of regional perfusion and graft patency after bypass graft surgery. Verani et al. demonstrated that coronary bypass surgery makes patients better but rarely makes them "normal" in consideration of their postoperative perfusion. Even after successful surgery, defects may be induced with stress that are much reduced compared with the preoperative study. This is another reason why a preoperative study may be valuable when applying scintigraphy to the determination of postoperative ischemia and graft patency.)

561. Lytle BW, Loop FD, Cosgrove DM, et al. Long-term (5-to-12 yr) serial studies of internal mammary artery and saphenous vein coronary bypass grafts. *J Thorac Cardiovasc Surg* 1985;89:248–258.
(The literature suggests that risk increases significantly 5 yr after saphenous vein grafts are placed. After that time, 15%–40% of patent grafts show abnormalities, ranging from luminal irregularities to significant stenoses, and an additional 20%–28% of grafts will be occluded, overall presenting an intermediate likelihood of significant ischemia at this time.)

562. Bateman TM, O'Keefe JH, Barnhart C. Prognostic value of exercise SPECT thallium-201 scintigraphy late after coronary artery bypass surgery. *J Am Coll Cardiol* 1992;19:703–705.
(After evaluation of treadmill exercise data, thallium-201 myocardial perfusion SPECT provided incremental prognostic information in such patients studied late after coronary artery bypass graft [CABG] [545] with results similar to those found in a general population using planar thallium imaging. In this study, the excellent prognostic value of stress perfusion imaging performed late [>5 yr] after CABG was demonstrated. However, after 10–15 yr, there was a somewhat increased event rate, even in those with normal stress images.)

563. Miller DD. Optimal imaging approaches for the evaluation of chest pain syndromes in women. *Cardiol Rev* 1997;5:279–284.
(Miller presents an elegant review of the problems faced in the evaluation of coronary disease in women and the tools to apply in its diagnosis and management.)

564. Travin MI, Johnson LL. Assessment of coronary artery disease in women. *Curr Opin Cardiol* 1997;12:587–594.
(When one considers the value of myocardial perfusion scintigraphy and other methods in women, the issue is compounded by concern regarding a sex bias in the application of diagnostic and therapeutic methods in coronary artery disease. Yet, the high diagnostic accuracy of the method and its unbiased application in women is presented in the review by Miller [563] and Travin and Johnson [564].)

565. Hendel RC, Berman DS, Iskandrian AS, et al. Diagnostic value of SPECT myocardial perfusion imaging utilizing attenuation correction with resolution compensation. Results of a multicenter trial. *Circulation* 1997;96:1719–1733.
(Some studies demonstrate an improved accuracy with a variety of attenuation correction methods, generally improving specificity if not sensitivity, with increased homogeneity in attenuation-corrected normal studies. However, in practice, sensitivity may suffer as well, and the methods may not yet be ready for general application.)

566. Hung J, Chaitman BR, Lam J, et al. Noninvasive diagnostic tests for the evaluation of coronary artery disease in women. A multivariate comparison of cardiac fluoroscopy, exercise electrocardiography, and exercise thallium myocardial perfusion scintigraphy. *J Am Coll Cardiol* 1984;4:8–14.
(This is 1 of many studies that demonstrate the diagnostic value of myocardial perfusion scintigraphy in women and its advantages compared with other methods.)

567. Van Train KF, Berman DS, Garcia EV, et al. Quantitative analysis of stress Tl-201 myocardial scintigrams. A multicenter trial. *J Nucl Med* 1986;27:1726–1735.
(In a multicenter study, Van Train et al. demonstrated similar sensitivity, specificity and normalcy in men and women.)

568. Iskandrian AS, Heo J, Nguyen T, et al. Assessment of coronary artery disease using SPECT with thallium-201 during adenosine induced hyperemia. *Am J Cardiol* 1991;67:1190–1194.
(Iskandrian et al. also found a similar sensitivity and normalcy for myocardial perfusion scintigraphy in men and women.)

569. Chae SC, Heo J, Iskandrian AS, et al. Identification of extensive coronary artery disease in women by exercise single photon emission tomographic (SPECT) thallium imaging. *J Am Coll Cardiol* 1993;21:1305–1311.

(In a group of 243 women evaluated for coronary artery disease, multivariate analysis identified the exercise heart rate and the number of reversible perfusion defects as the 2 predictors of high-risk, multivessel disease.)

570. Amanullah AM, Kiat H, Friedman JD, Berman DS. Adenosine technetium-99m sestamibi myocardial perfusion SPECT in women: diagnostic efficacy in detection of coronary artery disease. *J Am Coll Cardiol* 1996;27:803–809.

(Amanullah et al. found adenosine technetium-99m sestamibi SPECT to be an accurate and effective protocol for the detection of coronary artery disease [CAD] in women and was equally sensitive in women presenting with nonanginal symptoms. Sensitivity was maintained and similar in those with high or intermediate likelihood of CAD.)

571. Amanullah AM, Berman DS, Hachamovitch R, et al. Identification of severe or extensive coronary artery disease in women by adenosine technetium-99m sestamibi SPECT. *J Am Coll Cardiol* 1997;80:132–137.

(Using the same methodology as in their 1996 article, these authors found a sensitivity of 91% and specificity of 70% for the specific diagnosis of severe or extensive coronary artery disease.)

572. Marwick TH, Shaw LJ, Lauer MS, et al. The noninvasive prediction of cardiac mortality in men and women with known or suspected coronary artery disease. Economics of Noninvasive Diagnosis (END) Study Group. *Am J Med* 1999;106: 172–178.

(This large study conducted at 6 sites examined the prognostic value of stress myocardial perfusion scintigraphy [MPS] among 5009 men and 3402 women with symptomatic or suspected coronary artery disease undergoing exercise [7486] or pharmacologic [925] stress MPS. After adjustment for exercise variables, the number of abnormal territories was the strongest correlate of mortality in women undergoing exercise MPS. Such large multicenter studies, performed with attention to clinical detail, have contributed much to outcomes research and helped establish the prognostic value of MPS.)

573. Hachamovitch R, Cacciabando JM. Stress myocardial perfusion SPECT in women: is it the cornerstone of the noninvasive evaluation [editorial]? *J Nucl Med* 1998;39: 756–759.

(In the associated editorial written in reference to the article by Santana-Boada et al. [*335*] and based on its findings, Hachamovitch and Cacciabando present 2 approaches to the evaluation of coronary artery disease [CAD] in women and men: an anatomic approach based on the gold standard anatomical diagnosis of CAD and a physiologic, prognostic approach, based on scintigraphic findings that are employed to assess related risk and the need [if demonstrating moderate to severe defects] for coronary angiography.)

574. Gallup Survey. *Perceived Health Risks in Women.* New York, NY: Gallup, Inc.; 1995.

575. American Heart Association. *Heart and Stroke Facts Statistical Supplement.* Chicago, IL: American Heart Association; 1996.

576. Wenger NK. Coronary heart disease in women. An overview (myths, misconceptions and missed opportunities). In: Wenger NK, Speroff L, Packard B, eds. *Cardiovascular Health and Disease in Women.* Greenwich, CT: LeJaque Communications; 1993: 24–41.

(574–576: Among other things, this poll [*574*] assessed the perception of women about their own health problems. When asked which illness presented the greatest mortality threat, women identified cancer and breast cancer, specifically. However, cardiovascular disease, most prominently coronary artery disease, was then and is still the leading cause of death among women, exceeding by a factor of 2 the likelihood of death from cancer and responsible for the loss of 500,000 women each year and one-third of all deaths in women [575,576].)

577. Lerner DJ, Kannel WB. Patterns of coronary artery disease morbidity and mortality in the sexes: a 26-year follow-up of the Framingham population. *Am Heart J* 1986; 111:383–390.

(In general, symptoms were found to occur 10 yr and infarction 20 yr later in women than in men. Anginal symptoms developed earlier in women but were more benign, but there was a higher infarct-related fatality rate when events did eventually occur in older women. Similarly, women have higher perioperative morbidity and mortality at coronary artery bypass graft, probably as a result of greater age, concomitant illnesses and possibly the more advanced state of coronary artery disease [CAD] at the time of surgery. There is much evidence, however, that myocardial perfusion scintigraphy brings CAD diagnosis and prognosis in women and men to near equality with a high level of success.)

578. Tobin JN, Wassertheil-Smoller S, Wexler JP, et al. Sex bias in considering coronary bypass surgery. *Ann Intern Med* 1987;107:19–25.

(Some early studies suggested that the less frequent and later diagnosis and less aggressive treatment of coronary artery disease in women than in men is the result of a sex-related referral bias, with more frequent testing and subsequent cardiac catheterization of men than women with apparent similar clinical and risk profiles.)

579. Bicknell NA, Pieper KS, Lee KL, et al. Referral patterns for coronary artery disease treatment: gender bias or good clinical judgement? *Ann Int Med* 1992;116:791–797.

(To determine whether a gender bias exists in the referral of patients with documented coronary artery disease [CAD] to coronary artery bypass graft [CABG], 5795 patients presenting with angiographic CAD from 1969–1984 were studied. When risk of hard events was considered, men at low risk were somewhat more likely [1.24:1] to be referred. However, among high-risk patients most likely to benefit from surgery, women were at least as likely [1.18:1] to undergo CABG. These trends were most common in the recent years of the study, when women were seemingly treated more appropriately than men.)

580. Khan SS, Nessim S, Gray R, et al. Increased mortality of women in coronary artery bypass surgery: evidence for referral bias. *Ann Intern Med* 1990;112:561–567.

(A consecutive population of 2297 [21% women] patients who had coronary artery bypass graft [CABG] between 1982 and 1987 was studied to determine whether referral differences were related to the higher incidence of operative mortality among women. In fact, it was the functional class and age that most influenced surgical outcome. This seemed to be the result of referral of women to CABG later in the course of their illnesses.)

581. Fiebach NH, Viscoli CM, Horwitz RI. Differences between women and men in survival after myocardial infarction: biology or methodology? *JAMA* 1990;263:1092–1096.

(The impact of gender on survival after infarction was retrospectively studied in 332 women and 790 men. In fact, survival was related to differences in known postinfarction risk factors—not sex.)

582. Ayanian JZ, Epstein AM. Differences in the use of procedures between men and women hospitalized for coronary heart disease. *N Engl J Med* 1991;325:221–225.

(Gender differences in the utilization of major diagnostic tests and therapeutic procedures was retrospectively studied in 49,623 discharged patients. Women hospitalized for coronary artery disease have lower angiographic and revascularization rates. Although this was true for those who had recent infarctions, it may represent an appropriate care level given the clinical state of the patient, which was not studied here.)

583. Steingart RM, Packer M, Hamm P, et al. Sex differences in the management of coronary artery disease. *N Engl J Med* 1991;325:226–230.

(The application of anti-ischemic interventions was studied in a group of 2231 patients [389 women, 1842 men] with left ventricular ejection fraction <40% after myocardial infarction. Although women had greater functional disability, men more often underwent coronary angiography. However, women underwent revascularization with similar frequency.)

584. Shaw LJ, Miller DD, Romeis JC, et al. Gender differences in the noninvasive evaluation and management of patients with suspected coronary artery disease. *Ann Intern Med* 1994;120:559–566.

(Among 840 patients [47% women; 53% men] referred for outpatient stress testing with or without myocardial perfusion scintigraphy, women with suspected coronary artery disease [CAD] had fewer additional tests than men after an initial abnormal stress test, in spite of a higher incidence of angina and CAD risk factors.

579–584: These are part of the extensive literature that has evaluated sex-related differences in test utility and post-test angiography, as well as relative mortalities after cardiac events in men and women.)

585. Mark DB, Shaw LK, Delong DR, et al. Absence of sex bias in the referral of patients for cardiac catheterization. *N Engl J Med* 1994;330:1101–1106.

(The authors reported the lower referral rate of women to coronary angiography compared with the rate for men. Although some investigators who view the findings superficially consider them illustrative of a sex-related bias in the diagnosis and management of coronary artery disease, a deeper analysis of this and several other studies have found that such sex-related differences are appropriate when corrected for baseline group differences and the results of myocardial perfusion scintigraphy.)

586. Lauer MS, Pashkow F, Snader CE, et al. Gender and referral for coronary angiography after treadmill thallium testing. *Am J Cardiol* 1996;78:278–283.

(Lauer et al. prospectively evaluated the pattern and logic behind referral to angiography in both men and women. Women had a lower incidence of induced ischemia, coronary artery disease, angiography, mortality and overall end points than men. Again, gender-related differences in referral for coronary angiography after exercise perfusion imaging could be explained by the higher rate of abnormal tests in men.)

587. Travin MI, Duca MD, Kline GM, et al. Relation of gender to physician use of test results and to the prognostic value of stress technetium-99m sestamibi myocardial single photon emission tomography scintigraphy. *Am Heart J* 1997;134:73–82.

(The potential gender differences in the use and prognostic value of stress sestamibi imaging were studied in 1226 men and 1152 women. There was no difference in catheterization referral rates between sexes when normalized for defect size. Image defect size was an independent predictor of events. For both men and women, image findings were strongly correlated with prognosis, with event rates associated with abnormal images that were similar in men and women, 19.6% and 18.2%, respectively. Conversely, normal images were related to low event rates in both men [1.7%] and women [0.8%.] In a larger study, Hachamovitch et al. [19] demonstrated a strong and appropriate relationship between findings on stress myocardial perfusion scintigraphy and subsequent management in women.)

588. Hachamovitch R, Berman DS, Shaw LJ, et al. Relative role of history of coronary artery disease and patient sex on cardiac risk and referral to catheterization [abstract]. *J Nucl Med* 1997;38:164P.

(The sex-related bias in referral to angiography may favor women or men, not based on gender but on the presence of known coronary artery disease and also on the degree to which the physician involved is concerned about the diagnosis and dynamic nature of the disease process.)

589. Chowdhry SN, McGowan CM, Alaswad K, et al. Referral to coronary angiography after myocardial perfusion imaging: potential existence and significance of a gender bias [abstract]. *Circulation* 1999;100:I-383.

(Recently, Chowdhry et al. evaluated the contribution of quantitative stress perfusion image findings to referrals to angiography in 11,063 consecutive men [7006] and women [4057], compared with the influence of other clinical and stress test findings. The severity and extent of image ischemia was the leading predictor of angiography but with a lower threshold for referral in men among all scan score grades. However, this seemed to relate to the fact that men were studied too often and at a rate not justified by the outcomes, rather than that there was an antifemale bias.)

590. Roeters van Lennep JE, Borum JJJ, Zwinderman AH, et al. No gender bias in referral for angiography after myocardial perfusion scintigraphy with technetium-99m tetrofosmin. *J Nucl Cardiol* 1999;6:594–604.

(These authors demonstrated that after correction for the presence and severity of stress myocardial perfusion scintigraphy defects, both men and women were referred for coronary angiography at a similar and proportional rate. There was no association between sex and the likelihood of referral to angiography but a strong relationship in both sexes between defect size and referral to angiography.)

591. Miller DD, Stratmann H, Shaw LJ, et al. Gender and myocardial perfusion: key cardiovasular outcome co-variables in a multicenter study of stable angina patients undergoing stress Tc-99m sestamibi myocardial tomography [abstract]. *Circulation* 1995;92:I-129.

(The authors present the results of a multicenter study evaluating the prognostic value of stress perfusion imaging in 314 women and 1262 men. Both men and women had low event rates in the presence of a normal scan: 1.4% and 0.6%, respectively. However, although the risk related to an abnormal scan was high in both groups, it was higher in women than men [10.9% versus 6.9%, respectively], presenting women with an 11-fold risk ratio compared with a negative test and a risk ratio of 6 for men.)

592. Hachamovitch R, Shaw LK, Kesler K, et al. Does nuclear testing yield incremental information for the prediction of death in patients with normal rest ECG [abstract]. *J Am Coll Cardiol* 1997;29:136A.

593. Boyne TS, Koplan BA, Parsons WJ, et al. Predicting adverse outcome with exercise SPECT technetium-99m sestamibi imaging in patients with suspected or known coronary artery disease. *Am J Cardiol* 1997;79:270–274.

(592,593: Hachamovitch et al. demonstrated that hard coronary events in women could be predicted by findings on stress perfusion SPECT modulated by the pretest likelihood of disease. Here, the 1-yr rate of death or infarction was 1% in association with normal scans and 4% with abnormal scans in a low likelihood group, but 1% and 12% when normal and abnormal scans were evident in women with a high pretest likelihood of coronary disease [see reference *21*].

This was again confirmed by Boyne et al. who studied the value of exercise technetium-99m sestamibi SPECT to predict events in a total of 229 patients with a "comparable" population of 114 men and 115 women. Again, the event rate related to a normal scan was 0.8% but that related to an abnormal scan was 5.4%/yr [$P < 0.005$].)

594. Hachamovitch R, Diamond GA, Kiat H, et al. Comparison of incremental prognostic value of nuclear testing in men and women [abstract]. *J Nucl Cardiol* 1995;2:S45.

(When used in a strategy incorporating clinical and exercise variables toward a prognostic end point, perfusion imaging cost less per patient in women than in men.)

595. Tofler GH, Stone PH, Muller JE, et al. Effects of gender and race on prognosis after myocardial infarction. Adverse prognosis for women, particularly black women. *J Am Coll Cardiol* 1987;9:473–482.

596. Becker RC, Terrin M, Ross R, et al. Comparison of clinical outcomes for women and men after acute myocardial infarction. *Ann Int Med* 1994;120:638–645.

597. Greenland P, Reicher-Reiss H, Goldbourt U, et al. In-hospital and 1-year mortality in 1524 women after myocardial infarction: comparison with 4315 men. *Circulation* 1991;83:484–491.

   (595–597: Presented are a variety of studies that evaluate clinical outcomes after infarction in relation to sex. When myocardial perfusion scintigraphy [MPS] is performed, patient management is strongly influenced by scintigraphic findings, in which the larger the reversible defect the more likely was angiography. Therefore, contrary to popular belief, but similar to other reports, MPS better stratifies coronary risk and appropriately affected management in females, whereas the same scintigraphic abnormality appeared to relate to a worse prognosis than in males.)

598. Hendel RC, Chen MH, L'Italien GH, et al. Sex differences in perioperative and long-term cardiac event-free survival in vascular surgery patients: an analysis of clinical and scintigraphic variables. *Circulation* 1995;91:1044–1051.

   (Hendel et al. studied 187 women and 380 men before vascular surgery. Perfusion defects indicated a 3.9 times increase in risk of short-term perioperative events in men compared with a 4.5 times increase in women, whereas the values for predicting long-term outcome were 11.8-fold in women and 14.8-fold in men.)

599. Amanullah AM, Berman DS, Erel J, et al. Incremental prognostic value of adenosine myocardial perfusion single-photon emission computed tomography in women with suspected coronary artery disease. *Am J Cardiol* 1998;82:725–730.

   (The authors established the prognostic value of the pharmacologic stress method with the assessment of outcomes in a population of 923 women. Stress perfusion imaging added significant prognostic information to clinical and physiologic variables in women.)

600. Marwick TH, Anderson T, Williams J, et al. Exercise echocardiography is an accurate and cost-effective technique for detection of coronary artery disease. *J Am Coll Cardiol* 1995;26:335–341.

601. Marwick TH, Willemart B, D'Hondt AM, et al. Selection of optimal nonexercise stress for the evaluation of ischemic myocardial dysfunction and malperfusion. Comparison of dobutamine and adenosine using echocardiography and Tc-99m-MIBI single photon emission computed tomography. *Circulation* 1993;87:345–354.

   (600,601: These articles represent 2 among several instances in which the literature found no difference or a superiority in sensitivity of stress echocardiography compared with stress testing. However, the stress echocardiographic method did appear to have better specificity than stress testing: 56% versus 80%, respectively. How can this be explained?)

602. Marwick TH, D'Hondt AM, Baudhuin T, et al. Optimal use of dobutamine stress for the detection and evaluation of coronary artery disease: combination with echocardiography or scintigraphy or both? *J Am Coll Cardiol* 1993;22:159–167.

   (This study of 217 patients established being female as a significant contributing predictor of false negative stress imaging studies performed by both modalities.)

603. Severi S, Picano E, Michelassi C, et al. Diagnostic and prognostic value of dipyridamole echocardiography in patients with suspected coronary artery disease. *Circulation* 1994;89:1160–1173.

604. Heupler S, Mehta RT, Lobo A, et al. Prognostic implications of exercise echocardiography in women with known or suspected coronary artery disease. *J Am Coll Cardiol* 1997;30:414–420.

   (603,604: The prognostic value of stress echocardiography in patients with known or suspected coronary disease has found limited development, as illustrated in these 2 articles.)

605. Beller, GA. Are you ever too old to be risk stratified [editorial]? *J Am Coll Cardiol* 1992;19:1399–1401.

    (Beller considered the application of coronary risk stratification in the elderly. Of course, chronological age is only 1 factor to consider. Pharmacologic stress imaging with a coronary dilator is safe and widely available, even in this population.)

606. Hilton TC, Shaw LJ, Chaitman BR, et al. Prognostic significance of exercise thallium-201 testing in patients aged greater than or equal to 70 years with known or suspected coronary artery disease. *Am J Cardiol* 1992;69:45–50.

    (Hilton et al. found that exercise myocardial perfusion scintigraphy with thallium-201 in patients aged 70 yr and older was accurate in identifying a high-risk population.)

607. Hachamovitch R, Diamond GA, Kiat H, et al. Noninvasive risk stratification of the elderly patient; use of nuclear testing to identify high risk patient populations [abstract]. *Circulation* 1994;90:I-102.

608. Iskandrian AS, Heo J, Decoskey D, et al. Use of thallium-201 imaging for risk stratification of elderly patients with coronary artery disease. *Am J Cardiol* 1988;61:269–272.

    (607,608: In a large population [607], exercise dual-isotope SPECT was successfully able to risk stratify patients aged 65 and older. Here, patients with normal scans had a >1% event rate over the first year of follow-up. In addition, the perfusion scan added incremental prognostic information over nonimaging variables, and the addition of myocardial perfusion scintigraphy to test strategies reduced the overall per-patient cost of testing. Similar stratification was achieved by others [557,608].)

609. Lauer MS, Pashkow F, Snader CE, et al. Age and referral to coronary angiography after an abnormal thallium treadmill test. *Am Heart J* 1997;133:139–146.

    (Lauer et al. demonstrated that increasing age was a factor that increased the clinical value of findings on myocardial perfusion scintigraphy and its influence on management. The size of image defects was predictive of death. However, age was inversely related to the likelihood of referral to coronary angiography after an abnormal stress perfusion image.)

610. Alkeylani A, Miller DD, Shaw LJ, et al. Influence of race on the prediction of cardiac events with stress Tc-99m sestamibi tomographic imaging in patients with stable angina pectoris. *Am J Cardiol* 1998;81:293–297.

    (The prognostic value of both normal and abnormal perfusion scintigrams was well preserved among 1086 Caucasian and African-American patients studied. Normal images related to an extremely low event rate and multivessel abnormalities to the highest event rate in both races.)

611. Schweikert RA, Pashkow FJ, Snader CE, et al. Association of exercise-induced ventricular ectopic activity with thallium myocardial perfusion and angiographic coronary artery disease in stable, low-risk populations. *Am J Cardiol* 1999;83:530–534.

    (Although exercise-induced ventricular ectopy has been found to be associated with a higher incidence of perfusion defects, there was no relationship with disease severity or short-term mortality.)

612. Kothari M, Sing VP, Amanullah AM, et al. Relation between QT dispersion and myocardial perfusion to survival in patients with life threatening ventricular arrhythmias [abstract]. *J Am Coll Cardiol* 1999;33:480A.

    (The authors used rest myocardial perfusion scintigraphy to study 38 patients with ventricular arrhythmias and left ventricular dysfunction. Large perfusion defect size combined with reduced left ventricular ejection fraction <30% and QT interval >50 msec to predict survival, where there was a 50% mortality over 3 yr. Any combination of 2 adverse values brought a survival rate approaching 0%, whereas when any of 2 adverse outcome markers were not present, the 3-year survival approximated 87%.)

conservatively and influenced an aggressive approach among 12 of 35 who went to angiography, only 7 with coronary disease. Overall, stress echocardiography was found to influence management in only 19 of 152 patients, or 12%! Here, most studies are, in fact, ordered by physicians who will profit from their performance. Yet, somewhat surprisingly, the method was not often useful in patient management, a situation that seems to expose other motivations for its performance! Unlike myocardial perfusion scintigraphy, in unselected patients evaluated for chest pain, stress echocardiography adds little information to conventional dynamic stress testing.)

645. Steingart RM, Wasserheil-Smoller S, Tobin JN, et al. Nuclear exercise tests reduce the perceived need for catheterization. *J Nucl Med* 1991;32:753–760.

(Not only do negative images reduce the incidence of angiography but, judging from current prognostic data, they do so safely.)

646. Miller TD, Milavetz JJ, Christian T, et al. A normal exercise thallium-201 image is associated with lower subsequent utilization of medical resources [abstract]. *J Am Coll Cardiol* 1999;33:447A.

(Miller et al. reported the relationship between the findings on myocardial perfusion scintigraphy [MPS] and subsequent utilization of medical resources in 2696 patients. A normal stress MPS study, well validated to relate to a low risk of coronary events, was shown to dramatically reduce the utilization of medical resources, from 15%–40%, including: hospitalization, angiography and all forms of revascularization over the ensuing 7 yr.)

647. Berman DS, Shaw LJ, Thompson TD, et al. Stress myocardial perfusion SPECT with angina pectoris: gatekeeper to the cath lab [abstract]. *J Nucl Med* 1999;40:155P.

(In a large group of 3096 patients with typical or atypical angina, the summed segmental score remained a highly significant predictor of outcome and coronary angiography after adjusting for clinical variables. This effort documented the full "gatekeeper" function of the method.)

648. Amanullah AM, Heo J, Iskandrian AE. Impact of exercise single-photon emission computed tomographic imaging on appropriateness of coronary revascularization. *Am J Cardiol* 1998;81:1489–1496.

(Among 816 patients with chest pain syndromes who underwent coronary angiography and myocardial perfusion scinitgraphy [MPS], Amanullah et al. demonstrated that the most powerful predictor of revascularization by multivariate analysis was the presence of reversibility on stress SPECT MPS.)

649. Amanullah AM, Heo J, Acio E, et al. Predictors of outcome of medically treated patients with left main/three vessel coronary disease by coronary angiography. *Am J Cardiol* 1999;83:445–448.

(Multivariate Cox survival analysis of medically treated patients with left main or triple-vessel disease revealed that adenosine SPECT thallium-201 myocardial perfusion scintigraphy [MPS] parameters were the only independent predictors of outcome over a 5-yr follow-up period. Although this angiographic subgroup is at highest risk overall, only stress MPS could substratify them.)

650. Gremillet E, Champailler A, Soler C. Identification of extensive multivessel CAD among negative scans in dual isotope myocardial SPECT with ECG gating [abstract]. *J Nucl Med* 1999;40:161P.

(Normal stress myocardial perfusion scintigraphy [MPS] in 75 patients studied using a dual-isotope rest thallium-201 stress sestamibi protocol were analyzed seeking cues for the identification of 6 with multivessel disease. Stress images were acquired fully 1 hr after stress tracer administration, and so, apparently, enlarged left ventricular [LV] cavities at stress imaging represent extensive subendocardial ischemia, rather than cavitary dilation. The ratio of stress-to-rest ventricular volumes and LV ejection fraction provides clues to the presence of significant coronary artery disease in those unusual cases in which stress MPS is normal.)

651. Amanullah A, Kiat H, Hachamovitch R, et al. The impact of myocardial perfusion single photon emission computed tomography on referral to catheterization of the very elderly: is there evidence of gender-related bias? *J Am Coll Cardiol* 1996;28:680–686.

(This study evaluated the impact on clinical management [referral to catheterization within 60 days] of stress myocardial perfusion scintigraphy [MPS] in 1006 consecutive patients older than 80 yr [511 men, 495 women] using exercise [401 individuals] or pharmacologic [605 individuals] stress. Overall referral rates to catheterization were similar in men and women. However, women with severe defects were more often referred to angiography and revascularization than men with the same defect size. This difference in referral rate may be appropriate, in view of the higher event rate in women than men with similar defect size documented in some studies.)

652. Nallamothu N, Pancholy SB, Lee KR, et al. Impact of exercise single-photon computed tomographic thallium imaging on patient management and outcome. *J Nucl Cardiol* 1995;2:334–338.

(651,652: In patients without previously documented coronary artery disease [CAD], the rates of referral to catheterization increased significantly as a function of the scan abnormality. This is an overview of the clinical value of exercise SPECT perfusion imaging and its influence on the diagnosis, prognosis and management of CAD. However, for any given scan result, the referral rate was greater in patients with a higher likelihood of CAD.

The ability to identify low-risk coronary patients is at the basis of the value of any method if it is to serve as the gatekeeper for more expensive procedures of greater risk. This ability has placed myocardial perfusion scintigraphy [MPS] in this role with a strong and appropriate impact on the performance of coronary angiography and revascularization. MPS image findings clearly and appropriately influence the performance of coronary angiography and revascularization. Scintigraphy clearly serves as the gatekeeper for these next-most expensive and dangerous steps, in which those with normal stress scintigrams have a 1%–3% rate of coronary angiography, even in the presence of a high likelihood of clinical disease.)

653. Shaw LJ, Heller GV, Travin MI, et al. Cost analysis of diagnostic testing for coronary artery disease in women with stable chest pain. *J Nucl Cardiol* 1999;6:559–569.

(Myocardial perfusion scintigraphy [MPS] has been shown to decrease costs without harm when used as the gatekeeper to angiography in women with chest pain syndromes. Outcomes data from 4638 women with stable chest pain studied with early coronary angiography [3375 women] or with abnormal stress MPS [1263 women with 539 to angiography] demonstrated that referral to angiography increased in women in parallel with increasing pretest likelihood of coronary artery disease. Cardiac death rates were without difference between management groups. However, the revascularization rate and cost per patient were higher among the angiography-first group, and normal coronary angiograms were far more common among those who went first to angiography.)

654. Terrin ML, Williams DO, Kleiman NS, et al. Two and three year results of the thrombolysis in myocardial infarction TIMI Phase II clinical trial. *J Am Coll Cardiol* 1993;22:1763–1772.

(Patients presenting with ischemic symptoms within 4 hr of onset and at least 1-mm ST elevation were assigned to aggressive, angiography-first [n = 1681] or conservative [n = 1658] management groups. The former went to immediate angiography and revascularization when appropriate anatomically. The latter were managed medically, unless evident spontaneous ischemia or ischemia on low-level stress testing brought invasive study and possible revascularization. Both management groups had the same favorable outcomes.)

655. Boden WE, O'Rourke RA, Crawford MH, et al. for the Veterans Affairs Non-Q Wave Infarction Strategies in Hospital (VANQWISH) Trial Investigators. Outcomes in patients

with acute non-Q wave myocardial infarction randomly assigned to an invasive as compared with a conservative management strategy. *N Engl J Med* 1998;338:1785–1792.

656. Bateman TM. Clinical decision making for patients with CAD: medical therapy vs invasive strategies. Symposium. Society of Nuclear Medicine; June, 1998; Toronto, Canada.

(655,656: Recent studies have compared anatomic with risk-based management approaches and found no increase or a reduced rate of interventions and events with risk-based management. Most such studies simply divided similar populations into 2 therapeutic groups, 1 sent early to angiography with treatment determined by the anatomic findings and another treated medically in the absence of progressive symptoms. Better yet might be a management strategy actually based on physiologic risk stratification, as offered by myocardial perfusion scintigraphy (MPS). Only the VANQWISH study [655] used MPS as the specific method to determine risk.)

657. Bateman TM, Case JA, Moutray K, et al. Comparison of outcomes in patients with reversible perfusion defects in a single coronary distribution: medical therapy versus revascularization [abstract]. *J Nucl Med* 1999;40:7P.

(Hard event rates were calculated in 2942 patients with stress perfusion defects in a single-vessel distribution. For each vessel distribution, death and myocardial infarction rate were substantially and significantly higher if treated with revascularization compared with medical therapy.)

658. Berman DS, Shaw LJ, Hachamovitch R, et al. Temporal changes in noninvasive test utilization and influence on patient outcome [abstract]. *Circulation* 1999;100: I–585.

(The study demonstrated an increasing and appropriate reliance on scintigraphic findings for management decisions. In 1991, a moderate defect was related to angiography and revascularization in 16.7% and 8.9%, respectively, whereas patients with severe defects saw angiography in 31.8% and 21.7% of cases, respectively. In 1996, the same numbers for moderate defects were 41.7% and 25.5%, whereas for severe defects these were 45.4% and 33.2%, respectively. Thus, there was no change in the event rates related to any scan score, and the catheterization and intervention rates related to normal scans remained unchanged at levels of ~2% and 0.5%, respectively.)

659. Shaw LJ, Hachamovitch R, Berman DS, et al. Integrating clinical history and stress perfusion variables into a scoring system [abstract]. *J Nucl Cardiol* 1997;4(suppl):S-86.

(The authors relate image findings to other important clinical parameters. Each is weighted to derive a prognostic score, an inclusive index for risk stratification.)

660. Bateman TM, Thompson TD, Case JA, et al. Management decisions in post-CABG patients referred for SPECT myocardial perfusion scintigraphy [abstract]? *J Am Coll Cardiol* 1999;33:448A.

(Examined in 2866 consecutive patients having SPECT myocardial perfusion scintigraphy [MPS] was the relationship of clinical and scintigraphic findings with the performance of angiography in patients after coronary artery bypass graft [CABG]. The single most important predictor of angiography in post-CABG patients is the summed difference score [SDS] using a 20-segment MPS model. The higher the SDS, the more likely the patient was to have angiography. MPS was the pivotal factor in patient management.)

661. Hachamovitch R, Berman D, Kiat H, et al. Incremental prognostic value of nuclear testing using adenosine stress. *Am J Cardiol* 1997;80:426–433.

(The authors examined the hard event rate and the rate of referral to cardiac catheterization among 1159 consecutive patients who underwent adenosine stress dual-isotope SPECT myocardial perfusion scintigraphy [MPS]. Kaplan-Meier analysis demonstrated the ability of MPS to further risk stratify both low and intermediate-to-high risk patients after clinical risk stratification, with risk increasing with worsening scan result. By multivariate analysis, the extent and severity of reversible stress MPS defect was shown to be the only predictor of physician referral to angiography, which occurred at a rate similar to those after exercise SPECT MPS, in spite of the greater risk of events with similar findings on pharmacologic stress.)

662. Scandinavian Simvistatin Survival Study Group. Randomized trial of cholesterol lowering in 4444 patients with coronary heart disease: the Scandinavian simvistatin survival study. *Lancet* 1994;344:1383–1389.

663. Byington RP, Jukema JW, Pitt B, et al. Reduction in cardiac events during pravastatin therapy; pooled analysis of clinical events of the pravastatin atherosclerosis intervention program. *Circulation* 1995;92:2419–2425.

664. Shepard J, Cobbe SM, Ford I, et al. Prevention of coronary heart disease with pravastatin in men with hypercholesterolemia. *N Engl J Med* 1995;333:1301–1307.
    (662–664: These are a few of the articles that demonstrate the beneficial impact of lipid management on the event rate in coronary artery disease.)

665. Manson JE, Stampfer MJ, Colditz GA, et al. A prospective study of aspirin use and primary prevention of coronary disease in women. *JAMA* 1991;266:527–535.
    (Aspirin, antioxidants [such as vitamin E] or certain dihydropridine calcium channel blockers may also benefit outcome via modification of the disease process.)

666. Pilote L, Miller DP, Califf RM, et al. Determinants of the use of coronary angiography and revascularization after thrombolysis for acute myocardial infarction. *N Engl J Med* 1996;335:1198–1205.
    (Several studies noted previously demonstrate that patients with little residual ischemia after myocardial infarction have a benign follow-up with a low event rate, regardless of whether they are treated medically or with revascularization. Its high predictive value when negative makes myocardial perfusion scintigraphy a valuable method in the evaluation of this population. Yet, currently, 70%–80% of these patients undergo coronary angiography and often revascularization.)

667. Mark DB, Naylor CD, Hlatky MA, et al. Use of medical resources and quality of life after acute myocardial infarction in Canada and the United States. *N Engl J Med* 1994;331:1130–1135.
    (This is 1 of 2 large post-thrombolytic trials [see reference *520*] that demonstrate no significant advantage of revascularization with an equally beneficial outcome among patients treated in Canada and the United States, although U.S. patients were revascularized at a 3-fold higher rate.)

668. Rogers WJ, Bourassa MG, Andrews TC, et al. For the ACIP Investigators. Outcome at 1 year for patients with asymptomatic cardiac ischemia randomized to medical therapy or revascularization. *J Am Coll Cardiol* 1995;26:594–605.
    (Here, survival was improved if medical treatment or percutaneous transluminal coronary angioplasty reduced the extent of exercise-induced scintigraphic ischemia.)

669. Pepine CJ, Cohn PF, Deedwania PC, et al., for the ASIST Study Group. Effects of treatment on outcomes in mildly symptomatic patients with ischemia during daily life: the Atenolol Silent Ischemia Study (ASIST). *Circulation* 1994;90:762–768.
    (Atenolol treatment reduced ischemia in daily life and was associated with reduced risk for adverse outcome in asymptomatic and mildly symptomatic patients, compared with placebo. Stress myocardial perfusion scintigraphy is a valuable method to uncover asymptomatic ischemia.)

670. The MIAMI Trial Research Group. Metoprolol in acute myocardial infarction (MIAMI): mortality. *Am J Cardiol* 1985;56:15G–22G.
    (Metoprolol reduced mortality in the highest-risk postinfarction group.)

671. Fallen EL, Nahmias C, Scheffel A, et al. Redistribution of myocardial blood flow with topical nitroglycerin in patients with coronary artery disease. *Circulation* 1995;91: 1381–1388.

672. Bottcher M, Czernin J, Sun K, et al. Effects of B1 adrenergic receptor blockade on myocardial blood flow and vasodilatory capacity. *J Nucl Med* 1997;38:442–446.

(671,672: Myocardial perfusion scintigraphy [MPS] has been widely applied to assess the effect of pharmacologic agents on myocardial blood flow. One of the strong points of the pharmacologic method using direct coronary dilators, well supported in the literature, is that it can be done while the patient is on anti-ischemic therapy without loss of sensitivity or ability to risk stratify! This seems to relate to the fact that these dilators act on the coronary flow supply rather than demands, whereas beta blockers affect demands. This relationship has recently been brought into question [see reference *301*]. However, beta blockers reduce myocardial oxygen demands at rest and reduce resting myocardial blood flow [*299*]. With the subsequent administration of coronary dilators, the coronary flow reserve increases in areas supplied by stenotic vessels. Although a similar effect must occur in the bed of normal vessels as a result of reduced baseline demands, this could potentially result in a relative reduction in the differential flow augmentation between stenotic and normal beds [*672*]. This could, in turn, result in an apparent reduction of the related induced defect, with a potential underestimation of related disease and risk [*301,302*].)

673. Hachamovitch R. Myocardial perfusion imaging for risk stratification in CAD. Extracting all the information. Paper presented at: Patient Selection for Nuclear Cardiology Procedures: Meeting the Demands of the Cardiologist in 1998; American Society of Nuclear Cardiology Symposium; 1998; Atlanta, GA.

(Hachamovitch makes a number of points and related suggestions designed to extract the most from the interpretation of the perfusion study.)

674. Shaw LJ, Hachamovitch R, Peterson ED, et al. Using an outcomes-based approach to identify candidates for risk stratification after exercise treadmill testing. *J Gen Intern Med* 1999;14:1–9.

(A recent analysis by Shaw et al. analyzed stress test, myocardial perfusion scintigraphy [MPS] and clinical data among 3620 medically treated patients [42% female] with an intermediate [2.5% mortality] poststress risk, to develop a hierarchical approach to coronary risk stratification after exercise. Symptomatic patients with an intermediate event likelihood after exercise testing will benefit from further evaluation with an exercise MPS [see references *780,781*].)

675. Narula J, Amanulla A, Acio E, et al. Predictors of outcome in hypertensive subjects with coronary artery disease [abstract]. *J Am Coll Cardiol* 1999;33:479A.

(Among 355 hypertensives [213 males; ages 62 ±10 yr], the 4-yr event-free survival [by Kaplan-Meier analysis] was 38% in patients with left ventricular hypertrophy [LVH] and large defects, 78% in those with either LVH or large defects and 90% in patients without either characteristic. The latter was similar to the 93% 4-yr event-free survival in 493 nonhypertensive patients with no or small defects studied and followed during the same period. In hypertensives, LVH and perfusion defect size are independent predictors of outcome. Yet hypertension, even without LVH or large defects, is still related to a higher event rate than those without hypertension.)

676. DiCarlo LA, Botvinick EH, Canhasi BS. Value of noninvasive assessment of patients with atypical chest pain and suspected coronary spasm using ergonovine infusion and thallium-201 perfusion scintigraphy. *Am J Cardiol* 1984;54:744–752.

(Here, thallium-201 perfusion scintigraphy was applied with injection during stimulated coronary vasospasm to actually identify the resultant ischemic zone in a coronary care unit setting. This provocation was performed safely in patients known to otherwise have normal coronary arteries.)

677. Glynn TP Jr, Fleming RG, Haist JL, Hunterman RK. Coronary arteriovenous fistula as a cause for reversible thallium-201 perfusion defect. *J Nucl Med* 1994;35:1808–1810.

(Although most reversible perfusion abnormalities relate to epicardial coronary disease, congenital coronary anomalies are among those nonatherosclerotic lesions that may cause true perfusion defects. They are to be especially considered when addressing possibly ischemic symptoms in the young.)

678. Iriarte M, Caso R, Murga N, et al. Microvascular angina pectoris in hypertensive patients with left ventricular hypertrophy and diagnostic value of exercise thallium-201 scintigraphy. *Am J Cardiol* 1995;75:335–339.

(Among 31 selected hypertensive patients with left ventricular hypertrophy, 21 had angina and induced thallium-201 abnormalities, 10 had none and normal stress images and all had normal coronary arteries. The coronary flow reserve after papaverine was 3.7 ± 0.8 among those with normal thallium images and 2.71 ± 0.96 among those [21] with abnormal scans, compared with 6.25 ± 1.4 in 5 normal controls. Stress-induced angina in some hypertensive patients probably relates to small-vessel disease and can cause image abnormalities.)

679. Cannon RO, Dilsizian V, O'Gara PT, et al. Impact of surgical relief of outflow obstruction on thallium perfusion abnormalities in hypertrophic cardiomyopathy. *Circulation* 1992;85:1039–1045.

(The perfusion scintigraphic method is of great value in the assessment of ischemia and coronary disease in the presence of myocardial hypertrophy. However, it may at times reflect the presence of myocardial ischemia unrelated to coronary disease.)

680. Bart BA, Shaw LK, McCants CB Jr, et al. Clinical determinants of mortality in patients with angiographically diagnosed ischemic or nonischemic cardiomyopathy. *J Am Coll Cardiol* 1997;30:1002–1008.

(An ischemic cause was itself an independent predictor of mortality among those with cardiomyopathy. The major predictor of outcome, however, was the extent of coronary artery disease. Not studied was the importance to risk stratification of the extent of myocardium at ischemic risk.)

681. Danias PG, Ahlberg AW, Messineo FC, et al. Exercise technetium-99m gated SPECT myocardial perfusion imaging differentiates non-ischemic from ischemic dilated cardiomyopathy [abstract]. *Circulation* 1997;96:I-735.

(Defect distribution, severity and reversibility all serve to predict the presence of coronary artery disease [CAD] in the presence of a cardiomyopathy. The authors demonstrated that the distribution of defects, their severity and reversibility all contribute to the likelihood of CAD in the presence of a congestive cardiomyopathy. The presence of CAD does not, however, indicate an ischemic origin to the overall condition.)

682. Yao S, Diamond GA, Chandra P, et al. Prospective validation of a quantitative method to differentiate ischemic versus nonischemic cardiomyopathy by Tc-99m sestamibi SPECT [abstract]. *J Nucl Med 1999*;40:125P.

(Simply, the presence of a dense perfusion defect >45% [ischemic/normal] was a hallmark, specific for ischemic cardiomyopathy among the 58 patients with noncoronary and the 31 coronary cardiomyopathy patients studied. Although this measure yielded a high specificity [≥90%], sensitivity was variable.)

683. Croon CD, Atsma DE, Dibbets P, et al. Gated SPECT myocardial imaging improves test accuracy in patients with persistent perfusion defects [abstract]. *J Nucl Med* 1999;40:163P.

(Gated SPECT can help to differentiate attenuation artifact from scar and also can differentiate an ischemic from a nonischemic cardiomyopathy, by the finding of dysfunctional but perfused myocardium.)

684. Lamich R, Ballester M, Martai V, et al. Efficacy of augmented immunosuppressive therapy for early vasculopathy in heart transplantation. *J Am Coll Cardiol* 1998;32:413–419.

(Here, 230 coronary angiograms [at 1 mo and yearly] and 376 perfusion studies [at 1, 3 and 6 mo and twice each year thereafter] were performed serially over 8 yr in 76 cardiac allograft recipients. Among 22 clinical episodes of vasculopathy, 20 were evident on myocardial perfusion scintigraphy and 9 of these were not evident on angiography or biopsy! There was a 68% regression rate with augmented immunosupression, higher if implemented early.)

685. Bocchi EA, Mocelin AO, de Moraes AV, et al. Comparison between two strategies for rejection detection after heart transplantation. Routine endomyocardial biopsy versus gallium-67 cardiac imaging. *Transplant Proc* 1997;29:586–588.

(Nothing has replaced endomyocardial biopsy as the method for identifying rejection.)

686. Alexander EL, Firestein GS, Weiss JL, et al. Reversible cold-induced abnormalities in myocardial perfusion and function in systemic sclerosis. *Ann Intern Med* 1986;105:661–668.

(A report of the perfusion scintigraphic findings in scleroderma heart disease is presented.)

687. Samuels B, Kiat H, Friedman JD, et al. Adenosine pharmacologic stress myocardial perfusion tomographic imaging in patients with significant aortic stenosis. Diagnostic efficacy and comparison of clinical, hemodynamic and electrocardiographic variables with age-matched control subjects. *J Am Coll Cardiol* 1995;25:99–106.

(Adenosine myocardial perfusion scintigraphy was found to be safe and diagnostically accurate in this study of 35 patients with moderate-to-severe aortic stenosis and valve areas of 0.84–0.16 cm^2. Regardless of the likely safety of the study, risk must always be considered, especially in patients with severe stenosis. However, with the proper indication, this is the noninvasive stress study of choice.)

688. Nigam A, Human DP. Prognostic value of myocardial perfusion imaging with exercise and/or dipyridamole hyperemia in patients with preexisting left bundle branch block. *J Nucl Med* 1998;39:579–581.

(Dipyridamole perfusion scintigraphy was demonstrated to be an excellent prognostic as well as diagnostic tool in patients with left bundle branch block [LBBB] in this study evaluating 96 patients with LBBB. This appears to relate most prominently to scintigraphic defects, often reversible, in the interventricular septum. However, in high-risk, high-likelihood populations, the great number of normal and benign exercise scintigrams in LBBB relate to a benign prognosis, and most scintigraphic abnormalities in this setting relate to true coronary arteries, with a similar sensitivity to that observed in the absence of LBBB.

Several studies have indicated the lack of specificity of myocardial perfusion scintigraphy compared with coronary angiography, in the setting of LBBB. This does not appear to be a significant factor in relation to vasodilator pharmacologic stress imaging. Still, even with exercise testing, the majority of induced defects, even in the septum, will relate to coronary lesions.)

689. Hirzel HO, Senn M, Nuesch K, et al. Thallium-201 scintigraphy in complete left bundle branch block. *Am J Cardiol* 1984;53:764–769.

690. Ono S, Nohara R, Kambara H, et al. Regional myocardial perfusion and glucose metabolism in experimental left bundle branch block. *Circulation* 1992;85:1125–1131.

(689,690: The mechanism for induced septal perfusion defects in left bundle branch block is not well documented but has been postulated to relate to relatively reduced septal flow demands. Here, microspheres confirmed this relative flow reduction [*689*], and PET perfusion and metabolism appeared to confirm it in an experimental model [*690*].)

691. Lucas JR, Agarwal P, Krishnan R, Zhu YY, et al. The relationship of diagnostic accuracy to the hemodynamic response on dipyridamole perfusion scintigraphy [abstract]. *J Clin Res* 1993;41:35A.

(155,156,691: These studies demonstrate a maintained diagnostic specificity for coronary disease in relation to pharmacologic stress in the presence of left bundle branch block, with agents such as dipyridamole or adenosine that primarily test the coronary flow reserve and do not greatly augment heart rate and the double product.)

692. Ragosta M, Beller GA, Watson DD, et al. Quantitative planar rest–redistribution thallium-201 imaging in detection of myocardial viability and prediction of improvement in left ventricular function after coronary bypass surgery in patients with severely depressed left ventricular function. *Circulation* 1993;87:1630–1641.

693. Massie BM, Botvinick EH, Brundage BH, et al. Relationship of regional myocardial perfusion to segmental wall motion: a physiologic basis for understanding the presence and reversibility of asynergy. *Circulation* 1979;58:1154–1162.

(692,693: These 2 articles, 1 early and 1 more recent, are among a growing number that demonstrate improved systolic function and functional class after revascularization in the presence of viable, "hibernating" myocardium, documented by conventional perfusion scintigraphy. The greater the number of scintigraphically viable segments, the greater the potential improvement in left ventricular function.

The presence of dysfunctional myocardium with significant perfusion at rest or with redistribution presents a high likelihood of functional restoration after revascularization. The larger this area of perfused but dysfunctional myocardium, the greater is the likelihood for improvement after revascularization [see reference *710*].)

694. Elefteriades JA, Iolis G, Levi E, et al. Coronary artery bypass grafting in severe left ventricular dysfunction: excellent survival with improved ejection fraction and functional state. *J Am Coll Cardiol* 1993;22:141–147.

(Analyzed were 83 consecutive patients who had coronary artery bypass graft with a left ventricular ejection fraction [LVEF] of 10%–30% [mean, 25%]. LVEF improved in 68 of 76 hospital survivors in whom the LVEF increased to 33%.)

695. Christian TF, Miller TD, Hodge DO, et al. An estimate of the prevalence of reversible left ventricular dysfunction in patients referred for coronary artery bypass surgery. *J Nucl Cardiol* 1997;4:140–146.

(Christian et al. found that roughly one-third of unselected patients having coronary artery bypass grafts with reduced left ventricular function, improve left ventricular ejection fraction >4% after surgery. This is not a small percentage and suggests that they are an important group to identify prospectively.)

696. Pohost GM, Zir L, Moore RH, et al. Differentiation of transiently ischemic from infarcted myocardium by serial imaging after a single dose of thallium-201. *Circulation* 1977;55:294–302.

(This classic article first presented the concept and clinical implications of delayed defect reversibility on thallium-201 perfusion imaging, during transient coronary occlusion in dogs and after exercise in patients.)

697. Brunken R, Tillisch J, Schwaiger M, et al. Regional perfusion, metabolism and wall motion in patients with chronic electrocardiographic Q wave infarctions: evidence for persistence of viable tissue in some infarct regions by positron emission tomography. *Circulation* 1986;73:951–963.

(PET imaging with ^{13}NH$_3$ and 18-fluorodeoxyglucose was performed in 20 patients with 31 chronic electrocardiographic [ECG] Q-wave infarctions. Criteria of PET "match"[scar] and "mismatch"[viability] were applied. Only 10 [32%] of the 31 Q-wave segments exhibited matched defects, criteria for completed infarction. Others suggested viability. Neither the severity of the associated regional wall motion abnormality nor the associated ECG ST–T changes reliably distinguished hypoperfused regions with metabolic viability from hypoperfused regions with completed infarction. PET metabolism was the only way to identify viability among dysfunctional segments with Q waves.)

698. Gropler R, Geltman E, Sampathkumaran K, et al. Functional recovery after coronary revascularization for chronic coronary artery disease is dependent on maintenance of oxidative metabolism. *J Am Coll Cardiol* 1992;20:569–577.

(PET with H$_2$^{15}O, carbon-11 acetate and 18-fluorodeoxyglucose [FDG] was performed in 16 patients with coronary disease before coronary artery bypass graft. Viability was determined by the response of dysfunctional segments after revascularization. Preoperatively, neither the severity of the resting wall motion abnormality nor the level of relative myocardial perfusion distinguished viable from nonviable dysfunctional segments. Rates of glucose utilization and acetate clearance were higher in viable segments. Nineteen of 24 [79%] PET segments with enhanced FDG uptake preoperatively were viable, whereas 24 of 29 [83%] with matched reduction of PET perfusion and metabolism were nonviable. Relative perfusion and the ratio of perfusion to glucose improved in viable segments after revascularization. PET appeared to determine viability by several mechanisms.)

699. Bodenheimer MM, Banka VS, Fooshee C, et al. Relationship between regional myocardial perfusion and the presence, severity and reversibility of asynergy in patients with coronary heart disease. *Circulation* 1978;48:789–795.

700. Foster E, O'Kelly B, LaPidus A, et al. Segmental myocardial viability can be inferred from combined analysis of echocardiographic function and scintigraphic perfusion: implications for 24-hour redistribution and PET scanning. *Am Heart J* 1994;129:7–14.

   (An early study [699] and 1 published more recently [700] support the poor relationship between the degree of wall motion abnormality and its viability and likelihood of restored function after revascularization.

   In 73 patients studied by rest echocardiography and stress perfusion scintigraphy [700], the 2 methods agreed widely in the presence and severity of abnormalities, and, in ~15% of segments that were either severely underperfused or akinetic, appeared to complement each other in the identification of regional viability. Planar perfusion methods were used, and no gold standard was applied.)

701. Bodenheimer MM, Banka VS, Hermann GA, et al. Reversible asynergy: histopathologic and electrocardiographic correlations in patients with coronary artery disease. *Circulation* 1976;53:792–796.

   (This study demonstrates the inability to predict functional reversibility, here tested with the functional response to sublingual nitroglycerin, by the presence of electrocardiographic Q waves.)

702. Rozanski A, Berman D, Gray R, et al. Preoperative prediction of reversible myocardial asynergy by postexercise radionuclide ventriculography. *N Engl J Med* 1982;307: 212–216.

   (Here, the presence of scintigraphic "redistribution" strongly supported myocardial viability and functional reversibility after revascularization.)

703. Brundage BH, Massie BM, Botvinick EH. Improved regional ventricular function after successful surgical revascularization. *J Am Coll Cardiol* 1984;3:902–908.

   (Brundage et al. demonstrated the relationship of resting thallium-201 uptake or redistributing stress-induced defects to regional viability and functional improvement after successful revascularization. The frequency and implications of dense fixed defects were not analyzed in this article employing planar methods, before the application of reinjection methods.)

704. Gutman J, Berman DS, Freeman M, et al. Time to completed redistribution of Tl-201 in exercise myocardial scintigraphy: Relationship to the degree of coronary artery stenosis. *Am Heart J* 1983;106:989–995.

   (This classic article demonstrated an almost linear relationship between the severity of coronary stenosis and the time to thallium-201 redistribution. It confirmed the fact that 4 hr was insufficient time for redistribution in a significant minority of viable but ischemic segments.)

705. Gibson RS, Watson DD, Taylor GJ, et al. Prospective assessment of regional myocardial perfusion before and after coronary revascularization surgery by quantitative thallium-201 scintigraphy. *J Am Coll Cardiol* 1983;1:804–815.

   (The improvement in ventricular function seen in some nonredistributing segments after revascularization gives eloquent testimony to the underestimation of regional viability related to early planar perfusion imaging studies.)

706. Cloninger KG, DePuey EG, Garcia EV, et al. Incomplete redistribution, in delayed thallium-201 single photon emission computed tomographic (SPECT) images. An overestimation of myocardial scarring. *J Am Coll Cardiol* 1988;12:955–963.

(This article demonstrated the further reversibility evident in some studies with 24-hr delayed imaging. Again, this supports the underestimation of myocardial viability in the 4-hr set.)

707. Kiat H, Berman DS, Maddahi J, et al. Late reversibility of tomographic myocardial thallium-201 defects: an accurate marker of myocardial viability. *J Am Coll Cardiol* 1988;12:1456–1463.

(Here, the value of late, 24-hr imaging is demonstrated, with its ability to increase recognition of viable segments by virtue of their reversibility on thallium-201 [^{201}Tl] imaging. Similar to the results in reference *202*, there was a significant inverse relation between the degree of coronary stenosis and the rate of ^{201}Tl defect reversibility.)

708. Yang LD, Berman DS, Kiat H, et al. The frequency of late reversibility in SPECT thallium-201 stress-redistribution studies. *J Am Coll Cardiol* 1990;15:334–340.

(Here, the frequency of thallium-201 late reversibility was assessed prospectively.)

709. Pagley PR, Beller GA, Watson DD, et al. Improved outcome after coronary bypass surgery in patients with ischemic cardiomyopathy and residual myocardial viability. *Circulation* 1997;96:793–800.

(The study retrospectively analyzed quantitative rest thallium-201 myocardial perfusion scintigraphy performed before coronary artery bypass in 70 patients with multivessel coronary artery disease and left ventricular ejection fracion <40%. Survival free of transplantation was significantly higher in those with a high "viability index.")

710. Mori T, Minamiji K, Kurogane H, et al. Rest-injected thallium-201 imaging for assessing viability of severe asynergic regions. *J Nucl Med* 1991;32:1718–1724.

(References *692* and *710* are 2 of several studies that document that regional defect reversibility and viability relate to improved image findings with delayed postrest imaging. Rest and delayed images are not necessarily the same if, in the setting of resting ischemia, postinfection images relate to the distribution of perfusion, whereas delayed images relate to the distribution of K+ space or the distribution of viable myocardium.)

711. Sharir T, Berman DS, Cohen I, et al. Incremental prognostic value of rest-redistribution thallium-201 SPECT for prediction of cardiac death [abstract]. *J Nucl Med* 1999;40:8P.

(Identification of a large amount of rest reversibility was an independent and incremental predictor of cardiac death beyond that related to the findings on stress and rest myocardial perfusion scintigraphy.)

712. Sciagraa R, Santoro GM, Bisi G, et al. Rest-redistribution thallium-201 SPECT to detect myocardial viability. *J Nucl Med* 1998;39:384–390.

(Functional recovery after revascularization was the marker of viability applied in 29 patients with ventricular dysfunction studied before revascularization. It was the relative regional activity at redistribution and also at rest [≥60% of peak], rather than evidence of redistribution, that was the best indicator of viability.)

713. Dilsizian V, Rocco TP, Freedman NM, et al. Enhanced detection of ischemic but viable myocardium by the reinjection thallium after stress-redistribution imaging. *N Engl J Med* 1990;323:141–146.

(The authors of this classic article studied 100 patients with coronary artery disease, using exercise thallium-201 [^{201}Tl] myocardial perfusion scintigraphy and a 2-mCi dose. Ninety-two patients had exercise-induced defects involving 260 segments, and 83 [33%] of these segments appeared irreversible at 4-hr delayed imaging. Yet 42 [49%] of these segments were improved or normal shortly after a second injection or reinjection, of 1 mCi ^{201}Tl. Among 20 patients restudied after percutaneous transluminal coronary angiography, 13 coronary vascular regions that were identified as viable among 15 that were thought nonviable on 4-hr redistribution imaging demonstrated improved or normal perfusion and improved regional wall motion. All 8 regions with persistent defects on reinjection continued to demonstrate abnormal ^{201}Tl uptake and regional wall motion. Reinjection technique was thus established as a method to optimize identification of viable myocardium.)

714. Bonow RO, Dilsizian V, Cuocolo A, et al. Identification of viable myocardium in patients with chronic coronary artery disease and left ventricular dysfunction: comparison of thallium scintigraphy with reinjection and PET imaging with ^{18}F-fluorodeoxyglucose. *Circulation* 1994;83:26–37.

(This classic article, described fully in the text, demonstrates that the reinjection technique maximizes thallium-201 "redistribution," reducing the need for 24-hr imaging, and that myocardial viability is identified by redistribution of a relatively high level of regional radioactivity, equal to 50% or more of the region with highest regional activity. These authors employed 3 SPECT scans in each patient in their study. The second delayed image was reviewed for defect normalization, and another scan was acquired postreinjection to determine defect reversibility. Reinjection could actually increase defect size if performed after defect redistribution. Probably related to ongoing resting ischemia, this might occur when a postreinjection image is acquired without reviewing or even acquiring the 4-hr image for redistribution. The reinjection dose reestablishes the heterogeneous rest perfusion pattern that was overcome and made homogeneous by the 4-hr period of redistribution. Again normalization can be optimized with the application of more time and the acquisition of a 24-hr delayed image.)

715. Brunken RC, Czernin J, Porenta F, et al. Can assessment of myocardial perfusion identify tissue viability in hypoperfused regions [abstract]? *J Nucl Med* 1992;33:857.

(In this animal study applying an occlusion–reperfusion model in dogs, the authors correlate regional viability with quantitative PET perfusion with ^{14}NH$_3$. The findings suggest only a modest relationship between regional perfusion and viability, rather than the close relationship suggested by conventional PET data using the reinjection technique. Here, absolute flow was measured in an animal model of infarcted and ischemic myocardium. Although viable regions demonstrated greater flow than infarcted regions, there was considerable overlap, indicating the lack of reliability of the flow marker alone to determine regional myocardial viability. This area remains the focus of active research.)

716. Bax JJ, Wijns W, Cornel JH, et al. Accuracy of currently available techniques for prediction of functional recovery after revascularization in patients with left ventricular dysfunction due to coronary artery disease: comparison of pooled data. *J Am Coll Cardiol* 1997;30:1451–1460.

717. Beller GA. Comparison of Tl-201 scintigraphy and low-dose dobutamine echocardiography for the noninvasive assessment of myocardial viability [editorial]. *Circulation* 1996;94:2681–2684.

(716,717: Bax et al. performed a meta-analysis of 37 studies thus far published. Taking the data at face value [which is the only choice available with meta-analysis], perfusion imaging appears to overestimate functional recovery, whereas low-dose dobutamine echocardiography has the highest overall predictive accuracy. However, the echocardiographic method is subjective and has poor reproducibility. It appears to underestimate functional recovery and has been relatively lightly tested. Further, the values taken for viability assume a fixed cut-off between normal and abnormal when, instead, regional perfusion presents a continuous scale and the quantitative values for the wall motion response vary from study to study and have not been well established. Issues related to analytic methods and blinded reading also exist. Finally, functional recovery is not the only determinant of benefit after revascularization.

What is the reason for this finding? Is the perfusion method *too* sensitive? Beller thinks not! Indeed, thallium-201 uptake marks regional viability.)

718. Bonow RO. Identification of viable myocardium. *Circulation* 1996;94:2674–2680.
    (References *718*, *753* and *764* are excellent editorial reviews and analyses of the viability literature. They present a particularly thorough analysis of the findings on and clinical implications of perfusion imaging for the assessment of myocardial viability in dysfunctional segments.)

719. Lee HH, Daavila-Romaan VG, Ludbrook PA, et al. Dependency of contractile reserve on myocardial blood flow: implications for the assessment of myocardial viability with dobutamine stress echocardiography. *Circulation* 1997;96:2884–2891.
    (PET was used with oxygen-15 water to quantitate perfusion and with fluoro-deoxyglucose to assess metabolism and viability in 19 patients with left ventricular dysfunction and coronary disease at rest, with incremental dobutamine infusion. Contraction reserve was found to depend on the ability to augment coronary flow with stress [the flow reserve]. Among segments defined as PET viable, 54% demonstrated no contractile reserve on dobutamine infusion.)

720. Bax JJ, Vanoverschelde JLJ, Cornel JH, et al. Optimal viability criteria on thallium-201 reinjection SPECT to predict improvement of function after revascularization [abstract]. *J Am Coll Cardiol* 1999;33:416A.
    (In this study, relatively normal segments and moderate and severe reversible defects demonstrated the greatest likelihood of functional improvement after revascularization. These results parallel those of Dilsizian et al. [*713*] but suggest less viability in fixed defects of moderate severity.)

721. Kitsiou AN, Srinivasan G, Quyyumi AA, et al. Stress-induced reversible thallium defects: are they equally accurate for predicting recovery of regional left ventricular function after revascularization? *Circulation* 1998;98:501–508.
    (Although mild-to-moderate fixed defects retain viability information, the identification of reversible thallium-201 defects more accurately predicts functional recovery.)

722. Bartenstein R, Hasfeld M, Schober O, et al. Tl-201 reinjection predicts improvement of left ventricular function following revascularization. *J Nucl Med* 1993:32:87–90.
    (Thallium-201 reinjection technique increases regional uptake and helps to maximize the assessment of myocardial viability. Here, that advantage permitted the identification of viable and dysfunctional segments more likely to improve after revascularization.)

723. Amanullah AM, Chaudhry FA, Heo J, et al. Comparison of dobutamine echocardiography, dobutamine sestamibi and rest-redistribution thallium-201 single photon emission computed tomography for determining contractile reserve and myocardial ischemia in ischemic cardiomyopathy. *Am J Cardiol* 1999;84:626–631.
    (A recent and thorough comparison was made between the response to low-dose dobutamine on echocardiography and sestamibi perfusion imaging, as well as the level of thallium-201 [^{201}Tl] uptake with 4-hr imaging, among the same 54 patients [45 men, 9 women] with severe ischemic cardiomyopathy defined as left ventricular ejection fraction [LVEF] of 24% ± 9%. Contractile reserve and ^{201}Tl uptake were more frequent among hypokinetic than akinetic or dyskinetic segments. Normal, mildly abnormal or reversible ^{201}Tl myocardial perfusion scintigraphy [MPS] as well as dobutamine MPS identified far more potentially viable segments than did dobutamine echocardiography. Included were 864 segments, of which 796 demonstrated wall motion abnormalities. Contractile reserve on echocardiography, gated MPS and ^{201}Tl uptake, was more common among those segments with hypokinesis than akinetic or dyskinetic segments. A significant incidence of contractile reserve was evident among normal, mildly abnormal and reversible ^{201}Tl segments. Here, measures of both function [65%] with gated sestamibi and perfusion [60%] with ^{201}Tl MPS were significantly more sensitive to the presence of contractile reserve than was dobutamine stress echocardiography [33%; $P < 0.001$]. Dobutamine sestamibi identified 518 of 796 [65%] ischemic segments, compared with only 265 of 796 [33%] by dobutamine echocardiography.)

765. Braunwald E, Kloner RA. The stunned myocardium: prolonged postischemic ventricular dysfunction. *Circulation* 1982;66:1146–1149.

766. Braunwald E, Rutherford JD. Reversible left ventricular dysfunction: evidence for the "hibernating myocardium." *J Am Coll Cardiol* 1986;8:1467–1470.
   (765,766: Hibernating myocardium may be seen with preserved perfusion and may be related to recurrent stunning. These are excellent early reviews on the subject and help give the perspective required to best understand hibernating myocardium.)

767. Dilsizian V, Bonow RO. Current diagnostic techniques of assessing myocardial viability in patients with hibernating and stunned myocardium. *Circulation* 1993;87:1–20.
   (Various protocols utilizing combinations of rest, redistribution and reinjection thallium imaging have been devised, validated and compared in order to optimally assess the presence of dysfunctional but viable myocardium. This review is an excellent summary of the field and its practical impact on imaging viability with SPECT.)

768. Udelson JE. Steps forward in the assessment of myocardial viability in left ventricular dysfunction [editorial]. *Circulation* 1997;97:833–838.
   (Udelson reviewed the clinical importance and methods of viability evaluation. An in-depth and insightful analysis is made of the definition of viable myocardium, the clinical importance of viability evaluation in dysfunctional myocardial segments and the methods designed to identify viable segments. Also assessed is the "gold standard" applied to confirm the presence of viability and its justification.)

769. Beller GA. Selecting patients with ischemic cardiomyopathy for medical treatment, revascularization or heart transplantation. *J Nucl Cardiol* 1997;4:S152–157.
   (Beller presented a review of the value of myocardial perfusion imaging for viability assessment in the evaluation and management of patients with heart failure.)

770. Sandler MP, Videlefsky S, Delbeke D, et al. Evaluation of myocardial ischemia using a rest metabolism/stress perfusion protocol with ^{18}FDG/^{99m}Tc-MIBI and dual isotope simultaneous acquisition SPECT. *J Am Coll Cardiol* 1995;26:870–878.
   (The authors sought to establish a dual-isotope single-acquisition SPECT protocol with an ultra-high-energy collimator to evaluate rest metabolism and stress perfusion with fluorine-18 fluorodeoxyglucose [^{18}F FDG] and technetium-99m [^{99m}Tc] sestamibi. After glucose loading, ^{18}F FDG was given intravenously. After a 35-min distribution phase, stress perfusion imaging was performed. A 20% window for both photopeaks and a ^{99m}Tc /^{18}F FDG concentration of 3.2:1 gave a 6% spillover of ^{18}F FDG into the ^{99m}Tc window. With a 70% lesion as diagnostic of coronary disease, SPECT sensitivity was 100%, specificity was 88%, positive predictive value was 93% and negative predictive value was 100%. Dual-isotope SPECT with FDG as the rest perfusion surrogate may provide an alternative cost-effective method to conventional PET flow-metabolism imaging or thallium-201 reinjection technique while providing state of the art data regarding both myocardium at ischemic risk and viability.)

771. Chen EQ, MacIntyre WJ, Go RT, et al. Myocardial viability studies using fluorine-18 FDG SPECT: a comparison with fluorine-18 FDG PET. *J Nucl Med* 1997;38:582–586.
   (The physical and imaging characteristics of SPECT, acquired using either a high-energy, general-purpose collimator or a special, ultrahigh [UH]-energy, 511-keV collimator, and PET methods for fluorine-18 fluorodeoxyglucose [^{18}F FDG] evaluation were analyzed and compared among 18 patients. PET was superior to SPECT in all physical imaging characteristics, especially sensitivity and contrast resolution, and regardless of the collimator applied. Nonetheless, application of the UH collimator reduced septal penetration and significantly improved both spatial and contrast resolution but reduced sensitivity. Although there was a high concordance in segmental viability information between PET and SPECT using either collimator, the agreement between PET and SPECT was statistically better when the UH collimator was employed. SPECT with special 511-keV collimation appears to serve as an alternative to PET FDG imaging for viability evaluation.)

772. Burt RW, Perkins OW, Oppenheim BE, et al. Direct comparison of fluorine-18 FDG SPECT, fluorine-18 FDG PET and rest thallium-201 SPECT for detection of myocardial viability. *J Nucl Med* 1995;36:176–179.

(The authors compared the accuracy of fluorodeoxyglucose [FDG] SPECT, FDG PET and rest thallium-201 [^{201}Tl] imaging methods in 20 patients with left ventricular dysfunction and fixed ^{201}Tl defects at rest. Although FDG metabolic imaging identified 13 additional viable segments among 60 dysfunctional segments with fixed defects on rest ^{201}Tl imaging, both SPECT and PET FDG imaging were equally accurate. Important is that roughly 4 of 5 dysfunctional segments were correctly classified by ^{201}Tl rest imaging, if indeed FDG was the "gold standard," was always correct and the criterion for lack of viability on perfusion images was a measure of the relative radiotracer uptake! Evaluation of function after revascularization was not included.)

773. Bax JJ, Visser FC, Blanksma PK, et al. Comparison of myocardial uptake of fluorine-18 fluorodeoxyglucose imaged with PET and SPECT in dysynergic myocardium. *J Nucl Med* 1996;37:1631–1636.

(Here, 20 patients with previous infarction and wall motion abnormalities were studied by fluorodeoxyglucose [FDG] metabolic imaging with both SPECT and PET methods under conditions of hyperinsulinemic glucose clamping. Each also was studied by rest thallium-201 [^{201}Tl] SPECT and nitrogen-13 [^{13}N] ammonia PET for regional perfusion evaluation. The agreement between ^{201}Tl/FDG SPECT and ^{13}N ammonia/FDG PET for detection of viable dysynergic segments was 76%. Among those 12 patients with left ventricular ejection fraction<35%, all SPECT and PET data were identical.)

774. Pilote L, Califf RM, Sapp S, et al. Regional variation across the United States in the management of acute myocardial infarction: GUSTO-I Investigators. Global Utilization of Streptokinase and Tissue Plasmogen Activator for Occluded Coronary Arteries. *N Engl J Med* 1995;333:565–572.

775. Guadagnoli E, Hauptman PJ, Ayanian JZ, et al.Variation in the use of cardiac procedures after acute myocardial infarction. *N Engl J Med* 1995;333:573–578.

(774,775: Myocardial perfusion scintigraphy may be unnecessary if patients come to angiography regardless of stress image findings. Today, >70% of patients, with regional variation, come to angiography early after infarction [774]. Are all of these interventions beneficial or necessary? It is tempting to then intervene and open the occluded vessel or bypass the heart with 3-vessel disease. Although this is widely done, there is little data to support this practice and an international sampling of practice demonstrates no mortality benefit or improved outcome to angiography and revascularization performed routinely days after infarction [775].)

776. Travin MI, Dessouki AMR, Cameron T, Heller GV. Use of exercise technetium-99m-sestamibi SPECT imaging to detect residual ischemia and for risk stratification after acute myocardial infarction. *Am J Cardiol* 1995;75:665–659.

777. Basu S, Senior R, Dore C, Lahiri A. Value of thallium-201 imaging in detecting adverse cardiac events after myocardial infarction and thrombolysis: a follow-up of 100 consecutive patients. *Br Med J* 1996;313:844–848.

(776,777: Much work presented earlier demonstrated that risk can be assessed by stress myocardial perfusion scintigraphy. Basu et al. demonstrated that 68% of post-thrombolysis patients had evidence of myocardium at ischemic risk. Among these, the incidence of subsequent death or reinfarction was 49%, compared with 13% in those without such evidence [$P < 0.001$].)

778. Michels KB, Yusuf S. Do PTCA in acute myocardial infarction affect mortality and reinfarction rates? A quantitative overview (meta-analysis) of the randomized clinical trials. *Circulation* 1995;91:476–485.

(This meta-analysis summarizes the data in a number of studies that evaluated the potential benefit of primary postinfarction percutaneous transluminal coronary angioplasty in otherwise uncomplicated myocardial infarctions. In summary, there

857. Poldermans D, Fioretti PM, Boersma E, et al. Long-term prognostic value of dobu-tamine-atropine stress echocardiography in 1737 patients with known or suspected coronary artery disease. *Circulation* 1999;99:757–762.

(The long-term prognostic value of dobutamine-stress echocardiography was evaluated in a consecutive group of 1737 patients studied over a 9-yr period [<200/yr]. Both rest and stress-induced wall motion abnormalities related to risk where a normal study related to a 1.3% hard event rate, and the advantage of normal image findings compared with other methods was not presented. Although an ischemic result significantly increased the ratio of documented cardiac death or [re]infarction, there was a significant number of patients with rest wall motion abnormalities that bore a similar prognostic value. Although a normal study carried a relatively low event rate, the origin and nature of this low-risk population are not delineated and its pretest likelihood of coronary artery disease [CAD] is not calculated!

852–857: Examination of the current literature documented a significant diffi-culty or inability of the normal stress echocardiogram to identify populations with a low event rate, low risk and a good prognosis. Because of the well-documented predictive value of myocardial perfusion scintigraphy for the presence and extent of myocardium at ischemic risk for cardiac death and nonfatal infarction, the reduced sensitivity of stress echocardiography and its variable and subjective nature raise concern for a possible deficiency in its ability to identify patients at risk for cardiac events. Brown's review [14] addressed this question.

Among 9 available studies [351,754,851–857], 6 with dobutamine and 3 with exercise stress, the annualized rate of death and nonfatal myocardial infarction in 751 patients with known CAD and a negative stress echocardiogram is 6%/yr, a high event rate using the Unstable Angina Guidelines [31] and not different from the hard event rate in the same studies among patients with known CAD and a positive stress test [8%].)

858. Marcovitz PA, Shayna V, Horn RA, et al. Value of dobutamine stress echocardiogra-phy in determining the prognosis of patients with known or suspected coronary artery disease. *Am J Cardiol* 1996;78:404–408.

(In a study not included in the Brown review [14], Marcovitz et al. studied the prognosis over a mean of 15 mo after the performance of clinically requested ["indicated"] dobutamine stress echocardiography to a maximum 40 μg/kg/min dose. Although an abnormal response related to a 7.9 odds ratio for hard cardiac events and the fixed response [a rest wall motion abnormality unchanged with dobu-tamine] had a 6.1 odds ratio compared with the normal response, multivariate analy-sis revealed only a "mixed" or biphasic functional response [increased wall motion at low dose and decreased motion at high dose] to be statistically significantly re-lated [$P = 0.03$] to hard events in the follow-up period. Of course, 185 among 291 study patients had rest wall motion abnormalities, and 23 of 29 hard events occurred in those with rest abnormalities, which themselves were predictive of events!)

859. Krivokapich J, Child JS, Walter DO, Garfinkel A. Prognostic value of dobutamine stress echocardiography in predicting cardiac events in patients with known or suspected coronary artery disease. *J Am Coll Cardiol* 1999;33:708–716.

(The medical records of 558 consecutive patients [338 men and 220 women] undergoing dobutamine stress echocardiography were reviewed. The overall cardiac event rate was 34% if the study was positive and 10% if negative. There was a 10% myocardial infarction rate and an 8% death rate with a positive image, but rates were 3% for each if the test was negative. A negative stress echocardiogram gave no assurance. Interesting was the fact that the presence of rest wall motion abnormal-ities was the most useful variable in predicting events, with 25% with rest wall motion abnormalities having events compared with 6% with normal wall motion. Stress testing added little, and the method was unable to risk stratify among those with abnormal rest wall motion.)

860. McCully RB, Roger VL, Mahoney DW, et al. Outcome after normal exercise echocardiogram and predictors of subsequent cardiac events: follow-up of 1325 patients. *J Am Coll Cardiol* 1998;31:144–149.

861. Sawada SG, Ryan T, Conley MJ, et al. Prognostic value of a normal exercise echocardiogram. *Am Heart J* 1990;120:49–55.

862. Colon PJ, Mobarek SK, Milani RV, et al. Prognostic value of stress echocardiography in the evaluation of atypical chest pain patients without known coronary artery disease. *Am J Cardiol* 1998;81:545–551.

    (860–862: Some recent studies appear to attest to the high predictive value of a negative stress echocardiogram. Although 2 of the 5 [*860,861*] show a relatively low event rate in association with a normal stress echocardiogram, the other 3 [*351,603,862*] have event rates of 1.6% and 3%/yr, well above the 1% value generally taken as the upper limit of the low risk subgroup. These have an 8-fold or greater hard event rate compared with SPECT perfusion studies published in the same time frame, in spite of the selection of much lower-risk study cohorts. Further, the total event rates are much greater in the echocardiographic studies, strongly suggesting that progressive coronary artery disease is clearly missed.)

863. Olmos LI, Dakik H, Gordon R, et al. Long-term prognostic value of exercise echocardiography compared with exercise Tl-201, ECG and clinical variables in patients evaluated for coronary artery disease. *Circulation* 1998;98:2670–2686.

    (The study showed that exercise echocardiographic and thallium-201 myocardial perfusion scintigraphy variables were of equal predictive value for ischemic events or death.)

864. Davar JI, Brull DJ, Bulugahipitya S, et al. Prognostic value of negative dobutamine stress echo in women with intermediate probability of coronary artery disease. *Am J Cardiol* 1999;83:100–102.

    (The authors reported on follow-up among 332 women who had dobutamine stress echocardiography over a 2-yr period. Among 43 studies with evidence of induced ischemia, 9 [21%] had revascularization. Among the remaining 289 without evidence of ischemia, 72 [25%] with an intermediate coronary artery disease [CAD] likelihood but without evidence of reversible ischemia at ≥85% maximal predicted heart rate for age [MPHR] were in the study group. Excluded were those 227 patients with similar normal studies at a high rate but with high [or low] CAD likelihood, those with negative studies who did not reach 85% MPHR and those with fixed abnormalities. Mean age of participants was 60. The study reduced the probability of CAD from 49% to 14%. Although death, myocardial infarction and revascularization did not occur during the 13-mo follow-up, 27 angiograms were performed, 5 identifying CAD.)

865. Pozzoli MMA, Fioretti PM, Salustri A, et al. Exercise echocardiography and technetium-99m MIBI single photon emission computed tomography in the detection of coronary artery disease. *Am J Cardiol* 1991;67:350–355.

866. Galanti G, Sciagra R, Comeglio M, et al. Diagnostic accuracy of peak exercise echocardiography in coronary artery disease: comparison of thallium-201 myocardial scintigraphy. *Am Heart J* 1991;122:1609–1616.

867. Salustri A, Pozzoli MMA, Hermans W, et al. Relationship between exercise echocardiography and perfusion single photon emission computed tomography in patients with single vessel coronary artery disease. *Am Heart J* 1992;124:75–83.

868. Hoffmann R, Lethen H, Kleinhaus E, et al. Comparative evaluation of bicycle and dobutamine stress echocardiography with perfusion scintigraphy and bicycle electrocardiogram for identification of coronary artery disease. *Am J Cardiol* 1993;72: 555–559.

869. Forester T, McNeill AJ, Salustri A, et al. Simultaneous dobutamine stress echocardiography and technetium-99m isonitrile single photon emission computed tomography in patients with suspected coronary artery disease. *J Am Coll Cardiol* 1993;21:1591–1596.

870. Simeck CL, Watson D, Smith WH, et al. Dipyridamole thallium-201 imaging versus dobutamine echocardiography for the evaluation of coronary artery disease in patients unable to exercise. *Am J Cardiol* 1993;72:1257–1262.

(865–870: Many studies [see references *122* and *602*] performed by echocardiography advocates using a variety of stress techniques nonetheless demonstrate the higher sensitivity of the scintigraphic method. It is often claimed that such accuracy relates only to single-vessel disease and that the specificity of stress echocardiography is equal or superior to that of the scintigraphic method for identification of multivessel CAD. Of course, less sensitive tests may more specifically see disease with more extensive and severe involvement. Yet, the literature strongly demonstrates the superior sensitivity of the scintigraphic method for the identification of multivessel, high-risk disease in ~66%–72% of such patients, compared with 50% by stress echocardiography.)

871. Roger VL, Pellikka PA, Oh JK, et al. Identification of multivessel coronary artery disease by exercise echocardiography. *J Am Coll Cardiol* 1994;24:109–114.

(Attention must also be given to methods of studies claiming diagnostic or prognostic advantage. Sensitivity must be assessed with reference to the population studied and the methods applied. The study by Roger et al. seems to demonstrate the value of stress echocardiography for the identification of multivessel coronary artery disease [CAD], but the diagnosis actually relates as well to the rest ejection fraction. Here, a rest left ventricular ejection fraction [LVEF] <40% was well correlated with multivessel disease, whereas an LVEF >40% was related to the absence of multivessel disease. The stress study was unnecessary for this differentiation! In fact, contrary to its contention, this study indicates the extreme difficulty of the echocardiographic diagnosis of multivessel CAD in the presence of normal wall motion and is compounded by the general rule to stop the stress test with the appearance of the first new wall motion abnormality.)

872. Bates J, Ryan T, Rimmerman C, et al. Color coding of digitized echocardiograms: description of a new technique and application in detecting and correcting for cardiac translation. *J Am Soc Echocardiol* 1994;7:363–369.

(The influence of cardiac motion on stress echocardiography is addressed but not resolved. In fact, no methods to counter the effects of cardiac motion are applied.)

873. Sciari R, Varga A, Picano E, et al. Comparison of combination of dipyridamole and dobutamine during echocardiography with thallium scintigraphy to improve viabiltiy detection. *Am J Cardiol* 1999;83:6–10.

(Thallium-201 [^{201}Tl] uptake was the most sensitive indicator of viability. The functional responses to dobutamine [or dipyridamole] were not so sensitive. Combining dipyridamole and dobutamine brought the sensitivity of the wall motion response for viability to the level seen with ^{201}Tl. Such polypharmacy is often needed for the functional response to compare with the perfusion response. Why would anyone apply this multiple pharmaceutical method? Only if they seek to profit by the application of their modality. Echocardiography advocates might wish to apply multiple agents, but more sensible and more rewarding is the simple assessment of viability with a simple safe perfusion evaluation.)

874. Zoghbi WA, Barasch E. Dobutamine MRI: a serious contender in pharmacologic stress imaging [editorial]? *Circulation* 1999;99:730–732.

(This is an editorial by echocardiography enthusiasts. The authors comment on the article by Nagel et al. [*875*].)

875. Nagel E, Lehmkuhl HB, Bocksch W, et al. Noninvasive diagnosis of ischemia-induced wall motion abnormalities with the use of high dose dobutamine stress MRI: comparison with dobutamine stress echocardiography. *Circulation* 1999;99:763–770.

(The authors studied 172 patients with both methods. Fully 11% of patients were excluded with each test: from MRI because of claustrophobia and obesity, and from echocardiography because of suboptimal image quality. Yet MRI exceeded stress echocardiography in sensitivity [88.7% versus 74.3%, respectively;

$P < 0.05$] and specificity [85.7% versus 69.8%, respectively; $P < 0.05$]. This was thought to be the result of superior image resolution on MRI, in which image quality was at least "good" in 82% of those imaged [not excluded], whereas only 51% had such high quality echocardiograms! Here, the sensitivity and specificity of dobutamine echocardiography did not approach the values quoted for the method when performed by enthusiasts. The nature of the intervention, the stress end point and the disadvantages of the imaging methods make the most appealing method one not considered here: pharmacologic myocardial perfusion scintigraphy with a coronary dilator! None of this is noted in the editorial, which looks at MRI as a possible threat to the application of echocardiography for pharmacologic stress.)

876. Rogers WJ, Kramer CM, Geskin G, et al. Early contrast-enhanced MRI predicts late functional recovery after reperfused myocardial infarction. *Circulation* 1999;99: 744–750.

    (Other methods of MRI assess regional perfusion and coronary flow reserve.)

877. Hoffmann R, Lethen H, Marwick T, et al. Analysis of interinstitutional observer agreement in interpretation of dobutamine stress echocardiograms. *J Am Coll Cardiol* 1996;27:330–336.

    (As shown here in references *877* and *329*, the reproducibility of stress echocardiography image interpretation, even among expert readers in stationary dobutamine studies, is poor and compares poorly with that of stress perfusion scintigraphy. Quantitation is rarely performed and is subjective, and quantitative methods have not undergone an in-depth evaluation of reproducibility. This deeply restricts the ability of the method to address risk stratification. Only recently has a qualitative, visual impression of a stress-induced increase in end-systolic volume been reported to relate to a poor prognosis.)

878. Lattanzi F, Picano E, Adamo E, Varga A. Dobutamine stress echocardiography; safety in diagnosing coronary artery disease. *Drug Safety* 2000;4:251–262.

    (Contrary to the title, this review of 35 studies, each with more than 100 patients, as well as 2 multicenter trials, tabulated the too frequent and too severe complications of dobutamine infusion in 26,438 tests.)

879. Ciati C, Mantaldo C, Zedda N, et al. New noninvasive methods for coronary flow reserve assessment. Contrast-enhanced transthoracic second harmonic echo Doppler. *Circulation* 1999;99:771–778.

    (Contrast-enhanced second harmonic imaging improved the ability to measure flow and flow reserve with dobutamine in left anterior descending coronary vessels. The method compared well with intracoronary Doppler measurements and is promising for the noninvasive measurement of coronary flow reserve.)

880. Feigenbaum H. Evolution of stress testing [editorial]. *Circulation* 1992;3:1217–1218.

881. Maddahi J, Gambhir SS. Cost-effective selection of patients for coronary angiography. In: Maddahi J, Iskandrian A, eds. Nuclear cardiology and managed care: from challenge to opportunity. *J Nucl Cardiol* 1997;4(suppl):S141–S151.

    (Maddahi and Gambhir present a mathematical model for the cost-effective application of perfusion imaging for the diagnosis of coronary disease and its prognostic assessment.)

882. Beller GA, Zaret BL. Wintergreen panel summaries. *J Nucl Cardiol* 1999;6:93–155.

    (Summaries from the Wintergreen Symposium topical panels, interactive exchanges of ideas between leading researchers and practitioners of nuclear cardiology and industry, review the current state of nuclear cardiology and goals for future work.)

883. Wackers FJTh, Fetterman RC, Mattera JA, Clements JP. Quantitative planar thallium-201 stress scintigraphy: a critical evaluation of the method. *Semin Nucl Med* 1985;15:46–58.

884. Verzijlbergen JF, Cramer MJ, Niemeyer MG, et al. ^{99m}Tc sestamibi for planar myocardial perfusion imaging; not as ideal as the physical properties. *Nucl Med Commun* 1991;12:381–386.

885. Taillefer R, Lambert R, Essiambre R, et al. Comparison between thallium-201, technetium-99m sestamibi and technetium-99m-teboroxime planar myocardial perfusion imaging in detection of coronary artery disease. *J Nucl Med* 1992;33: 1091–1097.

886. Verzijlbergen JF, van Oudeusden D, Cramer MJ, et al. Quantitative analysis of planar technetium-99m sestamibi myocardial perfusion images. Clinical application of modified methods for the subtraction of tissue crosstalk. *Eur Heart J* 1994;15:1217–1223.

887. Plachcinska A, Kusmierek J, Kosmider M, et al. Quantitative assessment of technetium-99m methoxyisobutylisonitrile planar perfusion heart studies: application of multivariate analysis to patient classification. *Eur J Nucl Med* 1995;22:193–199.

888. Maddahi J, Kiat H, Van Train KF, et al. Myocardial perfusion imaging with technetium-99m sestamibi SPECT in the evaluation of coronary artery disease. *Am J Cardiol* 1992;19:484–462.

889. Jamar F, Topcuoglu R, Cauwe F, et al. Exercise gated planar myocardial perfusion imaging using technetium-99m sestamibi for the diagnosis of coronary artery disease: an alternative to exercise tomographic imaging. *Eur J Nucl Med* 1995;22:40–46.

890. Berman DS, Kiat HS, Van Train KF, et al. Myocardial perfusion imaging with technetium-99m sestamibi. Comparative analysis of available imaging protocols. *J Nucl Med* 1994;35:681–688.

891. Rigo P, Bailey IK, Griffith LSC, et al. Stress thallium-201 myocardial scintigraphy for the detection of individual coronary arterial lesions in patients with and without previous myocardial infarction. *Am J Cardiol* 1981;48:209–215.

892. Starling MR, Dehmer GJ, Lancaster JL, et al. Comparison of quantitative SPECT vs planar thallium-201 myocardial scintigraphy for detecting and localizing segmental coronary artery disease. *J Am Coll Cardiol* 1985;5:531–538.

893. Gerson MC, Lukes J, Deutsch E, et al. Comparison of technetium-99m Q12 and thallium-201 for detection of angiographically documented coronary artery disease in humans. *J Nucl Cardiol* 1994;1:499–506.

894. Sporn V, Balino NP, Holman BL, et al. Simultaneous measurement of ventricular function and myocardial perfusion using the technetium-99m isonitriles. *Clin Nucl Med* 1988;13:77–83.

895. Van Train KF, Garcia EV, Maddahi J, et al. Multicenter trial validation for quantitative analysis of same-day rest stress technetium-99m-sestamibi myocardial tomograms. *J Nucl Med* 1994;35:609–615.

896. Berman DS, Kiat H, Friedman JD, et al. Separate acquisition rest thallium-201/stress technetium-99m sestamibi dual-isotope myocardial perfusion single-photon emission computed tomography: a clinical validation study. *J Am Coll Cardiol* 1993;22:1455–1463.

897. Heo J, Wolmer I, Kegel J, et al. Sequential dual-isotope SPECT imaging with thallium-201 and technetium-99m-sestamibi. *J Nucl Med* 1994;35:549–555.

898. Sridhara BS, Braat S, Rigo P, et al. Comparison of myocardial perfusion imaging with technetium-99m tetrofosmin versus thallium-201 in coronary artery disease. *Am J Cardiol* 1993;72:1015–1019.

899. Heo J, Cave V, Wasserleben V, et al. Planar and tomographic imaging with technetium-99m-labeled tetrofosmin: correlation with thallium-201 and coronary angiography. *J Nucl Cardiol* 1994;1:317–327.

900. Rigo P, Leclercq B, Itti R, et al. Technetium-99m-tetrofosmin myocardial imaging: a comparison with thallium-201 and angiography. *J Nucl Med* 1994;35:587–593.

901. Sridhara B, Sochor H, Rigo P, et al. Myocardial single-photon emission computed tomographic imaging with techentium-99m tetrofosmin: stress-rest imaging with same-day and separate-day rest imaging. *J Nucl Cardiol* 1994;1:138–143.

902. Takahasi N, Tamaki N, Tadamura E, et al. Combined assessment of regional perfusion and wall motion in patients with coronary artery disease with technetium 99m-tetrofosmin. *J Nucl Cardiol* 1994;1:29–38.

903. Zaret BL, Rigo P, Wackers FJTh, et al. Myocardial perfusion imaging with ^{99m}Tc tetrofosmin. Comparison to ^{201}Tl imaging and coronary angiography in a phase III multicenter trial. Tetrofosmin International Trial Study Group. *Circulation* 1995;91:313–319.

904. Mahmood S, Gunning M, Bomanji JB, et al. Combined rest thallium-201/stress technetium-99m-tetrofosmin SPECT: feasibility and diagnostic accuracy of a 90-minute protocol. *J Nucl Med* 1995;36:932–935.

905. Yong TK, Chambers J, Maisey MN, et al. Technetium-99m tetrofosmin myocardial perfusion scan: comparison of 1-day and 3-day protocols. *Eur J Nucl Med* 1996;23:320–325.

906. Sullo P, Cuocolo A, Nicolai E, et al. Quantitative exercise technetium-99m tetrofosmin myocardial tomography for the identification and localization of coronary artery disease. *Eur J Nucl Med* 1996;23:648–655.

907. Montz R, Perez-Castejâon MJ, Jurado JA, et al. Technetium-99m tetrofosmin rest/stress myocardial SPECT with a same-day 2–hour protocol: comparison with coronary angiography. A Spanish-Portuguese multicentre clinical trial. *Eur J Nucl Med* 1996;23:639–647.

908. Benoit T, Vivegnis D, Foulon J, et al. Quantitative evaluation of myocardial single-photon emission tomographic imaging: application to the measurement of perfusion defect size and severity. *Eur J Nucl Med* 1996;23:1603–1612.

909. He ZX, Iskandrian AS, Gupta NC, et al. Assessing coronary artery disease with dipyridamole technetium-99m-tetrofosmin SPECT: a multicenter trial. *J Nucl Med* 1997;38:44–48.

910. Cuocolo A, Sullo P, Pace L, et al. Adenosine coronary vasodilation in coronary artery disease: technetium-99m tetrofosmin myocardial tomography versus echocardiography. *J Nucl Med* 1997;38:1089–1094.

911. Sacchetti G, Inglese E, Bongo AS, et al. Detection of moderate and severe coronary artery stenosis with technetium-99m tetrofosmin myocardial single-photon emission tomography. *Eur J Nucl Med* 1997;24:1230–1236.

912. Takeishi Y, Takahasi N, Fujiwara S, et al. Myocardial tomography with technetium-99m-tetrofosmin during intravenous infusion of adenosine triphosphate. *J Nucl Med* 1998;39:582–586.

913. Boomsma MM, Niemeyer MG, van der Wall EE, et al. Tc-99m tetrofosmin myocardial SPECT perfusion imaging: comparison of rest-stress and stress-rest protocols. *Int J Cardiol Imaging* 1998;14:105–111.

914. Acampa W, Cuocolo A, Sullo P, et al. Direct comparison of technetium 99m-sestamibi and technetium-99m tetrofosmin cardiac single photon emission computed tomography in patients with coronary artery disease. *J Nucl Cardiol* 1998;5:265–274.

915. Matsuda J, Miyamoto N, Ikushima I, et al. Stress technetium-99m tetrofosmin myocardial scintigraphy: a new one-hour protocol for the detection of coronary artery disease. *J Cardiol* 1998;32:219–226.

916. Kim Y, Goto H, Kobayashi K, et al. A new method to evaluate ischemic heart disease: combined use of rest thallium-201 myocardial SPECT and Tc-99m exercise tetrofosmin first pass and myocardial SPECT. *Ann Nucl Med* 1999;13:147–153.

917. Iskandrian AS, Hakki AH, Kane-Marsch S. Prognostic implications of exercise thallium-201 scintigraphy in patients with suspected or known coronary artery disease. *Am Heart J* 1985;110:135–143.

918. Wackers FJTh, Russo DJ, Russo D, et al. Prognostic significance of normal quantitative planar thallium-201 stress scintigraphy in patients with chest pain. *J Am Coll Cardiol* 1985;6:27–30.

919. Wahl JM, Hakki AH, Iskandrian AS. Prognostic importance of silent myocardial ischemia detected by intravenous dipyridamole thallium myocardial imaging in asymptomatic patients with coronary artery disease. *J Am Coll Cardiol* 1989; 14:1635–1641.

920. Heo J, Thompson WO, Iskandrian AS. Prognostic implications of normal exercise thallium images. *Am J Noninvasive Cardiol* 1987;1:209–212.

921. Koss JH, Kobren SM, Grunwalk AM, et al. Role of exercise thallium-201 myocardial perfusion scintigraphy in predicting prognosis in suspected coronary artery disease. *Am J Cardiol* 1987;59:531–534.

922. Bairey CN, Rozanski A, Maddahi J, et al. Exercise thallium-201 scintigraphy and prognosis in typical angina pectoris and negative exercise electrocardiography. *Am J Cardiol* 1989;564:282–287.

923. Stratmann HG, Mark AL, Walter KE, et al. Prognostic value of atrial pacing and thallium-201 scintigraphy in patients with stable chest pain. *Am J Cardiol* 1989;64: 985–990.

924. Brown KA, Atland E, Rowen M. Prognostic value of normal Tc-99m sestamibi myocardial perfusion imaging [abstract]. *J Nucl Med* 1993;34:55P.

925. Burns RJ, Romagnuolo J, Mehta SL, et al. Low likelihood of coronary events in young patients with normal thallium-201 SPECT [abstract]. *J Nucl Med* 1993;34:54P.

926. Herman SD, Santos-Ocampo CD, McClellan JR, et al. Dipyridamole Tc-99m SPECT myocardial perfusion imaging-prognostic implications [abstract]. *J Nucl Med* 1993;34:85P.

927. Steinberg EH, Koss JH, Lee M, et al. Prognostic significance from 10-year follow-up of a qualitatively normal planar exercise thallium test in suspected coronary artery disease. *Am J Cardiol* 1993;71:1270–1273.

   (883–927: These references deal with the diagnostic accuracy of perfusion scintigraphy with various radiotracers and acquisition and analysis protocols represented in Tables 6A–E.)

Questions and Case Examples

1. You are told that a patient's perfusion study has been selected by the staff cardiologist for discussion at the cardiac catheterization conference, where catheterization results are discussed in the full clinical perspective. You are asked to bring the image for discussion and review. Further, you learn that there was an apparent discrepancy between the image findings and angiography, in which a grossly abnormal scan related to normal coronary arteries! The study is (not) shown in Figure 117. Describe the image findings. Can you suggest reasons why this case was selected? Characterize the discrepancy between scintigraphic and angiographic data, and select all choices that could explain how this could possibly have occurred.

   a. The cardiologist was very knowledgeable about the imaging study and wanted to present the findings.
   b. The cardiologist never saw the study but was told that the results were "poor" and thought that this meant a poor relationship to the angiogram.
   c. The cardiologist was a practitioner of nuclear cardiology and wanted to present this study to demonstrate its specific advantages.
   d. The cardiologist was skeptical of the scintigraphic method and wanted to demonstrate a failure of the method.
   e. The scintigram is nonexistent!

2. Consider these clinical terms. Match each to its most appropriate definition and the clarifying points offered thereafter.

   A. Coronary "dominance"
   B. Left main disease
   C. "Culprit" vessel
   D. High-risk disease
   E. Hypertrophic cardiomyopathy
   F. Diastolic dysfunction
   G. Ischemia
   H. Myocardium at ischemic risk
   I. Congestive (dilated) cardiomy-
      opathy
   J. Ischemic cardiomyopathy
   K. Dysynergy
   L. Akinesis
   M. Dyskinesis
   N. Aneurysm
   O. Hypokinesis
   P. Tardokinesis
   Q. Coronary flow reserve
   R. ST elevation
   S. ST depression
   T. Angina
   U. Atypical pain
   V. Anginal equivalent

Figure 117

W. Viable myocardium
X. "Hibernation"
Y. "Stunning"
Z. New onset angina

With:

a. Without provocation, this is chronically dysfunctional myocardium at rest, but it is viable and potentially reversible with revascularization.
b. Left ventricular dysfunction based in coronary disease and often resembling the congestive variety. Myocardial viability may be important to determine in this population in order to assess the possible benefit from coronary bypass graft surgery.
c. Generally extensive coronary disease, subtending a large territory, related to a high subsequent event rate and thus managed aggressively
d. Generally perceived as ventricular stiffness or reduced compliance, leading to high left ventricular filling pressures and pulmonary congestion in the absence of coronary disease or in the presence of only limited coronary disease. There is preserved left ventricular systolic function, ie, left ventricular ejection fraction (LVEF)
e. A dilated, widely dysfunctional left ventricle with a low ejection fraction and heart failure. The condition may or may not be based in coronary disease. Myocardial viability may be important to determine in this population in order to assess the possible benefit from coronary bypass graft surgery.
f. Apparent systolic bulging in a ventricular segment
g. Ventricular dysfunction, often with a large diastolic component and hyperdynamic systolic function. It may bring ischemia in the absence of coronary disease and may cause pulmonary congestion in the presence of limited coronary disease and preserved LVEF.
h. Delayed ventricular inward systolic wall motion
i. The stenotic vessel, among several, which is the cause of ischemic symptoms. Scintigraphic findings permit performance of a selective "culprit" angioplasty with symptomatic and prognostic outcome rivaling a more generalized approach.
j. The absence of inward systolic wall motion
k. The ability of the coronary resistance vessels to accommodate increased flow under conditions of physiologic demand or induced pharmacologic dilation
l. Ischemic pain of recent onset, a form of unstable angina. The implication relates to its unestablished and unpredictable behavior and that of the underlying lesion. Such patients should be well evaluated, generally noninvasively, and carefully managed.
m. A segmental ventricular wall motion abnormality associated with dyskinesis or frank akinesis. It often suggests a coronary cause.
n. Reduced ventricular systolic wall motion.
o. The extent of myocardium that becomes ischemic with increased demands (or reduced supply). The former is better predicted than the latter. The parameter has an important relationship with prognosis.
p. The electrocardiographic (ECG) finding generally, but not specifically, related to an acute ischemic event, usually indicating transmural ischemia and often needing rapid intervention
q. An abnormally contracting ventricular segment.

   r. The ECG finding generally but not specifically related to subendocardial ischemia or nontransmural infarction

   s. An imbalance of myocardial oxygen supply and demand with insufficiency of the former

   t. Typical chest pain or pressure that is characteristic of a cardiac ischemic cause

   u. Some well-known symptom other than classic angina, such as shortness of breath, arm or jaw pain, that may occur with exertion and relate to myocardial ischemia

   v. Dysfunctional on an ischemic basis, but may be returned to a functional condition with time (stunning) or revascularization (hibernation)

   w. Significant coronary disease involving the left main coronary artery, subtending a large myocardial region and generally justifying aggressive revascularization treatment related to its high prognostic risk

   x. Suggests but does not clearly derive from an ischemic cause

   y. Widely applied to indicate the vessel that supplies the posterior aspect of the interventricular septum, most commonly the right coronary artery (RCA). This relates only indirectly and quite poorly to the extent of myocardium at ischemic risk.

   z. Postischemic myocardial dysfunction. Given time (sometimes months) and maintained perfusion, function will recover.

3A. Shown in the top 3 rows of the 2 panels of Figure 118 are short-axis single positron emission computed tomography (SPECT) images from apex (top panel, upper left) to base (bottom panel, upper right) acquired with thallium-201 (^{201}Tl) after exercise stress in a 53-yr-old woman with diabetes, atypical chest discomfort, a history of prior anterior infarction and a known anterior apical aneurysm. There was no induced chest pain, but ECG ST segment changes suggested induced ischemia. The delayed images (second rows of each panel) were acquired after the "reinjection" (RI) of an additional 1 mCi ^{201}Tl. The images reveal a reversible defect of the inferior wall with a large fixed apical, anterior and septal defect, associated with stress-related cavitary dilation. There was evidence of diverging distal myocardial walls on long-axis slices after stress but not in delayed images. Gating was not performed. Angioplasty of an RCA is contemplated, but bypass surgery would be performed if multivessel ischemia and viability in the left anterior descending coronary artery (LAD) region could be documented. What more could be done? Choose the 1 best answer.

   a. Inject another 1 mCi ^{201}Tl.

   b. Reimage at 24 hr.

   c. Nothing. The LAD distribution is scarred.

   d. Reimage with technetium-99m (^{99m}Tc) sestamibi.

   e. Gate the thallium study to determine the motion of the underperfused wall.

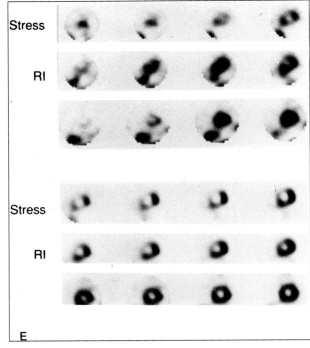

Figure 118

3B. Shown in Figure 118 and also in other figures in this section are examples of delayed 24-hr ^{201}Tl redistribution. What interventions or imaging tactics can be applied to enhance defect reversibility and identification of viable myocardium when applying the sequential rest ^{201}Tl/^{99m}Tc stress protocol? Choose all correct answers.

   a. (Re)inject 1 mCi ^{201}Tl and reimage at 4 hr in the ^{201}Tl window.
   b. (Re)inject 1 mCi ^{201}Tl at 4 hr and reimage at 24 hr in the ^{201}Tl window.
   c. (Re)inject 1 mCi ^{201}Tl at 24 hr and reimage in the ^{201}Tl window.
   d. Reimage at 24 hr in the ^{201}Tl window.
   e. Image at 24 hr after an additional injection of 1 mCi ^{99m}Tc sestamibi.
   f. Nitroglycerin may be given with the rest study to maximize uptake and viability evaluation.

4. Shown in the upper rows in each image set of the SPECT study in Figure 119 are exercise (stress) ^{99m}Tc sestamibi slices, and in the lower rows of each image set are rest ^{201}Tl slices in the short-axis (top 2 rows, from apex, left, to base, right), vertical long-axis (middle 2 rows, from septum, left, to lateral wall, right) and horizontal long-axis (bottom 2 rows, from anterior, left, to inferior, right) slices of the SPECT study acquired in a 72-yr-old man with a prior coronary history undergoing risk stratification after a traumatic fall. Working on a construction site, he apparently missed a step and fell off a tall ladder, sustaining multiple head, face and upper body fractures. He has a history of a remote myocardial infarction (MI) but has been active and asymptomatic for many years on minimal

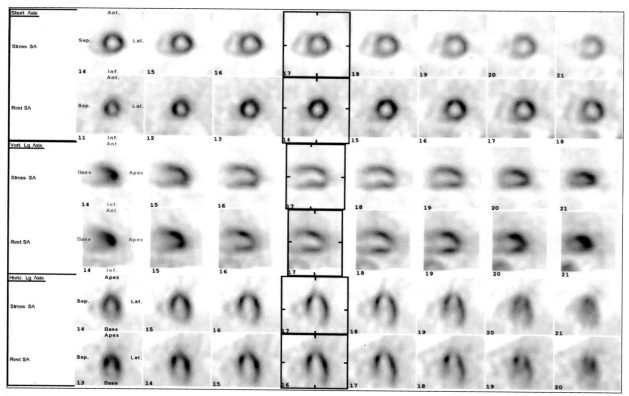

Figure 119

medications. In spite of his fractures, he was able to perform a vigorous exercise test to a high double product in the absence of ischemic symptoms or ECG changes. The study is read as showing modest fixed defects in the inferior-lateral and apical left ventricular wall without evidence of reversibility. The patient's coronary disease is treated conservatively with medications and he undergoes multiple, event-free orthopedic and plastic surgery procedures, He continues an active, event-free life. Thirteen months later, the patient feels ill while in his car and goes to a local emergency department (ED) where an ECG shows no acute changes. Nonetheless, he suffers irreversible sudden death and cannot be revived. At autopsy, the patient has evidence of the prior infarction and multivessel coronary involvement, but there is no evidence of acute infarction. The patient's prior studies are reviewed and a lawsuit is brought against the cardiologist who initially managed the patient at the time of trauma and the nuclear physician who read the scan >1 yr earlier. The prosecution expert witness states that the prior study showed inferior reversibility and cavitary dilation that predicted more extensive disease and a worse prognosis that were initially overlooked but should have alerted all to the occurrence of the final outcome. Which of the following is (are) true?

a. The initial reading was in gross error.
b. The initial image findings were more consistent with multivessel ischemia.
c. Image findings would support aggressive management and revascularization at the time they were performed.
d. The initial image reading was appropriate, as, probably, was the management.
e. The image shows a fixed defect but displacement of otherwise similar slices makes it appear as though dilation and reversibility were present.

5. A debilitated, arthritic 73-yr-old man with renal insufficiency, diabetes and hypercholesterolemia but no history or symptoms of coronary artery disease (CAD) has dipyridamole perfusion imaging for risk stratification before major peripheral vascular surgery. The rest ^{201}Tl/dipyridamole stress ^{99m}Tc sestamibi SPECT slices are shown in Figure 121A, according to a format similar to that applied in Figure 119. Here, short-axis slices are displayed from apex (left) to base (right), vertical long-axis slices are displayed from septal to lateral walls and horizontal long-axis slices are displayed from inferior to anterior walls. Shown in Figure 121B are polar maps of the radionuclide distribution in SPECT slices from this man compared with the normal, sex-matched data base, at stress and rest, as shown in Figure 120B. The LVEF calculation from gated perfusion images acquired after stress is shown in Figure 121C. In the vertical left panels are end-diastolic (left) and end-systolic frames in 3 short-axis slices, a midventricular horizontal long-axis slice and a vertical long-axis slice, from above downward. Polar maps, beginning at upper left and proceeding clockwise, plot perfusion, regional LVEF, wall thickening and wall motion. LVEF is reduced at 39%. Choose all that can be concluded from these image findings.

a. Modest reversible anterior apical and septal defects are accompanied by gross cavitary dilation and a reduced LVEF, the latter in the presence of a normal rest image and no prior infarction.

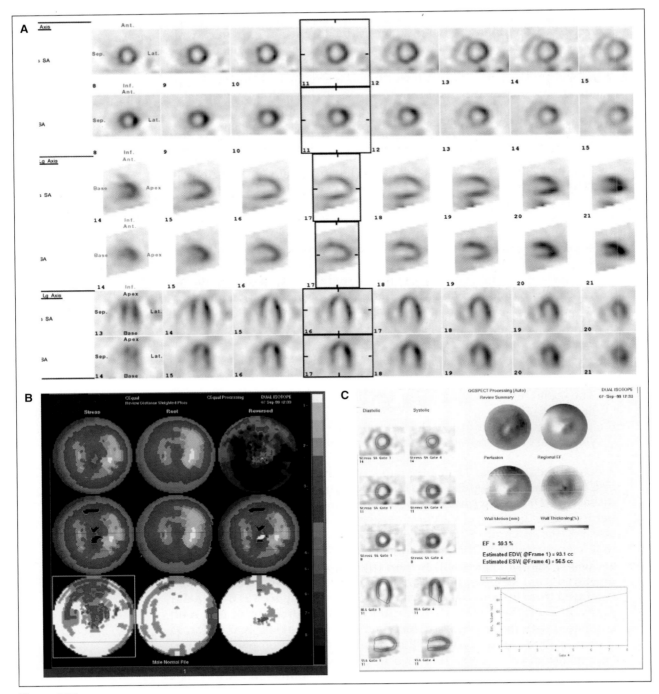

Figure 121

b. Depressed wall motion and LVEF suggest post-stress "stunning," adding gravity to the perfusion findings.

c. Cavitary dilation, better seen in black-and-white images, adds further prognostic import to the study.

d. Perfusion defects are modest and suggest a low surgical risk and a benign outcome.

e. The sum of image findings suggests a high perioperative risk.

6. A 60-yr-old woman is admitted to the hospital with rest pain and an abnormal ECG. An infarction is ruled out, and a dipyridamole ^{201}Tl SPECT perfusion scintigram is performed. Limited short-axis SPECT slices of the initial stress (first and third rows) and redistribution set (second and fourth rows) are shown in Figure 122A, whereas selected vertical and horizontal long-axis slices are shown in Figures 122B and continue in Figure 122C. They reveal reversible defects in a multivessel distribution, confirming the clinical suspicion. However, owing to a persistent defect, 24-hr images are requested. The latter are subsequently acquired, and alternating rows of selected short-axis slices at stress (top) are compared with 24-hr delay slices (bottom) in Figure 122D, and a similar comparison in selected vertical (top) and horizontal (bottom) slices are shown in Figure 122E. The patient is moved to the coronary care unit, because recurrent ischemic pain with related ECG changes is occurring at rest. Yet, surprisingly the 24-hr delayed image set now reveals no reversible component compared with stress. The reader now reverses his or her prior interpretation and, much to the chagrin of the cardiology team, states that all defects are "fixed." Yet, prior images demonstrate reversibility, and the clinical course is undeniably ischemic in this patient now demonstrated on angiography to have severe, multivessel coronary disease. In spite, not because of, the scintigraphic findings, bypass surgery is scheduled for the next day. Indeed, the nuclear cardiology team is puzzled, and the images are reviewed. Explain the findings. Are the conclusions correct or erroneous? Which of the following is (are) true?

   a. Indeed, the initial images showed reversible defects that were fixed on the delayed study.
   b. The change in delayed image findings relate to the interim occurrence of a silent infarction.
   c. The findings relate to a form of "reverse redistribution."
   d. The patient truly displays image evidence of induced ischemia, which is obscured by a technical flaw related to the display of the delayed image.
   e. The findings are classic for coronary spasm.
   f. The patient truly displays image evidence of induced ischemia, which is obscured by a technical flaw related to the acquisition of the delayed image.

7. Shown in Figure 123A according to the same format as the previous images are exercise stress ^{99m}Tc sestamibi and rest ^{201}Tl images acquired in a 55-yr-old man with atypical chest pain and multiple risk factors. The related polar maps are shown in Figure 123B, and the functional results of gated post-stress imaging are shown in Figure 123C, according to the formats applied previously. Global left ventricular systolic function was preserved with an anteroapical hypokinetic segment and an LVEF of 53%. The image findings include:

   a. Gross reversible defects that are compatible with extensive myocardium at ischemic risk.
   b. Cavitary dilation, cavitary photopenia and diverging walls in the stress study all indicate significant stress-induced ischemia with possible aneurysm formation.
   c. Cavitary dilation and aneurysm formation, which often indicate high-risk multivessel coronary disease and increased risk of subsequent coronary events
   d. A pattern related to multivessel coronary disease

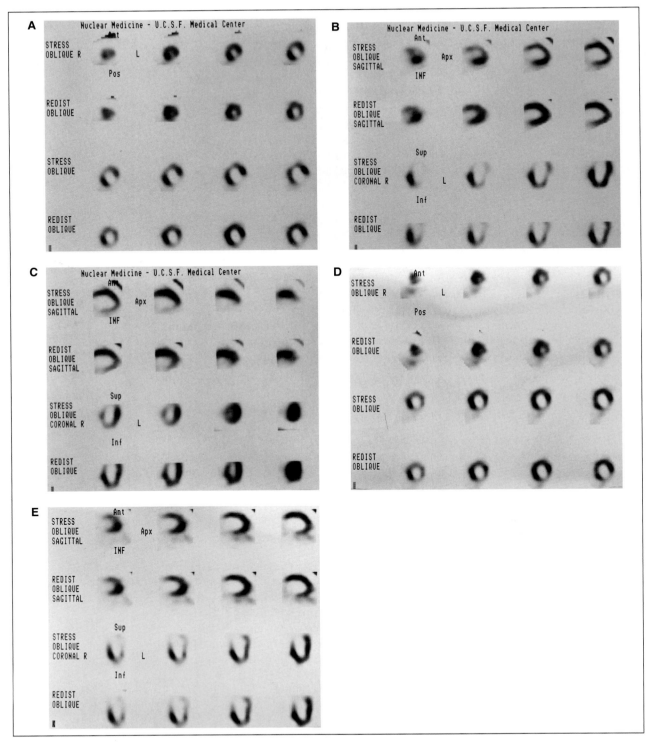

Figure 122

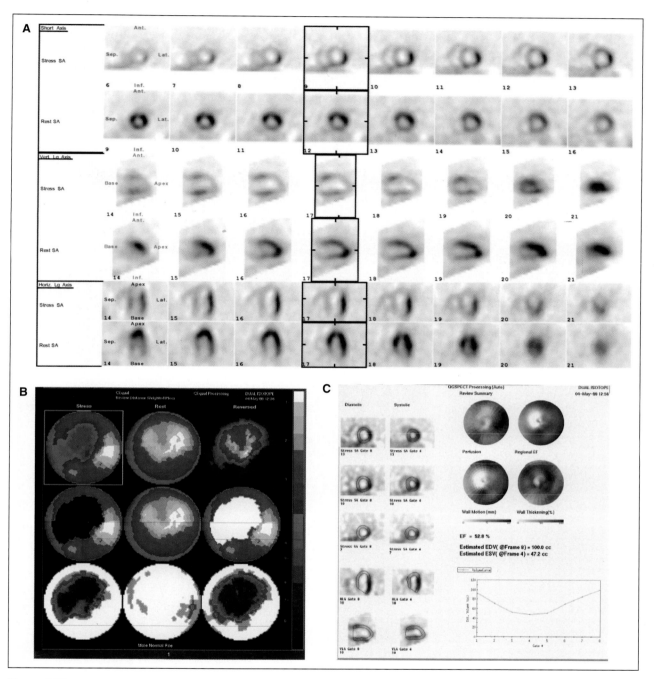

Figure 123

    e. Lung uptake, another nonperfusion marker for high-risk coronary disease, is easily seen in SPECT images and is well established in association with ^{99m}Tc sestamibi.

    f. An anterior apical wall motion abnormality is most likely the result of poststress "stunning."

8. A 48-yr-old bartender with agoraphobia, known CAD and prior infarction who had undergone acute percutaneous transluminal coronary angioplasty (PTCA) of the LAD 4 yr earlier, comes to the hospital with new chest pain at rest and with stress. An acute infarction is ruled out by enzymes. A prior rest ^{201}Tl/dipyridamole ^{99m}Tc sestamibi perfusion study performed soon after that prior angioplasty and shown, according to the previous format, in Figure 124A, with polar map in Figure 124B, demonstrated a subtle reversible lateral wall defect without fixed abnormalities. The patient is again scheduled for dipyridamole study. He complains of chest pain the morning of the test. The ECG is unchanged, and enzymes

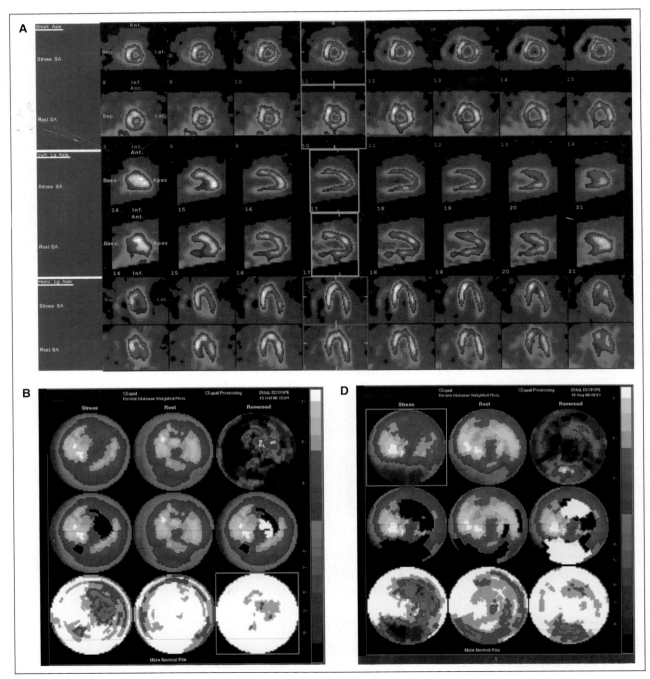

Figure 124

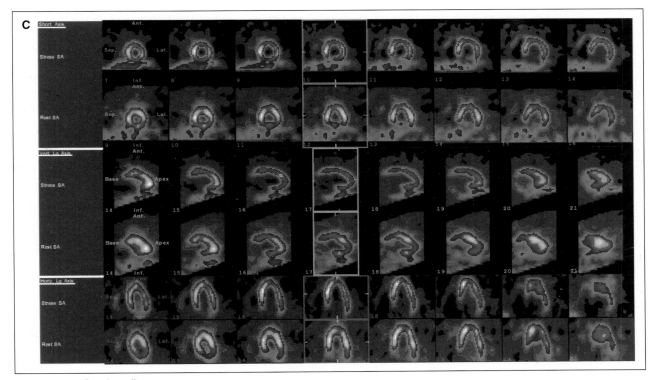

Figure 124 (*Continued*)

are again drawn. Stress testing brings no ECG changes and a good hemodynamic effect. Technically excellent images and the related polar maps are shown, according to the previous format, in Figures 124C and 124D, respectively. What can be said about the image findings and their clinical implications? Choose all correct answers.

a. The current images reveal continued presence of the reversible lateral defect.

b. The current images show a new fixed and partially reversible inferior defect.

c. The fixed defect on the current study suggests that the patient indeed suffered an acute infarction!

d. If the patient infarcted, it seems likely to have occurred with his morning pain, just before testing, because an infarct had been excluded previously.

e. The current image recommends conservative management.

f. Symptoms must be taken very seriously here, not only because of the cardiac history, but also because of the patient's psychological profile.

9A. A 76-yr-old woman with treated hypercholesterolemia, hypertension and left ventricular hypertrophy (LVH) on her EKG is to undergo major nonvascular surgery. She complains of severe, exercise-related shortness of breath, to the point of severe disability. Pulmonary function tests are normal, and there is no chest discomfort. What can be said of the patient's symptoms and their possible evaluation? Choose all correct answers.

a. Stress-related shortness of breath is an unlikely symptom of coronary disease.

b. Stress-related shortness of breath is a likely symptom of coronary disease.

   c. To evaluate ischemia associated with stress-induced shortness of breath, stress echocardiography must be applied, because a functional ischemic end point must be applied to identify a functional ischemic symptom.

   d. To evaluate ischemia associated with stress-induced shortness of breath, the same methods should be applied as would generally be applied to the evaluation of ischemia.

   e. Perfusion scintigraphy maintains its high diagnostic sensitivity in the setting of ischemic, anginal equivalents, such as stress-induced shortness of breath, as it does in association with asymptomatic ischemia

9B. The patient discussed in 9A undergoes an exercise perfusion study. She completes 6 min 30 sec of the standard Bruce protocol, achieving a high double product and stopping with shortness of breath and fatigue in the absence of chest pain or new ST changes. The technically excellent rest ^{201}Tl/stress sestamibi images are presented in Figure 125. Which is (are) true regarding the methods applied, the findings and their clinical applications?

   a. Exercise testing without imaging would have sufficed, because there were none of the nonspecific ECG changes expected in the setting of LVH.

   b. The image shows the typical features of soft-tissue attenuation.

   c. Cavitary dilation is impressive and, with defects in anterior, anteroseptal and lateral distributions, is reflective of extensive myocardium at ischemic risk in multiple vascular areas.

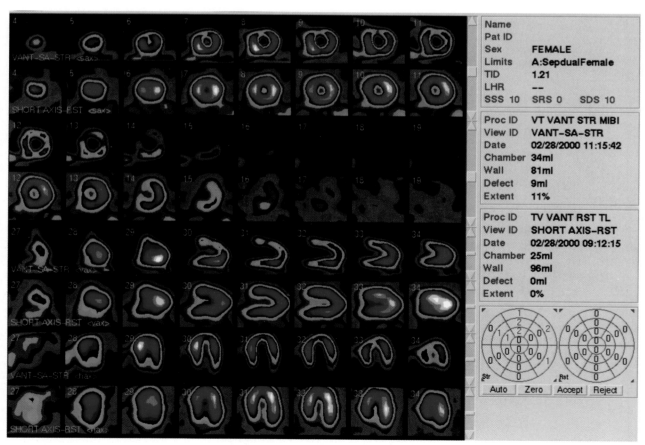

Figure 125

   d. The perfusion pattern is indicative of extensive myocardium at ischemic risk and high-risk multivessel coronary disease.

   e. The image findings are typical for LVH.

9C. What is the specific pathophysiologic cause of ischemia-related shortness of breath?

   a. Severe diffuse systolic dysfunction leads to a severe reduction in LVEF and reduced cardiac output.

   b. Associated right ventricular dysfunction affects pulmonary function.

   c. Ischemic-induced ventricular dysfunction leads to pericardial effusion, which causes underfilling of the left ventricle and low output.

   d. Multiple pulmonary emboli

   e. Ischemic-induced diastolic dysfunction leads to increased end-diastolic pressure, increased pulmonary venous and pulmonary capillary pressures and pulmonary congestion.

   f. Myocardial ischemia leads directly to hypoxia.

10. A 65-yr-old man has chest discomfort that is only sometimes related to exertion. There is a possible history of prior hypertension, and the patient did smoke in the past. A recent exercise test was negative to a high level of exertion, but continued symptoms brought re-evaluation with perfusion scintigraphy. Shown in Figures 126A–C are baseline, exercise and recovery tracings, respectively, associated with a moderate workload and high achieved double product (9 min of a standard Bruce protocol to a peak achieved heart rate of 147 bpm, 85% of maximal predicted heart rate for age [MPHR], and peak blood pressure of 180/80). There was shortness of breath but no chest discomfort. The related rest ^{201}Tl/stress ^{99m}Tc sestamibi images and polar maps are shown in Figures 126D and 126E in a format similar to that outlined in previous questions. Shown also are regional defect maps. Choose all correct answers.

   a. The treadmill test is positive for ischemia, with gross ST segment elevation during exercise.

   b. The treadmill test is negative for ischemia.

   c. The image reveals evidence of a large reversible defect in the LAD territory.

   d. The image findings, although impressive, recommend a conservative management approach in the presence of a high achieved workload and double product.

   e. The image findings, although impressive, indicate a low prognostic risk in the presence of a high achieved workload and double product, compared with the same defect elicited in relation to a low workload and achieved double product.

   f. The absence of stress-induced chest discomfort and the negative exercise test, taken to a high workload and double product, indicates that the image findings are not related to the patients symptoms and are of little diagnostic or prognostic import.

   g. Although associated with a high achieved workload and double product, the extent of the defect and associated cavitary dilation recommend an aggressive approach

   h. The absence of induced chest discomfort excludes any relationship between this image abnormality and the clinical syndrome.

Figure 126

i. Chest pain was variable clinically and, although absent with stress testing, does not reduce the clinical suspicion of coronary disease nor the significance of the image findings.

j. Although chest pain was absent, the shortness of breath noted could be an anginal equivalent.

k. Silent ischemia is related to a prognosis that is no different from the "noisy" variety.

l. The baseline ECG suggests a prior anteroseptal infarction with associated ST elevation, suggesting a related aneurysm.

11A. A 79-yr-old semiretired male physician notes a gradual loss of energy with some dyspnea on exertion. Over the last 3–6 mo, he has lost the stamina to play singles tennis, yet believes there is little wrong other than aging. There is no history of chest pain or other coronary risk factors, and he is on no cardiovascular medication. His cardiologist requests an exercise perfusion study. No rest image is performed. He exercises 12 min 18 sec of a modified Bruce Protocol (stage III), stopping with fatigue at a peak heart rate of only 104 (77% MPHR) and blood pressure of 140/75. His 12-lead ECGs at baseline, peak exercise and in recovery are shown in Figures 127A–C, respectively. Which of the following is (are) true regarding the stress test and ECG findings?

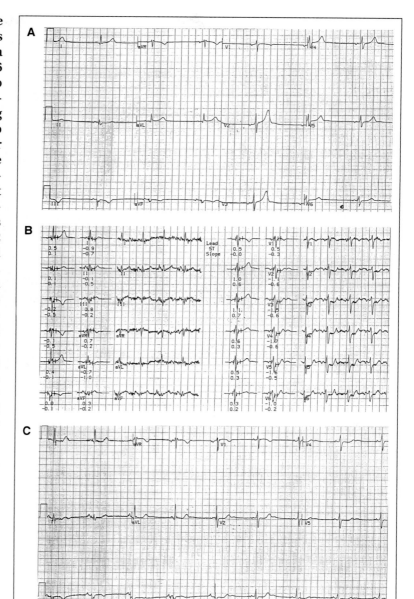

Figure 127

a. The absence of induced chest pain excludes coronary disease.
b. The test is normal.
c. The stress ECG reveals ischemic changes at a high heart rate and workload.
d. The stress ECG reveals ischemic changes at a modest achieved double product.
e. The heart rate response is inadequate and inappropriate.
f. The heart rate response is appropriate given the modest workload.
g. The exercise tracings demonstrate a junctional escape rhythm with apparent isorhythmic A-V dissociation and chronotropic incompetence.
h. The patient's diagnosis simply relates to an electrophysiologic condition that can be cured by a pacemaker.

11B. Shown in Figure 128 are the accompanying ^{99m}Tc sestamibi stress SPECT images from above downward in short-axis, from apex (left) to base (right), vertical long-axis, from septum (left) to lateral wall (right) and horizontal

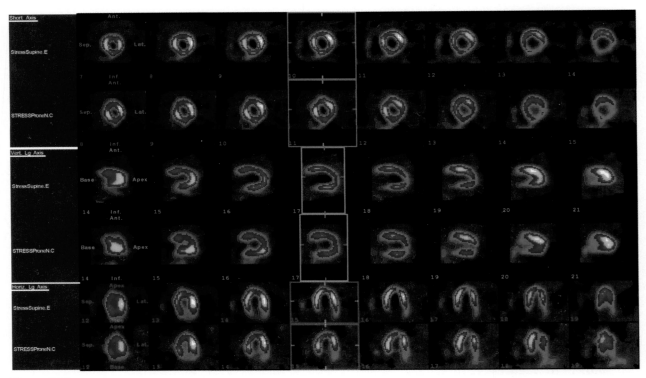

Figure 128

long-axis slices, from anterior (left) to inferior (right), with supine images above and prone images below in each view. The gated LVEF was 52% with normal wall motion. What are the image findings?

a. The images are normal, and so no rest study was performed.
b. The images demonstrate a gross anterior and septal defect.
c. The images reveal evidence of attenuation by the lateral wall.
d. The images are classic for upward creep.
e. The images demonstrate limited abnormalities of the apex as well as the basal inferior and lateral walls.

12. A hypertensive 62-yr-old woman, with a prior acute MI and immediate LAD PTCA 2 yr earlier, has recurrent chest pain and prior normal dipyridamole perfusion studies both 2 yr and 2 wk earlier. The patient presents with rest chest pain and is admitted. She is to go to angiography as her most recent perfusion study is reviewed. Shown in Figures 129A and 129B are the supine rest ^{201}Tl/stress ^{99m}Tc sestamibi and prone stress perfusion study shown in the same format as presented in previous questions. Figure 129C shows epicardial and endocardial outlines from the gated poststress images in anterior (left) and left anterior oblique (LAO) (right) projections. These reveal hyperdynamic left ventricular wall motion and an LVEF reported to be 91%. Which is (are) true regarding these images?

a. The study is normal.
b. The study clearly reveals the prior infarction.
c. The study shows no evidence of prior infarction.
d. The study makes coronary disease unlikely and relates to a good prognosis.
e. A normal study in this setting definitely excludes prior infarction.

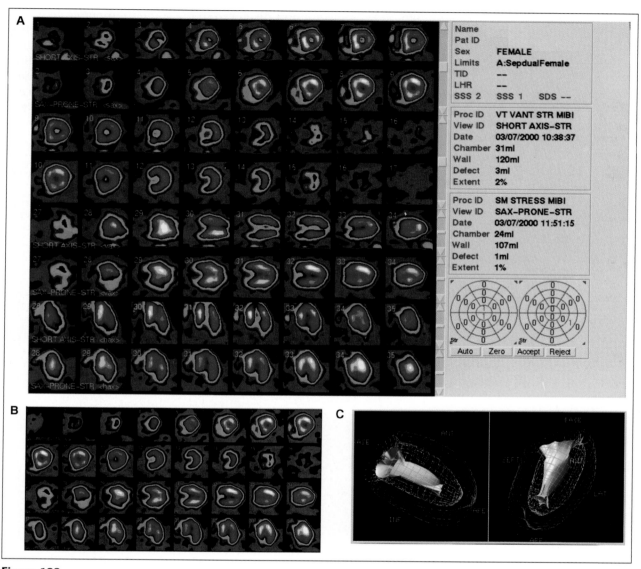

A

Name		
Pat ID		
Sex	FEMALE	
Limits	A:SepdualFemale	
TID	--	
LHR	--	
SSS 2	SSS 1	SDS --

Proc ID	VT VANT STR MIBI	
View ID	SHORT AXIS-STR	
Date	03/07/2000 10:38:37	
Chamber	31ml	
Wall	120ml	
Defect	3ml	
Extent	2%	

Proc ID	SM STRESS MIBI	
View ID	SAX-PRONE-STR	
Date	03/07/2000 11:51:15	
Chamber	24ml	
Wall	107ml	
Defect	1ml	
Extent	1%	

Auto | Zero | Accept | Reject

B

C

Figure 129

    f. A normal study in this setting suggests a limited infarction and successful prior angioplasty.

    g. The LVEF is quite accurate.

    h. The LVEF is likely overestimated because of an underestimated end-systolic volume.

13A. A 63-yr-old man with hypertension and increased cholesterol has no chest pain or shortness of breath. Although his rest ECG (Fig. 130A) has only minor ST-T irregularities, an exercise perfusion imaging study is requested. The patient completed 10 min 15 sec, reaching stage IV of a standard Bruce protocol, stopping with fatigue at a peak heart rate of 148 (90% MPHR) and blood pressure of 195/78. The immediate poststress ECG is shown in Figure 130B (AVF and V_6 not shown). Shown in Figure 130C according to the same format in previous questions are supine rest ^{201}Tl and stress sestamibi SPECT images, now displayed in the standard manner, in which horizontal long-axis slices progress from inferior (left) to anterior (right). Figure 130D presents polar maps of perfusion (above, center) at end-diastole (ED, left) and end-systole (ES, right) and function (below), with wall motion displayed at left and thickening at right. Figure 130E presents the end-diastolic (green mesh) and end-systolic (solid gray) endocardial and epicardial (red mesh) outlines of the stress gated study in the anterior (left) and LAO (right) projections. The stress prone image is unchanged. What can be said about the image findings? Choose all correct answers.

a. The findings can be explained well by diaphragmatic attenuation.
b. Supine perfusion images reveal a dense reversible inferior defect.

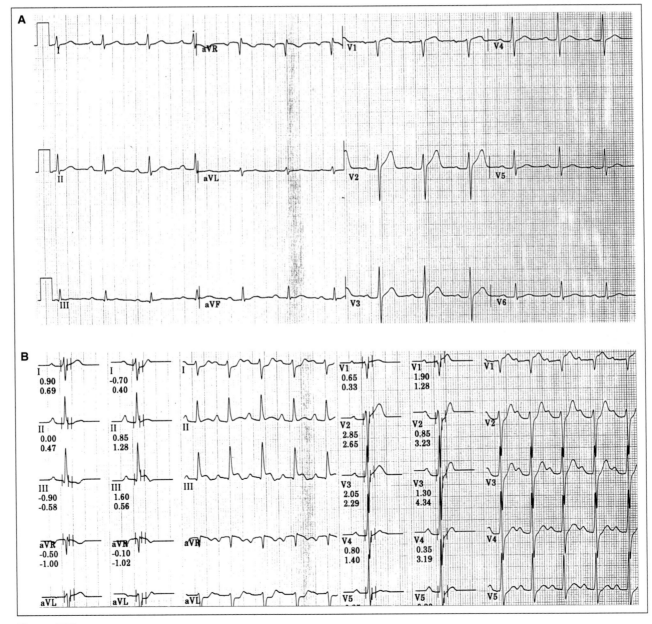

Figure 130

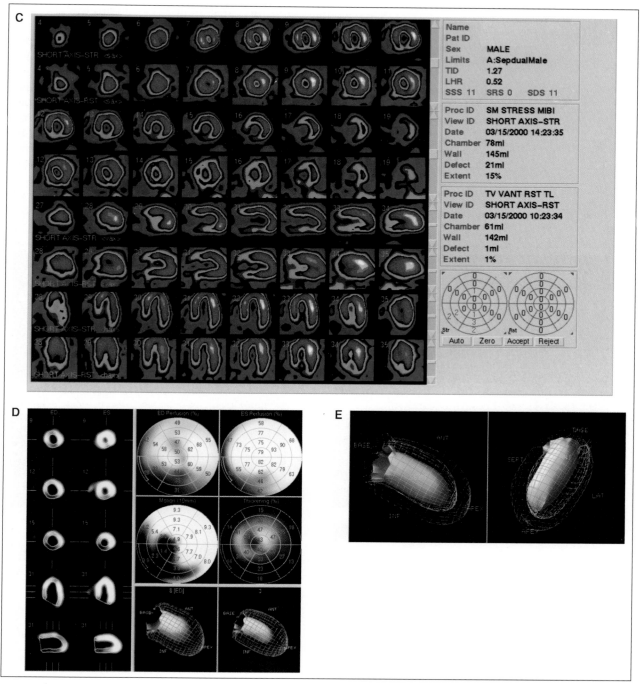

Figure 130 (*Continued*)

    c. A clear anterior defect is seen.

    d. The stress ECG demonstrates ST elevation in inferior leads with no Q waves at baseline and is specific for dense transmural inferior ischemia.

    e. Reduced inferior wall motion and thickening poststress in the presence of a normal rest image are likely evidence of induced "stunning."

    f. Left ventricular dilation in the stress image set adds to the gravity of image findings and their related prognostic risk.

    g. All image findings can be ignored, because the patient achieved a high workload and double product.

13B. The same 63-yr-old man shown in 13A undergoes exercise perfusion imaging when he presents with recurrent chest pain, only 4 days after placement of an RCA stent. Another rest–exercise perfusion study is performed and is shown in Figure 131A, with supine stress slices shown above supine rest slices in each panel. There were no induced ECG changes in 12 min of a Bruce protocol, with a heart rate of 174 (110% MPHR) and blood pressure of 185/80, and the patient was taking no anti-ischemic medications. In Figure 131B, the stress supine SPECT slices are presented above the stress prone set. Polar maps of stress perfusion in diastole and systole and

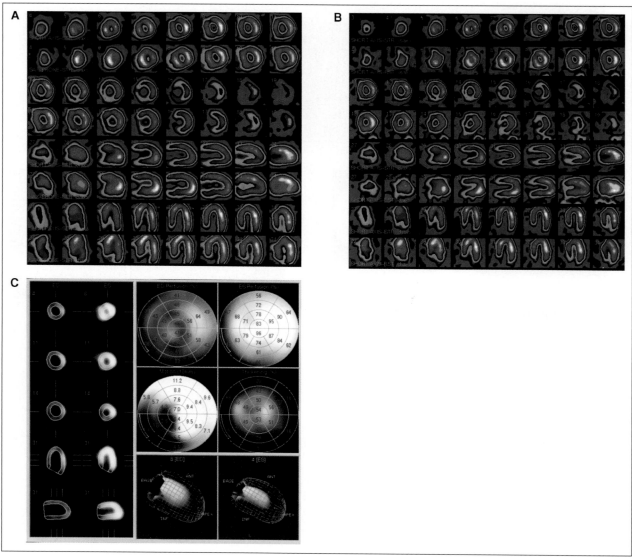

Figure 131

function, wall motion and thickening, as shown in Figure 130E are presented in Figure 131C. Which of the following choices best describe(s) the image findings?

a. The stent placement appears successful, because the RCA region is well perfused. However, an inferior wall motion abnormality persists.

b. The patient now has severe LAD ischemia.

c. A subtle reduction in stress-related apical activity may relate to the known limited LAD lesion.

d. There is evidence of new left circumflex artery (LCX) ischemic potential.

e. There is evidence of multivessel disease.

14A. A 49-yr-old man without obvious coronary risk factors is seen in the stress testing laboratory before performance of a requested exercise perfusion scintigram. He has recently experienced 2 episodes of exertion-related substernal chest pressure. Two days earlier, he played golf without pain, but drove a cart to avoid walking. Yesterday, he noted a brief period of rest pain. He is on no cardiac medication. Serial rest EKGs are presented for 2 yr (Fig. 132A) and 2 wk earlier (Fig. 132B) and on the day of study (Fig. 132C). Which is (are) true regarding these tracings and the clinical response to exercise?

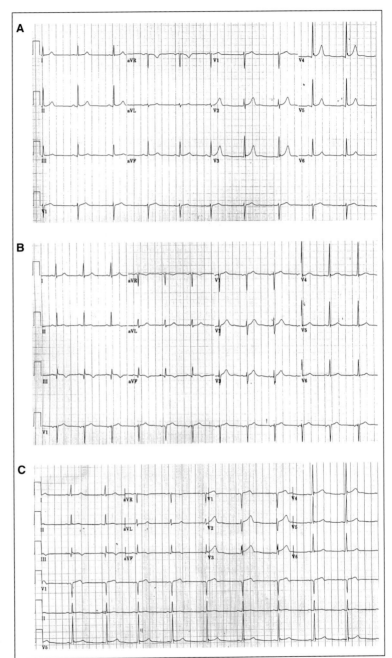

Figure 132

a. Apparent currently are inferior ST elevation with new Q wave in III, recent loss of R wave in V2, terminal T inversion in V1 and V2, with increased J point and ST elevation in right precordial leads.

b. The findings suggest a recent inferior infarction and possible evolving anteroseptal injury.

c. The findings demonstrate chronic abnormalities without significant change.

d. The tracings indicate possible ischemic events as recent as 2 wk, with continued evolution.

e. J point elevation noted is benign and not a cause for concern.

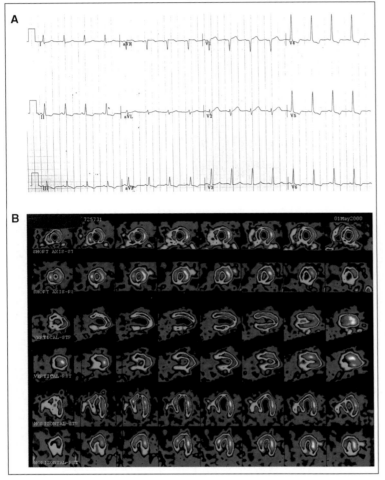

Figure 133

f. The history and ECG findings raise concerns about the safety of exercise testing and the consideration for coronary intervention.

g. The history and ECG present no concern for the safety of exercise testing.

h. The patient should go straight to coronary angiography.

14B. The rest ^{201}Tl study performed on the patient in 14A was benign, and dipyridamole stress was performed. There was an appropriate hemodynamic response with modest chest pressure, which were all reversed with aminophylline administered intravenously after radionuclide localization. The peak stress ECG is presented in Figure 133A. The rest and stress images were technically without flaw and are presented in the standard format in Figure 133B. Wall motion was preserved on the poststress gated acquisition, and the LVEF was normal. Which is (are) true?

a. The stress ECG showed no ischemic changes, and the images revealed no evidence of coronary disease.

b. Ischemic ECG changes were clear, along with reversible abnormalities in a multivessel distribution with cavitary dilation.

c. The scenario demonstrates the value and safety of dipyridamole study in patients with unstable angina.

d. The performance of dobutamine stress imaging would have been better advised.

e. This course of evaluation presents an approach superior to that of direct coronary angiography.

f. There was much lost in not immediately performing coronary angiography.

15. A 58-yr-old woman with hepatic failure has a history of prior LAD PTCA when she comes to stress dipyridamole perfusion imaging as part of her preoperative clearance before consideration for liver transplantation. Since angioplasty, she has had only a single episode of chest pain at rest several months earlier. The study was accompanied by an appropriate hemodynamic effect and was without ECG changes. Related rest ^{201}Tl and stress ^{99m}Tc sestamibi images were technically excellent (Fig. 134A) and showed normal regional perfusion with a transient ischemic dilation ratio of 1.51. Gated LVEF was 72% with normal wall motion (Fig. 134B), as

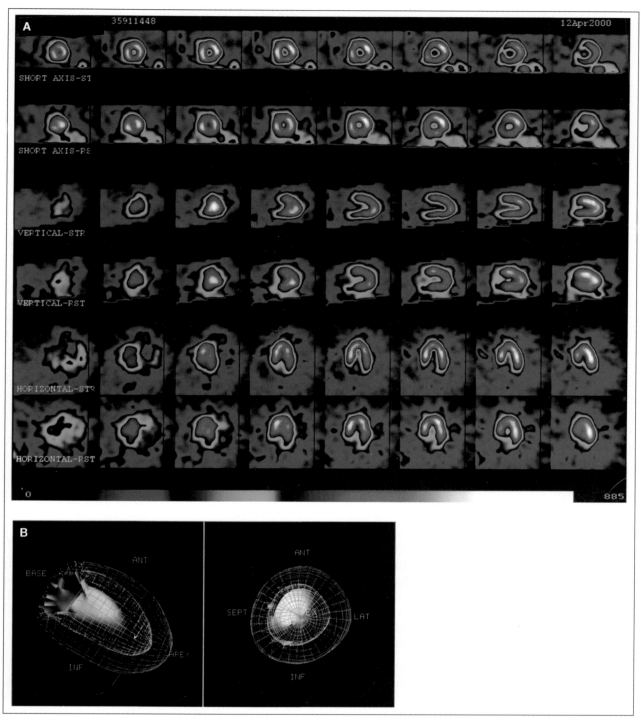

Figure 134

shown according to the prior illustrated standard format in anterior (left) and apical (right) projections. Nonetheless, she is readmitted for screening coronary angiography. On angiography, there is only a single lesion, a tight stenosis at the orifice of the left main. The catheter pressure blunted with each engagement of the left main, which was unchanged with intra-coronary nitroglycerin. No aortic root injection was seen. The patient is, for now, no longer a hepatic transplant candidate and is being considered for coronary bypass graft surgery. How can the images and the angiogram be reconciled? How could lesion severity be further established?

a. Transient ischemic dilation suggests global ischemia that might be balanced and so unseen.
b. The apparent left main lesion was less severe than apparent.
c. The left main lesion was based in spasm with catheter placement and would have been resolved with an aortic root injection.
d. The study demonstrates the imperfection of the scintigraphic method.
e. Intracoronary ultrasound and Doppler study could help establish lesion severity.
f. Dipyridamole brought an insufficient vascular response.

16A. A 50-yr-old Asian business man with no prior history of CAD but with multiple coronary risk factors, including hypertension, smoking and hyper-cholesterolemia, developed substernal chest discomfort and palpitations on a Saturday while doing his usual gardening. He stopped work immediately, and symptoms resolved only 20 min later. When symptoms recurred later the same day at rest, he came to the ED. He formerly noted no impairment of his exercise tolerance or stress-related pain. Physical examination, ECG (with and without pain) and routine lab tests were normal. He was admitted to the hospital to rule out an MI, and remained pain free there. Serial troponins were normal, and the ECG showed no changes. Which would be the most appropriate next step?

a. Refer immediately to coronary angiography.
b. Refer for a regular (nonimaging) exercise test.
c. Discharge to follow as an outpatient.
d. Treat for angina and discharge if symptom free on ambulation.
e. Refer for stress test with exercise or dilator stress pharmacologic perfusion imaging.
f. Refer for dobutamine pharmacologic stress perfusion imaging.

16B. It was a weekend and both test availability and physician preference dictated that a dipyridamole stress test be performed at the bedside of the patient in 16A. Dipyridamole infusion brought no change in heart rate, blood pressure or the 12-lead ECG. However, the patient complained of agonizing chest pain until the effects were reversed with aminophylline. Which is (are) true about the stress test?

a. In this scenario chest pain is diagnostic of ischemia.
b. The absence of a hemodynamic response makes test results unreliable.
c. Dipyridamole infusion should be augmented to provide a hemodynamic effect.
d. The sensitivity of the monitored ECG has the same sensitivity for coronary disease detection with dipyridamole or adenosine infusion as with an exercise test.
e. Absent ECG changes suggest circumflex disease.
f. A negative test would totally exclude coronary disease and assure immediate discharge.

16C. Rest and stress perfusion images in this same patient are shown in Figure 135A according to the standard format with the associated polar maps in Figure 135B. Where is the coronary lesion?

    a. LAD
    b. RCA
    c. In a ramus intermedius branch
    d. LCX
    e. In the left main coronary artery

17A. A 79-yr-old man with no coronary history but with multiple coronary risk factors is admitted to the coronary care unit with acute ECG changes consistent with an acute lateral wall infarction. The patient received intravenous thrombolytic therapy and was treated medically. He underwent dipyridamole pharmacologic stress testing for risk stratification. There were no symptoms or ECG changes, with an appropriate hemodynamic response. Gated images indicate extensive systolic wall motion abnormalities and an LVEF of 37%, as shown in Figure 136A. A rest echocardiogram demonstrated an LVEF of 55% with an isolated wall motion abnormality of the lateral wall. The rest ^{201}Tl/stress sestamibi images are shown according to the standard format in Figure 136B, with related polar maps in Figure 136C. Which is (are) true regarding the stress perfusion images?

    a. There is a fixed lateral wall defect consistent with the recent infarction.
    b. There are dense fixed anterior, septal and inferior defects.
    c. There are extensive reversible defects in the anterior, septal, lateral and inferior walls.
    d. Reduced wall motion in the stress gated image, in association with preserved perfusion at rest, suggests poststress "stunning."
    e. Reduced wall motion in the stress gated image, in association with preserved wall motion at rest by echocardiography, supports poststress "stunning."
    f. Based on the image findings, the incidence of recurrent infarction or death is >4%/year.
    g. Based on the image findings, the incidence of recurrent infarction or death is <1%/year.
    h. Poststress "stunning" indicates significant induced ischemia on dipyridamole infusion, in spite of the absence of ST changes.

17B. The same patient returns 4 mo later, after multivessel coronary artery bypass graft (CABG) with recurrent chest pressure. An infarct is ruled out, and the patient is sent for exercise stress perfusion imaging. At exercise, the patient completed 15 min of the standard Bruce protocol and stopped at the end of stage V, with fatigue and a heart rate of 127 (90% MPHR) in the absence of chest pain or ECG changes. Rest and stress images are shown in the standard format in Figure 136D, with polar maps in 136E. Gated images reveal good systolic wall motion and an LVEF of 53%. Which is (are) true regarding the findings?

    a. The absence of poststress stunning and a negative stress test, with less extensive defects than on the prior study at a high workload and double product, probably places the patient in a better prognostic group compared with that in which he was placed by the prior test.

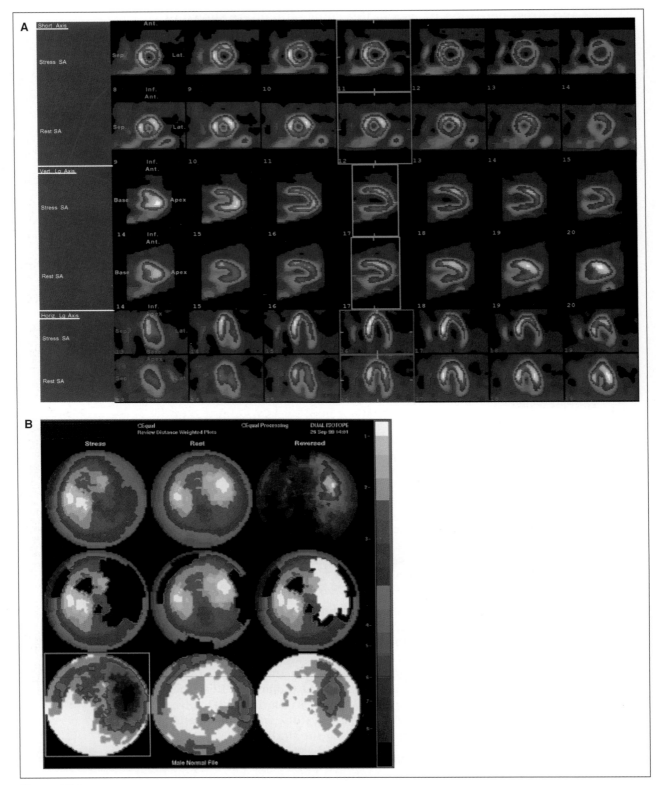

Figure 135

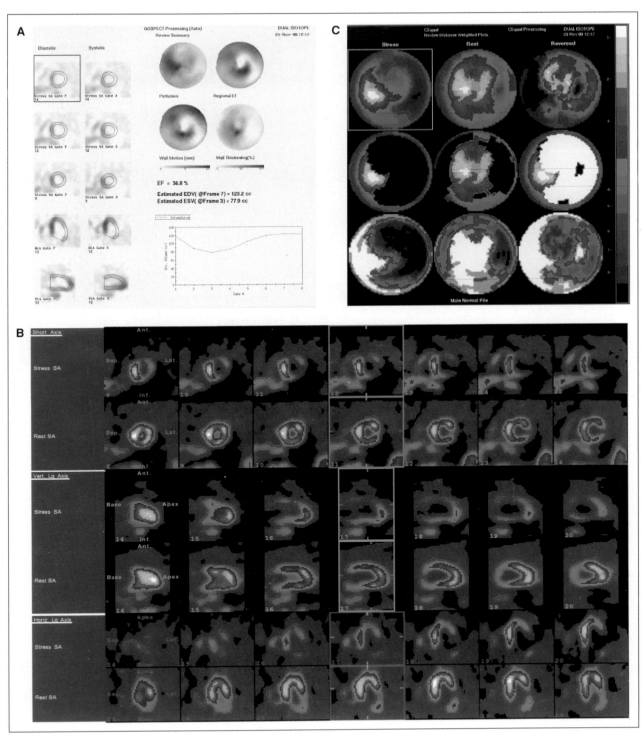

Figure 136

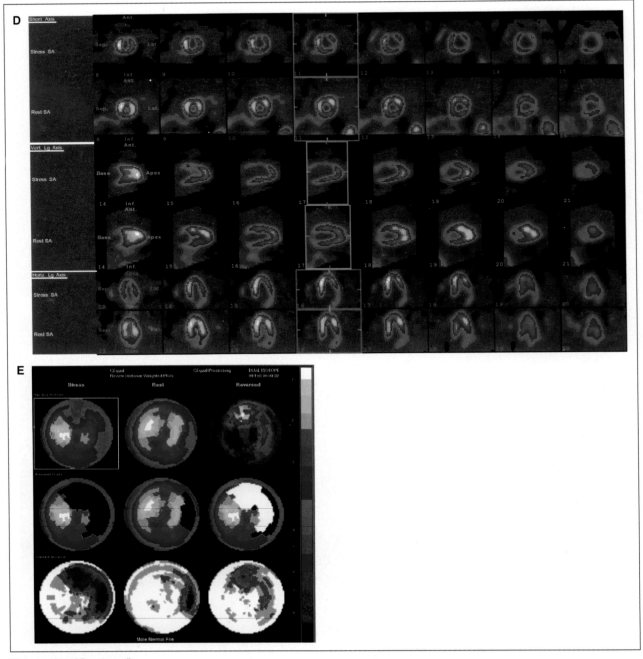

Figure 136 (*Continued*)

    b. The images present evidence of a patent left internal mammary (LIMA) graft.

    c. Reversible anterior and lateral defects are evident.

    d. Localized cavitary dilation is noted at the ventricular base, the region of most prominent induced ischemia.

    e. The findings, compared with the prior study, support a moderate ischemic burden and related risk, which may be successfully managed medically.

18. A previously well 56-yr-old African American woman is sent for pharmacologic rest ^{201}Tl/stress ^{99m}Tc sestamibi perfusion imaging to evaluate atypical chest pain that occurs both at rest and with stress and has become disabling over the last 4 mo. There is no history of a prior coronary event, and risk factors are minimal. Her rest ECG (Fig. 137A) is normal and unchanged for many years. ECGs have never been taken during pain, and antianginal medications have not been effective. The ECG at peak dipyridamole effect, when ^{99m}Tc sestamibi is administered ~8 min after infusion onset, is shown in Figure 137B, and related stress perfusion images and polar maps are shown in Figures 137C and 137D,

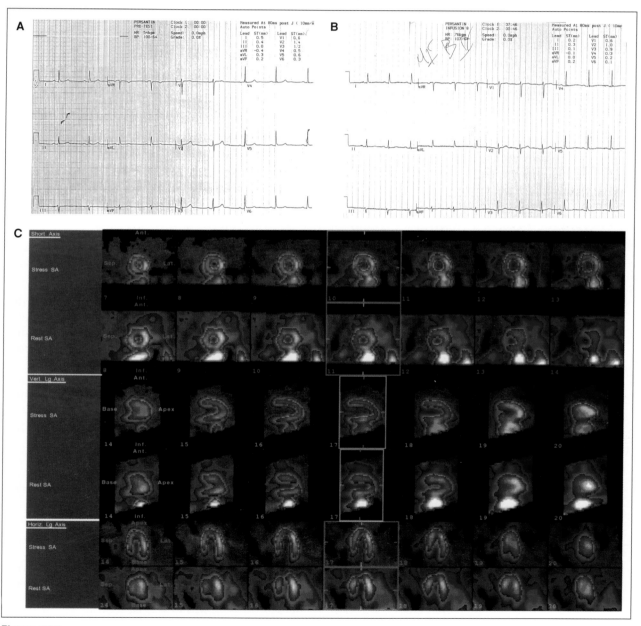

Figure 137

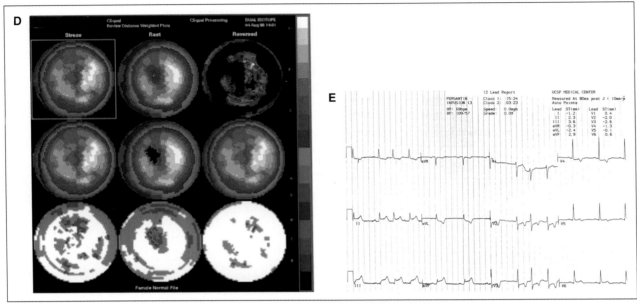

Figure 137 (*Continued*)

respectively. The stress ECG shows nonspecific T flattening with an expected increase in rate, and the images are normal. As always and according to laboratory policy, aminophylline, here 75 mg, is given intravenously 3–5 min after radionuclide administration, to reverse dipyridamole effects. Five minutes after the end of the test and aminophylline administration, the patient develops severe, progressive substernal pressure. An ECG performed at 15 min, 3 min after chest pain onset, is shown in Figure 137E. What conclusions should be reached and management implemented? Choose all correct answers.

a. The post-test ECG reveals marked ST elevation in inferior leads, suggesting coronary spasm and insensitivity of the perfusion scintigram.

b. The post-test ECG reveals marked inferior ST elevation, suggesting coronary artery spasm and insensitivity of the pharmacologic stress ECG.

c. Coronary artery spasm is unpredictable, generally transient and not necessarily induced by either pharmacologic or dynamic stress testing or by aminophylline.

d. The post-test ECG reveals marked ST elevation, suggesting coronary artery spasm.

e. Dipyridamole clearly induced the ST changes.

f. The symptoms should be treated with additional aminophylline.

g. The symptoms should be treated with calcium channel blockers, nitrates and other agents to discourage coronary vasoreactivity.

h. Immediate repeat imaging of the initially administered dose would reveal evidence and site of spasm-related myocardial ischemia.

19. A 75-yr-old, diabetic, retired physician, with a history of prior inferior infarction and emergency RCA angioplasty and stent, has recurrent pain when he sees his cardiologist. An exercise perfusion study is performed. The patient completes 8 min of a modified Bruce protocol and stops in stage I, with fatigue and chest pain at a rate of 108 (75% of maximal

predicted rate for age) and blood pressure of 155/70. Rest ^{201}Tl and stress ^{99m}Tc sestamibi images are shown in Figure 138A and polar maps in Figure 138B, according to the standard format. Figures 138C and 138D present the standard baseline and peak stress 12-lead ECGs, respectively. The cardiologist is concerned about a finding on the stress ECG. What is it? What is the cause? Choose the single correct answer.

a. The ECG leads are inverted, resulting in an inverse progression and development of the R wave from V6 to V1.
b. A right shift in axis raises concern regarding a pulmonary embolus.
c. Baseline motion artifact makes the tracing illegible.
d. The achieved rate makes the test result insensitive.
e. Induced ST elevation in inferior and lateral leads raises concern regarding the severity of ischemia related to the reversible abnormality in the inferior-basal and apicolateral walls.

20. An 80-yr-old man with prior coronary bypass graft surgery 18 yr earlier is asymptomatic from a coronary viewpoint when he undergoes dipyridamole stress testing for risk stratification before major abdominal surgery. There were no ECG changes and an appropriate hemodynamic response in the presence of mild flushing. The stress sestamibi SPECT images are presented according to the standard format in Figure 139A. A rest study was not performed. Figure 139B presents the results of gated wall motion and thickening as shown previously. Figure 139C presents the end-diastolic and end-systolic endocardial (green mesh and solid yellow, respectively) and the epicardial outlines (yellow mesh) in anterior (left) and LAO (right) views. Which of the following is (are) true?

a. The stress perfusion image is normal.
b. The stress perfusion image reveals a gross septal defect with matching wall motion abnormality, suggesting a prior infarction.
c. The stress perfusion image reveals a moderate inferolateral defect.
d. LVEF, as well as systolic wall motion and thickening, are normal.
e. Septal wall motion is abnormal, but its thickening is preserved, and inferolateral wall motion and thickening are normal.
f. Septal and inferolateral wall motion and thickening are abnormal.
g. The findings suggest viability in the septum and a wall motion abnormality related to prior CABG.
h. The function of the inferolateral wall suggest that the stress-related defect is reversible.

21. A 55-yr-old man experienced an anterior and lateral infarction and an LAD stent 5 mo earlier. He now undergoes an exercise test with myocardial perfusion imaging to evaluate the recent onset of atypical chest pain. He completed 12 min 30 sec, reaching stage 5 of a standard Bruce protocol, stopping with fatigue and an "icy" chest pain at a heart rate of 153 (92% MPHR) and blood pressure of 172/90 in the presence of mild ST depression with T inversion in inferior leads and 1–2-mm horizontal ST depression in leads V2-V5. Rest and peak stress ECGs are shown in Figures 140A and 140B. Shown in Figure 140C are the rest ^{201}Tl and stress sestamibi SPECT images, according to the standard format,

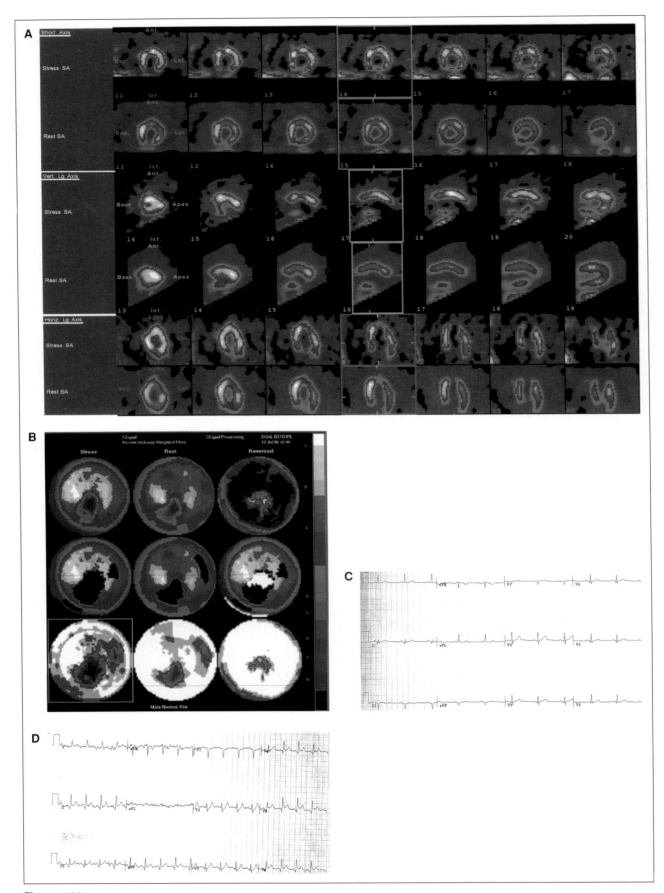

Figure 138

356

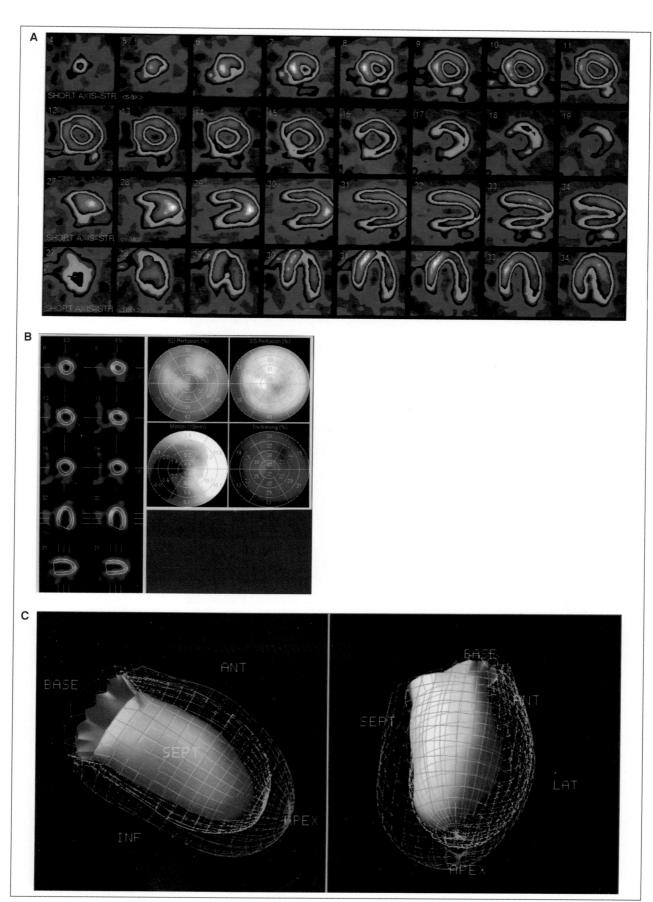

Figure 139

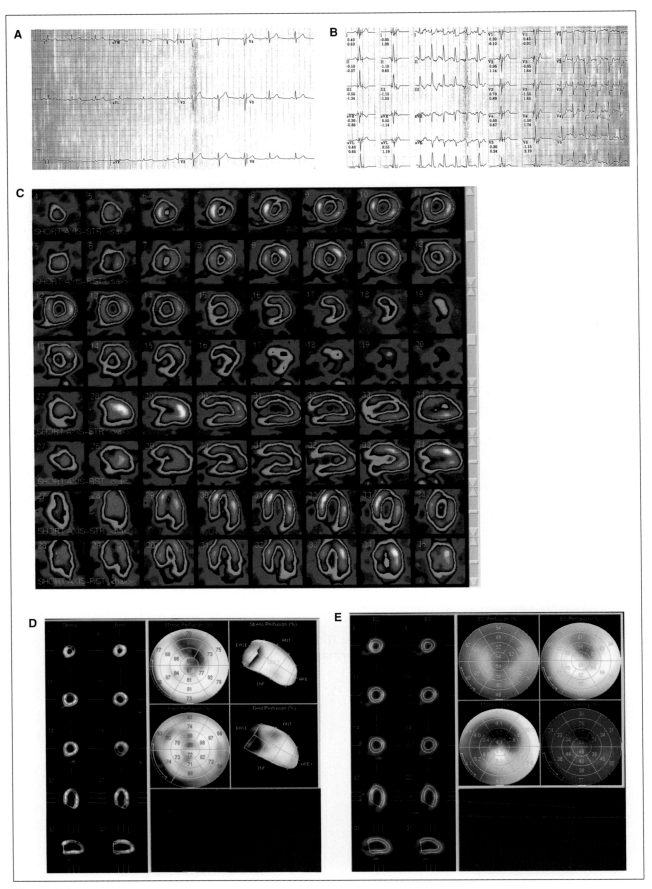

Figure 140

358

a. The images are normal. Proceed with surgery.
b. The images demonstrate limited myocardium at ischemic risk. Proceed with surgery.
c. The images demonstrate extensive myocardium at ischemic risk. Proceed with surgery.
d. The images demonstrate extensive myocardium at ischemic risk. Proceed with coronary angiography.
e. Proceed with surgery regardless of image findings. The images have no prognostic value.

26. A 45-yr-old man presents with symptoms of left heart failure in the presence of atypical chest pain. There are no other coronary risk factors. A rest

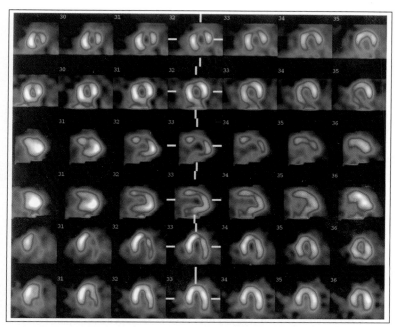

Figure 144

^{201}Tl/dipyridamole ^{99m}Tc sestamibi study is performed and shown in Figure 145A. The images are attenuation corrected. The related perfusion polar maps (Fig. 145B), wall motion and thickening polar maps (Fig. 145C), and endocardial and epicardial outlines in the anterior projection (Fig. 145D) are shown as well. The related LVEF was 31%. What is the nature of the pathophysiology?

a. The stress images demonstrate an enlarged left ventricle with diffuse and severe hypokinesis.
b. An apparent perfusion defect inferior in the rest image is no longer seen with stress.
c. Apparent reverse redistribution may be explained here by the fact that the inferior wall was attenuated but less so in the higher-energy ^{99m}Tc-based image.
d. Apparent reverse redistribution may be explained here by the fact that the inferior wall was attenuated but not so in these attenuation-corrected images.
e. The findings indicate that this is a noncoronary cardiomyopathy.

27. A 65-yr-old woman is admitted to the cardiology service with non-Q infarction. She is initially found to be in heart failure but quickly improves. She is risk stratified by stress dipyridamole perfusion imaging on the second hospital day. Rest ^{201}Tl/stress ^{99m}Tc sestamibi images (Fig. 146A) are shown with perfusion polar maps (Fig. 146B) and polar maps of perfusion during contraction, as well as wall motion and thickening polar maps (Fig. 146C) and outlines of endocardium and epicardium in end-diastole and end-systole in the anterior projection in the format previously presented (Fig. 146D). What can be said about the findings and their clinical implications?

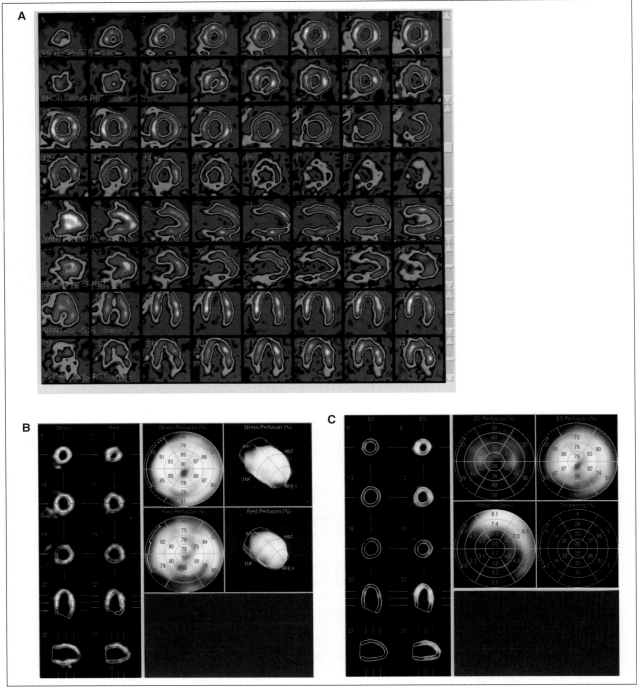

Figure 145

a. The images demonstrate evidence of a limited lateral basal infarction.
b. The images demonstrate extensive myocardium at ischemic risk.
c. There is stress-induced cavitary dilation.
d. There is a low LVEF, with diffuse wall motion and thickening abnormalities in the presence of widely preserved rest perfusion, suggesting poststress "stunning."

e. The image findings recommend aggressive revascularization in both cases.

f. Imaging was unnecessary, because the presence of heart failure suggested extensive disease and an aggressive management.

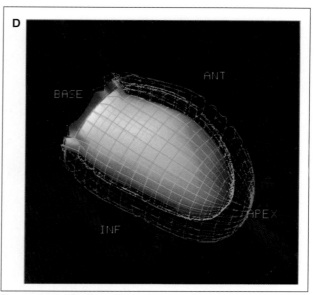

28A. A 70-yr-old man with severe congestive heart failure is studied with dipyridamole perfusion imaging. Rest ^{201}Tl/stress ^{99m}Tc sestamibi images are shown in Figure 147A, with polar maps in Figure 147B, and 24-hr images in the ^{201}Tl window are shown in Figure 147C, according to the standard format. The gated poststress study calculating the LVEF (8%) is shown in Figure 147D. Assess the findings and consider the clinical implications. Choose all correct answers.

Figure 145 (*Continued*)

a. The images show gross ventricular dilation at rest and stress.

b. There is relatively preserved perfusion of the lateral wall but with an ischemic component.

c. There is evident incomplete reversibility of stress defects in multiple vascular areas.

d. Twenty-four-hour imaging showed further relative improvement, especially in apical, anterior and septal regions.

e. The findings suggest extensive coronary disease, scar and myocardium at ischemic risk.

f. The findings suggest that revascularization would be high risk and with little chance of functional improvement.

28B. Evaluate the positron emission tomography (PET) images performed in this patient. Compare them with the rest ^{201}Tl images. How do these findings influence management decisions? Choose all correct answers.

a. The PET study confirms the presence of extensive scar and recommends a conservative approach.

b. The PET study adds nothing to the perfusion images in 28A.

c. The PET study reveals best uptake in the septum, an area of reduced perfusion compared with the lateral wall, and suggests viability and the functional benefit of revascularization.

d. The PET study reveals best uptake in the lateral wall, the area of best perfusion, and adds little to the perfusion study.

e. With evidence of reversibility on conventional perfusion study and extensive LAD viability on PET, the benefits of revascularization are strongly suggested.

f. Septal uptake here suggests the presence of actively ischemic myocardium and much-needed revascularization.

29A. A 55-yr-old Asian American man who works as a security guard and has little insight into his medical condition, presents to the medical clinic with a complaint of chest pain of 3 wk duration. He denies symptoms of heart failure or a prior infarction. There is a strong family history of CAD,

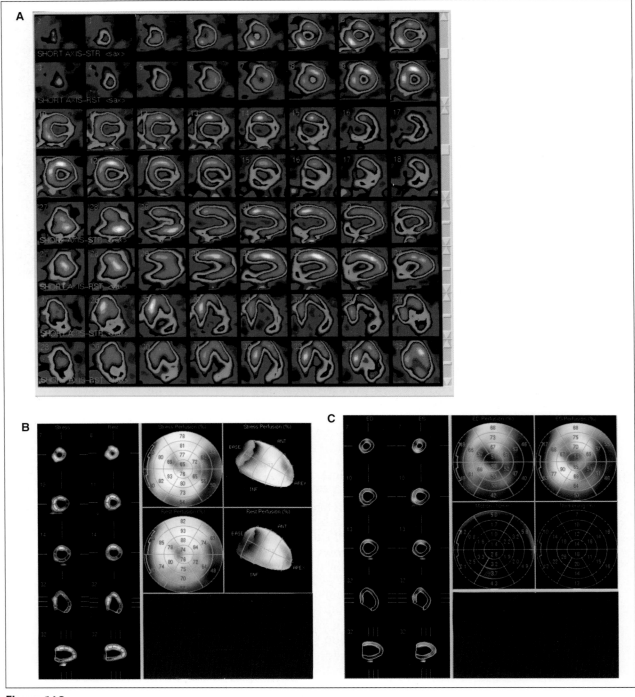

Figure 146

and he notes that his father died after CABG. An exercise test is requested to "assess the cause of chest pain." The patient presents to the laboratory on a very busy day when, with "add-on" studies, the imaging schedule is over capacity. For this reason, the nuclear medicine technologist, seeking to reduce image volume and accommodate all the patients, asks if we could do a stress-only ^{99m}Tc sestamibi perfusion study, omitting the rest study with a likelihood that it would be normal, or delay the rest study to another day. On further questioning, a history of classic exertional chest pain is elicited. A rest ECG is performed and the results are shown in Figure 148A. True or false: a rest study should be performed before stress.

a. True
b. False

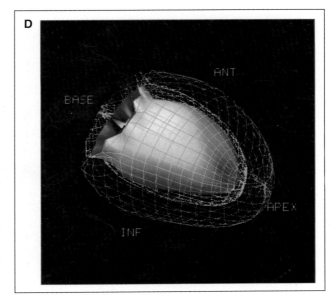

Figure 146 (*Continued*)

29B. A rest ^{201}Tl/exercise ^{99m}Tc sestamibi perfusion study is performed on the same patient presented in 29A. He exercises 7 min of a modified Bruce protocol, stopping with fatigue and chest pressure. The rest, baseline ECG, with limb leads shifted to the trunk to avoid motion artifact, and tracings at peak stress and in recovery are shown in Figures 148B and 148C, respectively. Which statement(s) best describes the ECG findings?

a. The baseline ECG shows a QS complex in leads V1–V4, suggesting the presence of a prior anteroseptal infarction.
b. With stress, there are ST elevations in V1–V4, indicating induced transmural anteroseptal ischemia.
c. The stress test is clearly positive for ischemia.
d. The ST elevations noted in V1–V4 are not specific for ischemia.
e. Evidence of left bundle branch block (LBBB) makes the interpretation of the stress test impossible.

29C. Rest ^{201}Tl/exercise ^{99m}Tc sestamibi perfusion scintigraphy in this same patient is displayed in Figure 148D, according to the same format in previous questions. Here, shown in the Autoquant (ADAC, Milpitas, CA) display are SPECT slices in short, vertical and horizontal long axes, from above downward, from the ^{99m}Tc sestamibi exercise stress (top rows in each image set) and the ^{201}Tl rest (bottom rows in each image set) perfusion study. In Figure 148E are the ventricular contours derived from the gated SPECT sestamibi slices, in which the epicardium is in orange mesh, the diastolic endocardium is in green mesh and the end-diastolic endocardium is in highlighted gray in anterior (left) and LAO (right) projections. Wall motion is generally reduced with severe systolic dysfunction in apical, anteroseptal, distal anterior and lateral regions, with an LVEF of 28%. Which is (are) true regarding the studies and the clinical management of this patient?

a. There are large rest defects that indicate prior infarction.
b. There are only fixed and no reversible defects. The damage has been done, and little can be offered other than medical therapy.
c. There are both rest and stress-induced defects, consistent with prior infarction and induced ischemia.
d. A 24-hr delayed ^{201}Tl acquisition is desired and could more fully indicate the extent of myocardium at ischemic risk.
e. A 24-hr delayed study would be of little value.

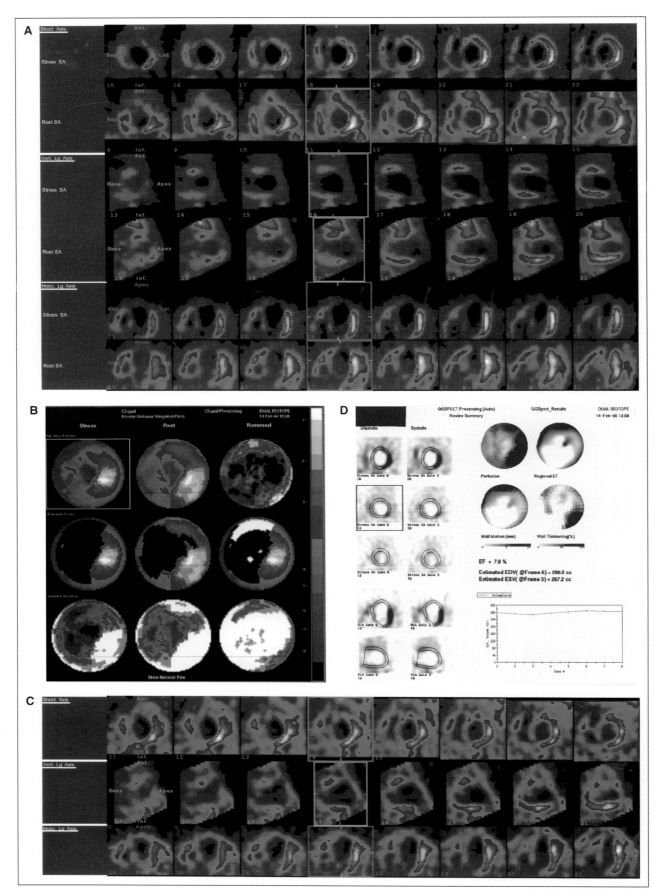

Figure 147

368

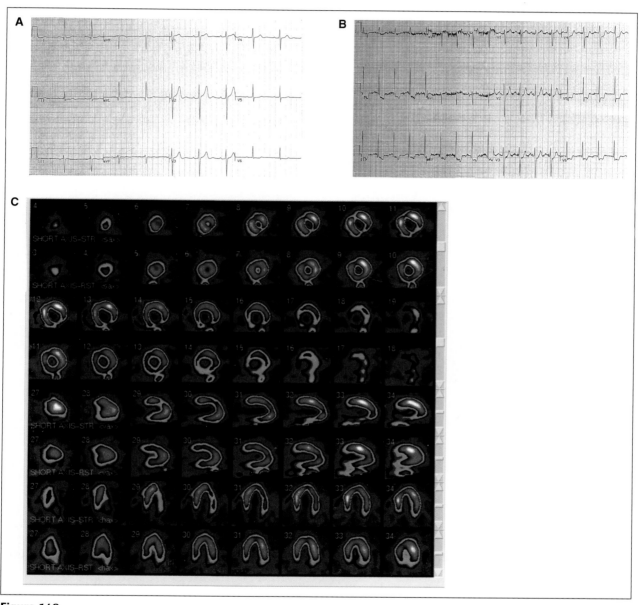

Figure 149

    c. Stress echocardiography has a lower sensitivity than stress perfusion imaging, and here the presence of widespread severe resting wall motion abnormalities make identification of decremental changes difficult.

    d. Left ventricular volume decreases with exercise.

    e. Left ventricular volume increases greatly with exercise.

    f. The presence of widespread severe resting wall motion abnormalities makes identification of the normal hyperdynamic response to exercise difficult.

32. **A 55-yr-old man with known multivessel CAD has atypical chest pain 4 mo after LAD PTCA and stent, when he is asked to participate in a**

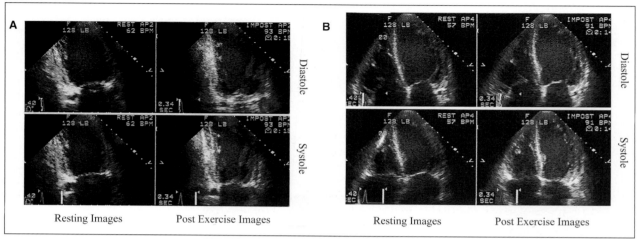

Figure 150

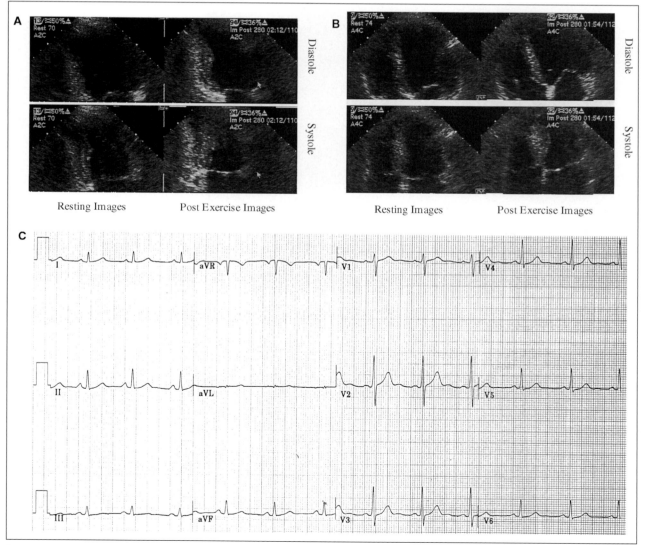

Figure 151

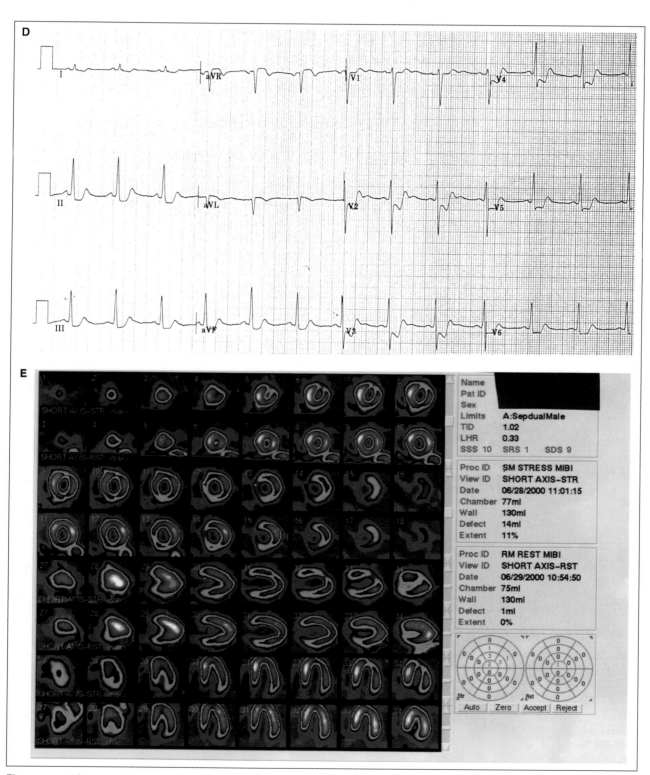

Figure 151 (*Continued*)

clinical trial for a new echocardiographic contrast agent. The agent is designed to opacify the left ventricular cavity and not specifically label the myocardium. The stress echocardiogram and stress scintigram are acquired at the same stress test. The rest scintigram is acquired the day after, using the same ^{99m}Tc-based agent. The echocardiogram, shown in Figure 151A and 151B in 2- and 4-chamber views, respectively, is normal, with normal augmentation of wall motion at a modest achieved double product. The ECGs at rest and early after stress are shown in Figures 151C and 151D, respectively. The stress test was abnormal with an ischemic ST response. The rest/exercise ^{99m}Tc sestamibi images are shown according to the standard format in Figure 151E. Read the perfusion images and choose all correct answers.

a. Echocardiographic contrast agents are well able to visualize the myocardial perfusion pattern.

b. Echocardiographic contrast agents have had some success in visualizing the left ventricular cavity.

c. The cost of a single intravenous dose of currently approved echo contrast agents to visualize the left ventricular cavity exceeds the dose cost of a radionuclide perfusion agent.

d. The scintigraphic study here supports the findings of stress-induced ischemia in anterolateral and lateral regions.

e. The echocardiogram shown is normal, with normal augmentation of wall motion.

f. The echocardiogram is grossly abnormal, with widespread induced wall motion abnormalities.

Answers and Critiques for Multiple Choice Questions

ITEM 1

Answer: b, d, e. The image was never acquired. The cardiologist in charge of the conference was anxious to demonstrate the inaccuracy of the method. He was told that the image results were "poor" and interpreted that to mean that there was evidence of a gross perfusion defect and ischemia in the presence of a normal coronary angiogram. However, there was, in fact, no study performed for the unique reason of "poor intravenous access," and Figure 117 is blank. When the case was presented at conference, a blank screen was projected. Yet, it was widely disseminated that the abnormal image was in error, because the coronary angiogram was normal. The case illustrates the importance of clinical correlation and follow-up. Further, it is not enough to simply validate findings by a phone call or a written report, but studies must be viewed and discussed in an open and unbiased manner if we are to understand the image information, its difference from the anatomy and its clinical relevance. When such discrepancies are identified, they must be fully investigated to learn and understand these differences and to identify insufficiencies of the method, as well as technical and interpretive errors in image reading. Occasionally, surprises like this will be discovered and represent important insights into professional attitudes. Today, with growing cardiologist acceptance of the method and active involvement in the field, this set of circumstances is less likely.

ITEM 2

Answer: A-y, B-w, C-i, D-c, E-g, F-d, G-s, H-o, I-e, J-b, K-q, L-j, M-f, N-m, O-n, P-h, Q-k, R-p, S-r, T-t, U-x, V-u, W-v, X-a, Y-z, Z-l.

ITEM 3A

Answer: b. Although functional evaluation of apparently fixed defects may give clues to viability, the density of the defect makes its function difficult to appreciate. Furthermore, the agent employed here,^{201}Tl, is given in low dosage and cannot be well gated. However, there could be a further yield of reversible defects, even after reinjection imaging, with 24-hr delayed image acquisition. In fact, the original publications dealing with reinjection studies first reviewed a 4-hr preinjection ^{201}Tl set. It was only with the finding of a fixed defect after 4 hr that reinjection was performed and subsequent images acquired (*748*). Reinjection optimally should be applied to determine the reversibility of defects noted to be fixed after 4 hr. Reversible defects should be assessed before reinjection. However, such a method will require the frequent performance of 3 SPECT image studies in a day! This is unacceptable to many labs. Subsequent studies have shown that reinjection with imaging early after redistribution may actually recreate a defect based in ongoing ischemia at rest (Dilsizian V, Bonow RO. Differential uptake and apparent 201Tl washout after thallium reinjection: options regarding late redistribution imaging before reinjection or late redistribution imaging after reinjection. *Circulation* 1992;85:1032–1038.) This may be true, because the initial post-injection ^{201}Tl distribution relates to the pattern of perfusion, whereas the delayed image distribution relates to viable intracellular (K+) space. Where the 2 are different, as in the setting of rest ischemia, reinjection can reestablish a defect that has already resolved over time. Such defects can nevertheless be normalized once again with subsequent delayed imaging. In this case, no 4-hr delayed image set was acquired before reinjection. Although most fixed defects imaged after reinjection are likely related to scar, a small but significant percentage of such fixed defects may be the result of the preceding reinjection rather than actual scar formation (Dae MW, Botvinick EH, Starksen NF, Zhu YY, LaPidus A. Do 4-hour reinjection thallium images and 24-hour thallium images provide equivalent information [abstract]? *J Am Coll Cardiol* 1991;17:29A). If clinically important and possibly ischemia-related, redistribution of such defects should be sought with 24-hr imaging (Bobba K, Botvinick EH, Dae MW, et al. Is there any advantage to the acquisition of 24-hour thallium images, in the presence of fixed defects at four hours after reinjection? *Eur J Nucl Med* 1998;25:509–514.)

Row 3 in each panel of Figure 118 shows short-axis stress ^{201}Tl SPECT slices in the same patient, in the same format, now imaged after 24-hr. The image defects are totally reversible! A clue to the potential for such reversibility was the absence of a dilated cavity on delayed images or other signs of marked ventricular dysfunction, such as diverging walls, on long-axis slices, in spite of an apparent large fixed defect and a history of aneurysm. The patient went to coronary bypass surgery, with subsequent normalization of perfusion and wall motion.

ITEM 3B

Answer: d, f. In the dual-isotope protocol, the full assessment of defect reversibility must be performed after adequate decay of ^{99m}Tc given with stress. Imaging must be performed in the ^{201}Tl window after 24 hr. Because the initial ^{201}Tl administration was made at rest, there is no evident advantage in adding a "reinjection" dose, which may, in fact, recreate a defect which resolved with time (Dilsizian V, Bonow RO. Differential uptake and apparent ^{201}Tl washout after thallium reinjection: options regarding late redistribution imaging before reinjection or late redistribution imaging after reinjection. *Circulation* 1992;85:1032–1038.) Nitroglycerin given with the rest injection has been shown to maximize uptake (*767,768*). In fact, imaging in the ^{201}Tl window after 24 hr demonstrated major improvement in defects illustrated in Figure 118 and others shown below.

ITEM 4

Answer: d, e. The initial reading was appropriate. However, it should be no surprise that the patient had coronary disease. This was known for years and was the reason for initial risk stratification. Pathologic study confirmed the disease but could well have overestimated it in vitro. Although coronary disease and probably multivessel involvement were present then, there was no image evidence of induced ischemia. In the absence of other compelling evidence, a conservative management could be recommended and was well accepted. The short-axis images are not well aligned, with stress short-axis slice 14 corresponding to rest slice 14 but actually matched with rest slice 11, likely leading to the misinterpretation of the later "expert witness." There is no evidence of "dilation" in long-axis slices, indicating the likely origin of the finding in technical factors unrelated to regional perfusion. The subsequent outcome was the worst possible. However, the clinical cause was never established, and it occurred after more than a full, active year. The event was not directly predictable from any current clinical marker. Even the excellent prognostic value of a normal scan does not provide indefinite protection or guarantee against adverse events (*342*). Certainly, this study, with a modest evident fixed defect, is indicative of coronary disease and always needs clinical judgment. Intervention with revascularization at that time might have averted the event or contributed to it! Intervention with revascularization was not suggested by any clinical measure, so its omission should not be considered erroneous. The corrected display, showing the same SPECT stress and rest sets, now properly aligned and without apparent dilation or reversible defects, is shown in Figure 120A, according to the same format. The related polar map is shown in Figure 120B. The upper row shows the distribution of perfusion, the bottom row shows the standard deviation (SD) of regional perfusion from the normal distribution in a sex-matched normal population. The middle row presents perfusion polar maps that highlight in black the few pixels with intensity >3 SD from the normal. In this display, the left column plots stress perfusion, the center column plots rest perfusion and the right column plots their difference. The SD color code, shown at right, is also applied to measure relative perfusion. The error in slice align-

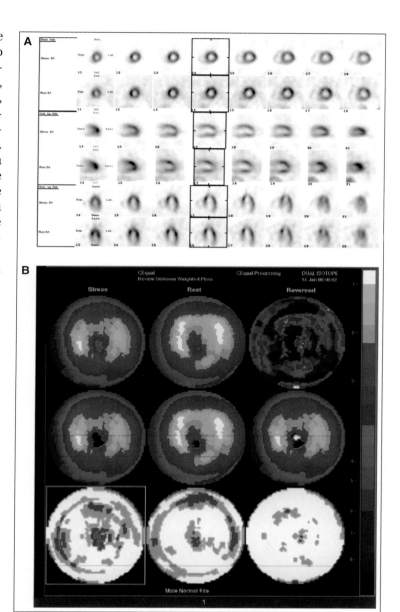

Figure 120

ment was demonstrated to the jury, and the findings of the prosecution were discredited. The defendants were found "not guilty," and no damages were paid. The history and trial summary is an account of a true case record.

ITEM 5

Answer: a, b, c, e. Slight differences in cavitary size may be explained by the imaging differences (*4,120,121,272,273*) related to the physical characteristics of the agents used. Here, the degree of cavitary dilation is clear, and changes in both internal and external dimensions exceed expected variation (*95,274,275*). Simply realigning these slices will not resolve the abnormality. This was objectively confirmed by the calculation of the change in computer-measured diameter that was documented here to exceed the range of acceptable variation of ~20%. In the presence of coronary disease, transient cavitary dilation is a well-documented indicator of severe and often extensive coronary disease and related high prognostic risk (*238*). Dilation may relate to subendocardial ischemia, presenting only an increase in the internal endocardial dimension, or gross cavitary dilation, with increase in the epicardial dimension, both evident here. In planar images, apparent dilation of the internal dimension may relate to ischemia in the overlying wall and may be projection related (*274*). However, the case presented is somewhat unusual, in that dilation is present in the absence of gross perfusion defects. The presence of transient dilation in the setting of a normal perfusion pattern often relates to a noncoronary diagnosis. Dilation of the left ventricle may be seen in the absence of coronary disease, in the presence of reduced functional reserve, as seen with myocardial or valvular heart disease. Nevertheless there were reversible defects here and the finding, with evidence of reduced function after stress, was taken as a sign of potentially serious CAD. (See Ziffer JA, Wells DE. Image of the month. *Newsletter of the American Society of Nuclear Cardiology* 1996;3[2]:9.)

Here, cavitary dilation and evidence of "stunning" are more evident than related perfusion defects. Perfusion is abnormal and accompanied by evidence of high-risk CAD. The managing cardiologists were informed but elected to proceed with noncardiac surgery, feeling the risk was acceptable and that the risks of full revascularization and CABG in this patient were high. Angiography and angioplasty were not performed. The patient went to surgery and suffered a large, perioperative MI.

ITEM 6

Answers: a, d. Image findings relating to vasospasm display patterns similar to those induced by stress but may resolve more quickly with recovery and vasodilation. An intervening large silent infarction would be an unexpected and unseen clinical event and was not here accompanied by new ECG, wall motion or hemodynamic changes. Also, once localized, the radionuclide would not be expected to dissipate, even in the face of a new ischemic event. Even if it did, that should not invalidate the initial findings. Acquisition of the delayed image was flawless.

Actually, the explanation was much simpler. The "24-hr" images were a duplication of the 4-hr redistribution set. Here, the defects are, in fact, smaller than when viewed immediately after stress but were totally unchanged at "24 hr." Images are like fingerprints, completely unique. When we find images that are exactly alike, it is because they are—the same, that is! Reformatted comparisons of the true poststress and 24-hr images revealed yet further reversibility and supported well the clinical management. This error can be avoided by display or computer codes that ask for confirmation when told to compare the same study with itself. Although the error was trivial and quite mechanical, the explanation to the requesting cardiologist was quite humbling and added significant distrust to the relationships and insecurity in the imaging method. It took months to rebuild that trust.

ITEM 7

Answers: a, b, c, d, f. The polar map demonstrates a dense, reversible defect in the LAD region. Cavitary dilation, lung uptake and basal uptake are among the "nonperfusion indicators" of extensive, high-risk coronary disease. Lung uptake is best appreciated with planar imaging or in projection images and is not often seen in or well correlated with the findings on ^{99m}Tc sestamibi studies as it is with ^{201}Tl studies. Cavitary dilation related at angiography, as it often does, to multivessel disease. Here it served also to indicate stress-induced dysfunction and aneurysm formation in the LAD territory, also evidence of a high prognostic risk (8,191,197,199). This dysfunction and related left ventricular deformity persisted into recovery, representative of "stunned myocardium." The patient went on to successful CABG.

ITEM 8

Answers: a, b, c, d, f. The patient's world is his bar and the apartment above. The very fact that he came to the hospital for help demonstrates the severity, if not the gravity, of symptoms, because he had to overcome significant fear simply to leave his apartment. Although unstable angina with "hibernation" could explain the image findings, the current study and the defect on rest images strongly suggests that the patient infarcted the morning of the test. Enzymes drawn before imaging, in fact, came back positive that afternoon. By that time, the image findings had already made the diagnosis and the patient had been to the catheterization laboratory. Unfortunately, or fortunately, the rest images were not reviewed before dipyridamole infusion. Testing was uncomplicated and gave important information regarding coronary risk. Regardless of whether indicative of infarction or hibernating myocardium, the rest image would itself likely have brought angiography in this clinical context. Even if after viewing the rest image, it was elected to proceed with testing, it would be with full knowledge of an acute dynamic ischemic condition. The LVEF on gated poststress perfusion imaging was 34% (Fig. 124E), significantly reduced from that at the time of prior study. Coronary angiography revealed an occluded RCA, which was opened and a stent placed. Always review the rest study, when available, before proceeding with stress testing. The study also illustrates the occurrence of infarction involving a vessel neither previously known to be significantly stenotic nor known to subtend significant ischemia. Of course, the prior study was 4 yr earlier. A subsequent rest ^{201}Tl/dipyridamole ^{99m}Tc sestamibi study performed 3 mo later was essentially normal, with a much improved LVEF on gated evaluation at 50%. The rest defect demonstrated in Figure 124C was, in fact, primarily ischemic in nature!

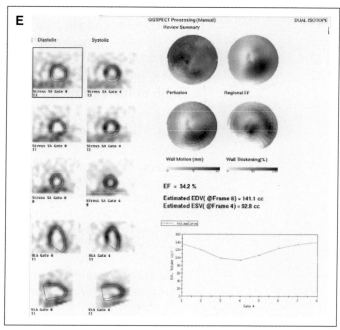

ITEM 9A

Answers: b, d, e. Of course, stress-related shortness of breath is a classic angina equivalent. Ischemia, whatever its manifestations, is evaluated well by perfusion scintigraphy. Stress echocardiography has no demonstrated advantage in the setting of such "functional" symptoms.

Figure 124

ITEM 9B

Answers: c, d, e. Imaging was critical here. The stress ECG could well have demonstrated nonspecific ST changes. However, the stress ECG was, in fact, false negative in the setting of gross ischemic image changes! The defect is reversible and involves the apex, anteroseptal and lateral walls. This, with gross exercise-related cavitary dilation makes artifact an unlikely cause of findings. Instead, high-risk multivessel coronary disease is evident and was confirmed at angiography. The findings on stress study are not the result of LVH. However, the rest pattern of a prominent left ventricle with preserved perfusion is strongly suggestive of increased left ventricular mass. The patient went on to successful CABG.

ITEM 9C

Answer: e. Although low output does not lead directly to shortness of breath but to easy fatigability and loss of energy, systolic dysfunction can lead to high filling pressures and diastolic dysfunction. Diastolic dysfunction is the earliest functional event in the "ischemic cascade." The other responses are unlikely or make no physiologic sense.

ITEM 10

Answers: b, c, e, g, i, j, k, l. Although defect size and density relate to prognosis (10,18–21,32), this is significantly and exponentially modulated by the augmentation of coronary flow demands, measured by the double product (10,29–33,179). The double product related to the induction of ischemia is the "ischemic threshold," the level of coronary flow demand that can be delivered before ischemia occurs. Exercise time, or workload, is another recognized predictor of risk in coronary disease. However, here an impressive, reversible defect, suggesting tight proximal LAD disease, recommends aggressive evaluation and therapy, even though related to a high workload and double product.

The absence of induced chest pain does not remove the possible relationship between the scintigraphic findings and the clinical syndrome. Certainly, the absence of related pain does not reduce the significance of scintigraphic findings.

The stress EKG is negative for ischemia in the presence of baseline J point and ST elevation. Nonetheless, this finding should not and did not discourage pursuit of an ischemic cause, even after a prior negative stress test performed without imaging. A baseline QS complex in leads V1–V3 supports the diagnosis of an anteroseptal infarction and suggests that associated ST elevation relates to an anterior aneurysm. However, there was no image evidence of aneurysm at rest, and baseline wall motion was normal. This case demonstrates the variability of noninvasive diagnostic data, in which all ischemic indicators do not necessarily or even usually point in the same direction. Although this makes evaluation more difficult, it demonstrates the importance of clinical judgment, which here uncovered a tight proximal and potentially life-threatening LAD lesion with normal left ventricular wall motion on subsequent cardiac catheterization, in spite of a host of negative and ambiguous clinical cues. The absence of induced pain reduces diagnostic certainty, and the high achieved double product modulates the risk. The rest ECG was also misleading. However, neither can support ignoring the impressive scintigraphic findings that brought angiography and revascularization.

ITEM 11A

Answers: d, e, g. Obviously, chest pain need not be present on stress testing in coronary disease. The achieved workload was much reduced, in view of the recent manifest vigor and activity of this 79-yr-old man. The stress ECG shows clear ischemic ST changes at a low achieved heart rate and modest double product. The rate is inappropriate and limited by chronotropic incompetence, an inability to raise heart rate. Although a bit noisy, the exercise training shows a junctional escape rhythm and isorhythmic dissociation, where A-V dissociation is seen in the presence of the competing junctional rhythm at a rate similar to the sinus rate.

ITEM 11B

Answer: e. Image abnormalities, although relatively limited in extent, related to a low achieved double product and so to a higher prognostic importance and event rate. Taken in the clinical context with evident induced ST depression and rhythm abnormality in this vigorous and otherwise well, although elderly, man, an aggressive approach was well justified. A rest study was not performed, because there was no history of infarction, left ventricular systolic function was normal and the coronary and electrophysiologic problems were clear. Angiography performed the next day revealed 3-vessel CAD. CABG was performed and a pacemaker placed. Although it is unclear what aspect of the intervention specifically brought improvement, both were indicated. The patient has regained vigor and energy beyond his expectations. He is back at work and playing limited tennis, less than 3 mo after surgery!

ITEM 12

Answer: a, c, d, f, h. This normal study shows no infarction, makes significant CAD unlikely and relates to a good prognosis. Unlike thrombolytic therapy, timely acute angioplasty often relates to normal perfusion images. This likely relates to the speed and sufficiency of reperfusion. The LVEF is probably exaggerated, because the edge-defining algorithm may underestimate end-systolic dimensions in small ventricles, as here shown in Figure 129D. The coronary angiogram was normal, and the patient is being treated for hypertension while other causes of chest pain are being sought. Other sources of error in the calculation of LVEF from perfusion studies include the failure to find the endocardium in the presence of severe underperfusion or an inability of the edge-detection algorithm to find the endocardium in the presence of high extracardiac uptake. Figure 129E shows epicardial and endocardial edges applied to gated poststress ^{99m}Tc sestamibi images in a patient with severe underperfusion in the setting of a large anterior infarction. Figure 129F shows edges "pulled" to a region of high extracardiac subdiaphragmatic background (upper left) in another patient. The perfusion images from which these are derived are shown in Figures 129G, with a dense defect, and 129H, with high paracardiac background.

ITEM 13A

Answer: b, d, e, f. The defect appears reversible in the supine images and persists in the prone image set. It is not the result of an attenuation artifact. Unlike

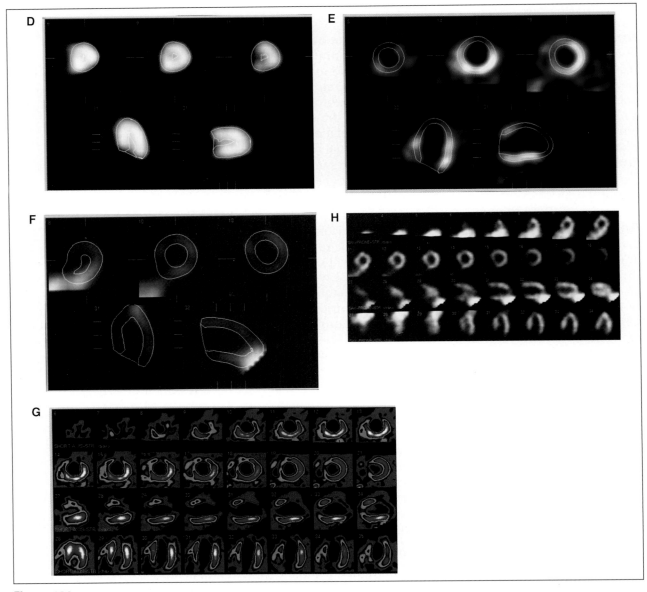

Figure 129

ST depression, ST elevation in leads without Q waves at rest is specific for transmural ischemia, with high localizing ability. In leads with Q waves the finding may relate to ischemia or may be a nonspecific finding related to an underlying aneurysm. The normal rest study suggests normal wall motion at rest, and so dysfunction is likely stress induced. Although exercise duration and the double product at ischemia modify the image-related prognostic risk (10), nonetheless ST elevation and impressive image findings are dominant in determining risk, even with the high exercise time and double product achieved. Inferior hypokinesis likely relates to post-stress "stunning." Angiography revealed a tight right coronary lesion and a 50% LAD narrowing. RCA angioplasty was performed, and a stent was placed.

ITEM 13B

Answer: a, c. Although improved compared with the prior supine stress study and acquired at a higher double product, subtle diminution of inferior activity is clarified by comparison with the normal rest image. Prone imaging is normal. Yet, inferior and posteroseptal wall motion is reduced and may take time to resolve. The LAD region presents minor stress-related diminution of activity in the anterior wall and septum. Although not evident previously, possibly because of the dense related inferior defect, it is subtle and conforms with that expected with the 50% LAD narrowing. This case is an example of the general value of perfusion scintigraphy in the assessment of ischemic symptoms after PTCA—even early after the intervention. It will be the rare case that demonstrates reversible image defects in the presence of a successful intervention. However, perfusion imaging is not recommended in asymptomatic patients early after the intervention. This patient was managed medically and did not have repeat angiography.

ITEM 14A

Answers: a, b, d, f. The history and ECG changes raise great concern for unstable angina and possible infarction. However, prolonged rest pain was not present, and the current state, distribution and risk of the suspected ischemic process were unclear. Further J point elevation was present 2 yr ago, and the upward concave ST segments were of unclear origin. The patient's physician was contacted and was aware of the prior tracings but not the current ECG or most recent symptoms. Although concerned, he felt that stress perfusion imaging was the best way to evaluate the condition, provided there was no evidence of acute infarction. The stress laboratory physician recommended that they go ahead with the test but perform a dipyridamole stress sestamibi study after review of the rest ^{201}Tl study. If the former was grossly abnormal, consideration would be made to send the patient directly to angiography with subsequent stress testing as needed.

ITEM 14B

Answers: b, c, e. Transient ST elevation in V2 suggest transmural anteroseptal ischemia with lateral ST depression and T inversion. In fact, with the finding of induced ischemia in multiple vascular beds and a study presenting a high coronary risk in the absence of infarction, the patient was admitted to the hospital. Troponins were negative, and the patient was treated briefly for ischemia and then sent to angiography. Here, extensive 3-vessel disease was found, and the patient was scheduled for coronary bypass surgery. Early angiography could have resulted in similar management but could have brought an acute angioplasty of a severe stenosis without image documentation of full regional viability or other pathophysiology. Imaging also permitted angiography to be performed without surprise. Here, the interventional approach could be planned based on the probable, image-based findings and related prognosis rather than face a potential surprise. The evaluation of left ventricular function made the left ventriculogram unnecessary. Dipyridamole was safe in even this evolving ischemic setting, but the infusion of high-dose dobutamine would be problematic in this scenario and in many cases of advanced and dynamic coronary disease where stress image evaluation is needed most.

ITEM 15

Answer: All may be correct. Isolated left main stenosis is unusual. Although dilation was visually unimpressive, the transient ischemic dilation was high and could support the presence of unseen ischemia. However, such "balanced ischemia" is actually rare, generally seen with extensive 3-vessel disease, not seen here, and was not accompanied here by ECG changes, chest pain or reduced LVEF. Intracoronary ultrasound would show fine-lesion anatomy and dimensions, and Doppler could measure flow reserve. However, it might not be prudent to repeatedly instrument and occlude a left main lesion. Although the lesion may not have been as tight as visually evident, it was tight enough to keep the patient from liver transplantation. Could the lesion have been based in spasm? All must be done to disprove that possibility. Beyond these considerations, it must be realized that the case is essentially that of an asymptomatic left main lesion, which for obvious reasons has not been well studied in the literature.

ITEM 16A

Answer: e. Although some would accept answer a, this could too often bring unnecessary instrumentation of coronary imperfections not necessarily pathophysiologically significant or even related to the symptomatology. A normal ECG during pain reduces the likelihood that a simple stress test will provide the diagnosis or lesion localization. The patient presents with possible new onset angina, a form of unstable angina. Although discharge with medical therapy may be appropriate in some cases, it would be inappropriate to discharge him without a more certain diagnosis and risk stratification. A stress perfusion study would best permit diagnosis and prognosis and present the best guide to therapy and angiography, if performed. Either exercise or dilator pharmacologic stress would be acceptable. Dynamic exercise would relate ischemic findings to activities, although dilator pharmacologic stress could be somewhat safer in this setting (*31,413*). Dobutamine stress testing is not as sensitive as dilator pharmacologic stress. Even with perfusion scintigraphy and delivery of the agent in high doses it is not prudent in this patient with possible unstable angina.

ITEM 16B

Answer: None of the answers presented is correct. Chest pain may occur with dipyridamole or adenosine infusion without ischemia, possibly because of the role of adenosine as a mediator of chest pain. Severe or agonizing chest pain has not been well evaluated, but it may be more diagnostic for an ischemic cause. The absence of a hemodynamic response does not reduce test sensitivity. There is no good evidence in the scintigraphic literature that an augmented dipyridamole dose will be more effective. Although some researchers advocate an augmented dipyridamole infusion with stress echocardiography, the prescribed dose already provides maximum dilation, and the method has not been well accepted beyond its sphere of origin. Of course, the ECG rarely reflects ischemic potential, because vasodilator stress does not increase coronary flow demands and so creates flow heterogeneity without induced ischemia. For these reasons, a negative ECG cannot be taken as evidence of absent coronary disease. Even with an exercise test, absent ST changes cannot be presumed to exclude (nor include) electrically silent circumflex disease. A negative stress test still leaves clinical judgment in the hands of the managing cardiologist.

ITEM 16C

Answer: d. Poststress LVEF was 49% in gated images. Cavitary dilation and a gross reversible lateral defect are seen. With this finding, related to the dramatic clinical progression and rest symptoms, the patient went to angiography, where a tight proximal LCX lesion was found and stented.

ITEM 17A

Answer: a, c, d, e, f, h. The limited fixed and extensive reversible defects suggest a significant ischemic risk (32). At the same time, these image findings suggest that the poststress gated LVEF may be indicative of postischemic dysfunction, "stunning" rather than scar. This is supported by the fact that a rest echocardiogram demonstrated generally preserved wall motion with an LVEF of 55%. Such evidence of stunning also supports the severity of the related perfusion defects and the likelihood of induced ischemia. The findings suggest a significant prognostic risk, probably made worse by the integration of data regarding left ventricular function (214).

ITEM 17B

Answer: All are correct. Preserved apical perfusion presents evidence of a patent LIMA graft. The perfusion pattern, although abnormal, is improved compared with the preoperative study at a high double product. This, with an improved, poststress LVEF, limited anterior and lateral ischemia and a negative stress test at a high workload and double product, suggest a low-to-moderate ischemic risk and support a trial of medical therapy.

ITEM 18

Answer: c, d, g. Apparently, we have fortuitously demonstrated the cause of the patient's pain in coronary spasm. Neither the stress ECG or image related to dipyridamole infusion should be expected to demonstrate abnormalities related to spasm that had not yet developed when the stress test was performed. There is no evidence of spasm induced by dipyridamole or aminophylline, and spasm related to exercise has been reported but is extremely uncommon. Spasm is best treated with calcium channel blockers and nitrates, which were given here with first ECG evidence of ST elevation and with subsequent ECG and pain resolution. Figure 137F shows the rest ECG made when completely pain free after 34 min. Even had [201]Tl

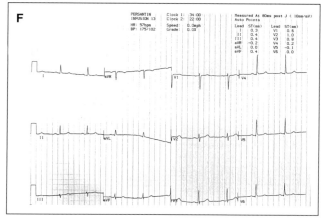

Figure 137

rather than sestamibi been applied for stress imaging, repeat imaging with short-lived ischemia after localization of the radionuclide would demonstrate no changes.

ITEM 19

Answer: e. ECG ST elevation in leads with Q waves may represent ischemia or electrophysiologic changes related to scar and underlying aneurysm. Here, the image findings clearly demonstrate induced reversible ischemia as well as infarction. The relatively low achieved double product adds to the gravity of the finding.

ITEM 20

Answer: c, e, g, h. Again the intensities in the thickening polar map are blunted, but numerical values confirm generally well-preserved thickening throughout. Here again, the combination of wall motion and thickening help to better interpret the findings on perfusion study. The active lateral wall motion suggests absent scar, with ischemic potential of the inferolateral wall imaged only at stress. Preserved thickening of the septum with vigorous systolic anterior motion of the myocardium (epicardium) indicates that the septal wall motion abnormality was more apparent than real and is likely the effect of increased cardiac mobility after CABG, a well-known finding often seen on echocardiography.

ITEM 21

Answers: a, c. This is another study that demonstrates the valuable interaction of function and perfusion in a single study. Clearly, the reduced anterior intensity in the perfusion image is clinically significant, because it relates to a contraction abnormality. No evidence of prior infarction was seen on perfusion imaging, and the patient was taken to angiography, where another LAD stent was placed distal to the initial stent.

ITEM 22

Answers: b, d. The area of intense regional extracardiac uptake could not be identified on computed tomography (CT) of the thorax, performed the next day. However, the patient was soon diagnosed with a squamous cell carcinoma of the head and neck. Repeat CT scan 5 mo later revealed multiple rib, soft tissue and lung masses. Metastatic cancer was first seen on perfusion imaging but was soon inoperable. As with all scintigrams, the full field of view and all images acquired must be evaluated. Sometimes an important finding may be evident where we least expect to see it.

ITEM 23

Answers: b, e. The ascites is evident as a clear (black) area below the heart and surrounding the liver in both projection images.

ITEM 24

Answers: a, c, d, e. The case testifies to the clinical value and safety of vasodilator pharmacologic stress perfusion imaging in even the most threatening clinical setting. The patient had right ventricular tachycardia, and the focus was ablated.

ITEM 25

Answers: c, d. Although most patients with even extensive myocardium at risk survive major surgery without infarction, the risk can be great, as high as a 20%–40% hard event rate in some studies. Although one study suggests that beta blocker prophylaxis would be as protective of coronary events during noncardiac surgery as CABG, the study contained limited selected patients and had no control group (Lee TH. Reducing cardiac risk in noncardiac surgery [editorial]. *N Engl J Med* 1000;341:1838–1840). The risk related to the stress segmental score is well established (*17,19–21,32,33,129,131,210,330–335,597,691,706,825*) and is ignored with peril. The best rule to apply is to recommend coronary revascularization before noncardiac surgery, based on stress perfusion imaging findings, as one would outside the preoperative setting. If one would not recommend revascularization based on the stress image findings outside the surgical setting, it should not be recommended preoperatively. In the latter case, beta blockers and other monitoring and protective measures are most important. Should trouble come, the image could then serve a useful guide to intervention. The patient had angiography, in which multivessel CAD was found. Left ventricular function was normal. PTCA was not possible, and the patient refused CABG. After nephrectomy, he had 2 non-Q infarctions and heart failure requiring intubation. He is now recovering with an LVEF of 45% and will have CABG before aortic aneurysm resection.

ITEM 26

Answer: All are correct. Angiography revealed normal coronary arteries. Here, the stress image has been attenuation corrected with specific software. The prone image performed after stress also demonstrated resolution of the inferior wall defect, which was clearly attenuation based. Differential attenuation in the dual-isotope protocol and technical factors such as attenuation and motion are the most likely causes of reverse redistribution. Here, left ventricular dilation and diffuse wall motion abnormalities are associated with a homogeneously perfused ventricle, suggesting a noncoronary cause. Even the presence of a limited reversible defect would not change the major diagnosis, because limited coronary disease may be associated with a noncoronary cardiomyopathy but not be the cause of gross left ventricular dilation and dysfunction.

ITEM 27

Answer: All are correct. The study shows extensive defects and high stress-segmental scores (Fig. 146A) with reversible anterolateral and inferolateral defects and a fixed lateral basal defect. There is stress-induced cavitary dilation. There are stress-induced apical and anterior as well as inferior and inferolateral defects and a low LVEF with poor wall motion, likely evidence of poststress "stunning." The patient came to angiography with the finding of multivessel CAD and went on to CABG. She is doing well. Risk stratification of uncomplicated non-Q infarction appears safe and cost effective (685,825). Although the patient initially presented with heart failure, it was elected to risk stratify and assess regional myocardium at risk noninvasively. In this case, multivessel disease was evident both noninvasively and confirmed invasively. This is not always the case. The imaging study provided a guide to the anatomical study and a pathophysiologic measure of the prognostic risk. If imaging had been benign, a different management course may have been set.

ITEM 28A

Answers: a–e. The poststress ejection fraction certainly discourages further study, because improvement is unlikely with gross dilation and values in this range. However, other evaluations at rest indicate 15%–20% as the baseline value. Perhaps the value here reflected poststress "stunning"? Reversibility in virtually all vascular regions brought further evaluation with PET fluordeoxyglucose viability study performed after glucose loading, from which short-axis and horizontal long-axis slices are shown in Figures 147E and 147F, respectively.

ITEM 28B

Answers: c, e, f. In the postprandial state normal myocardium should metabolize fatty acids, and ischemic myocardium should take up glucose. The LAD region was seen to be viable and grossly ischemic on PET scanning. With this information and the findings on perfusion imaging, and in spite of the measured LVEF, the patient went to CABG. He survived, recovered and is now symptomatically improved. LVEF has not yet been remeasured.

ITEM 29A

Answer: True. A stress-first protocol may always be performed. However, when desired on the same day as the stress study, the rest study should best be performed with a larger dose after a delay to permit some decay of the stress dose. This would leave a low dose for the most important stress study. Of course, this would not save camera time on this busy day in the nuclear cardiology laboratory. Most expeditious for scheduling would be to perform a stress study with a rest study performed the next day only if needed. Best would be to apply this protocol to those unlikely to need a rest study. However, this patient has classic angina of new onset, a form of unstable angina. It is unlikely that the stress study will be normal. Further, the rest ECG suggests a prior infarction. It would be important to see the rest study before performing an exercise study.

ITEM 29B

Answers: a, c, d. Although not representing standard leads, the findings cannot be discounted and a prior anterior infarction is a possibility. Stress-induced ST elevation is generally diagnostic of transmural ischemia and localizes to the leads affected—but not here. The presence of Q waves in leads with ST elevation indicates regional infarction and makes the ST elevation ambiguous, indicative of transmural ischemia or simply related to infarction and aneurysm formation (Dunn RF, Bailey IK, Uren R, Kelly DT. Exercise-induced ST-segment elevation. Correlation of thallium-201 myocardial perfusion scanning and

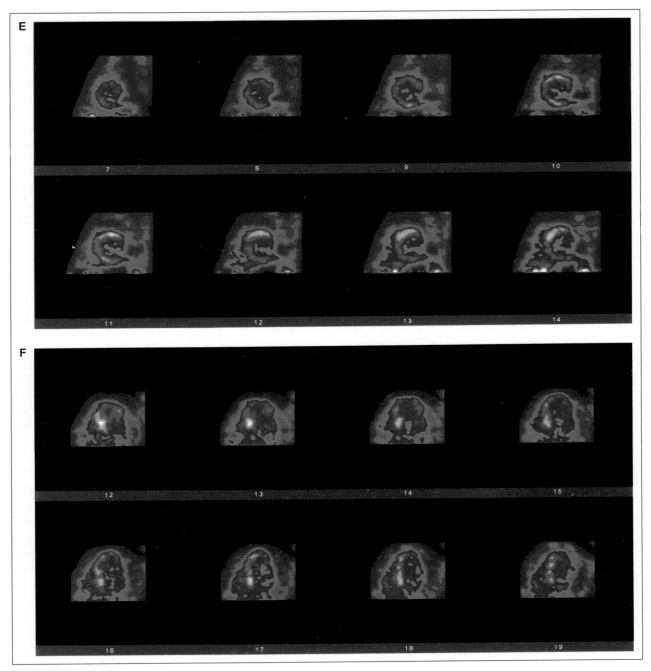

Figure 147

coronary arteriography. *Circulation* 1980;61:989–995). Stress-induced horizontal ST depression in V5 and V6 is diagnostic for ischemia. LBBB is not present.

ITEM 29C

Answers: c, d, f. The rest defects do not necessarily indicate prior infarction, because they could well improve on delayed imaging and represent hibernating myocardium—dysfunctional but viable myocardium unrelated to a clear preceding ischemic insult. Although first glance may suggest that defects are more extensive at rest than with stress, the higher intensity of uptake at rest in posteroseptal, anterolateral, distal anterior and lateral regions indicates extensive induced ischemia as well as possible infarction. The inferolateral region may well demonstrate "reverse redistribution." In the absence of evident artifact, this finding may indeed relate to a prior non-Q infarction. However, prone images demonstrated improvement in this region, the result, at least in part, of attenuation and other technical factors. A 24-hr delayed image may be critically important to this patient and give evidence of more extensive uptake and myocardial viability. Systolic dysfunction may here relate to poststress stunning, or, in the presence of widespread rest perfusion defects, to hibernating myocardium. A rest evaluation of wall motion would be important, because evidence of improved wall motion would suggest poststress stunning and added coronary-related risk (Taillefer R, Cohade C, Gagnon A, Lajeunesse S, Benjamin C. Is the left ventricle post-stress stunning a frequent finding on gated SPECT myocardial perfusion imaging [abstract]? *J Nucl Med* 2000;41:6P).

ITEM 29D

Answer: b, d, e, f. Widespread improvement at 24 hr suggests that defects seen at rest are related to viable, "hibernating" myocardium and that wall motion abnormalities are likely reversible with reperfusion. The extensive nature of reversible and fixed defects suggests multivessel disease and the likelihood of CABG. Although the LVEF is severely reduced after stress, the chance of significant functional benefit in the absence of symptoms of heart failure suggests that such surgery may be worth the risk. Although fearful because of the fate of his father, the patient is encouraged to go on to coronary angiography, not in spite of but because of the family history. Angiography is performed and shows severe, extensive 3-vessel CAD. There are prominent collaterals that help to explain the extensive preservation of myocardium in the setting of extensive disease and myocardium at ischemic risk. Figure 148G shows SPECT slices in this patient at stress (^{99m}Tc sestamibi), rest and 24 hr later (^{201}Tl) from above downward, in short- (upper 3 rows), vertical long- (lower 3 rows, at left) and horizontal long-axis (lower 3 rows, at right) slices. Figure 148H is a frame from the patient's selective coronary angiogram and shows severe RCA disease and prominent RCA-to-LAD collaterals. Figure 148I demonstrates the collateralization of the RCA (bottom) after injection of the LAD (top).

ITEM 30

Answers: b, c. Both stress test and image findings suggest severe and extensive coronary disease with a high related coronary risk. This man had come for evaluation of hypertension and coronary risk factors, in the presence of an atypical heart "awareness," and was treated aggressively based on the findings on exercise perfusion scintigraphy. Coronary angiography revealed severe 3-vessel CAD, as shown in Figures 149D, a frame of the cine made after left main coronary injection, and 149E, a frame made after RCA injection.

ITEM 31

Answers: c, d, f. The end-diastolic left ventricular volume appears to be reduced with (after) exercise, a normal response. However, the findings will vary

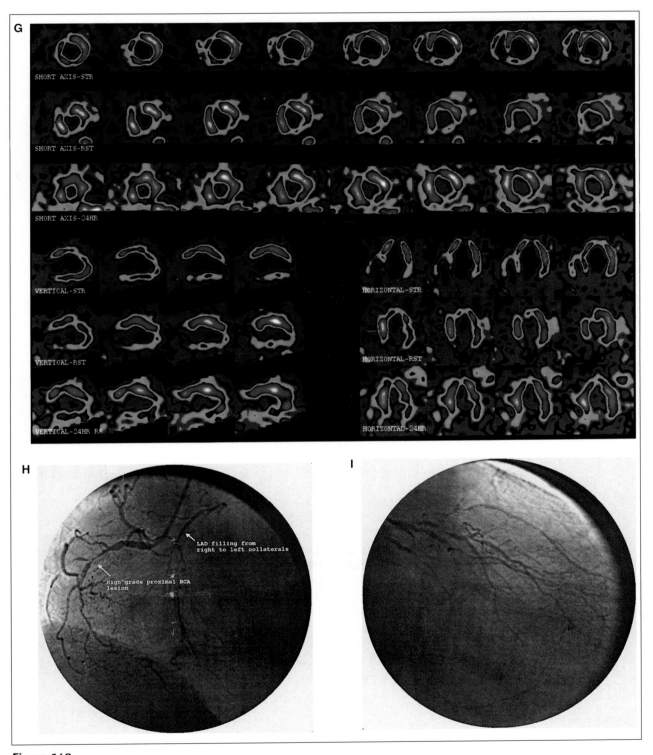

Figure 148

with the time delay between exercise and imaging, the ability to reproduce the baseline angulation, the state of postexercise volume depletion and the ability to visualize the endocardium, as well as other factors. The image is read as showing diffuse rest wall motion abnormalities with a normal response to

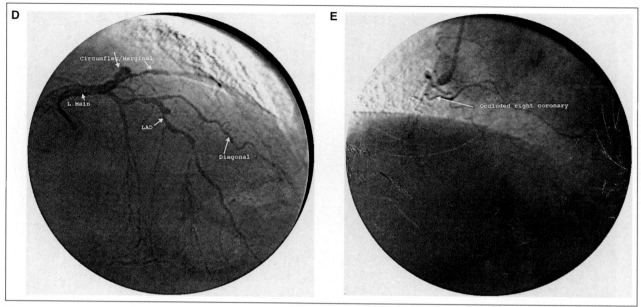

Figure 149

stress, consistent with a noncoronary cardiomyopathy. Yet, the history, ECG, stress test and scintigraphy all suggest CAD. The presence of widespread severe resting wall motion abnormalities make it difficult to identify both incremental and decremental wall motion changes with stress. Some laboratories refuse to study such patients, because of the lack of sensitivity and specificity in such a setting. Of course, some labs will study all such patients. However, how will the reader interpret the findings in the presence of such wall motion abnormalities? Will they be able to recognize decremental function? Will they be able to recognize incremental motion? With what level of objectivity or assurance? The echocardiogram was read as negative for ischemia. Shown in Figure 150C, from above downward in each axial set, are rest ^{201}Tl, exercise ^{99m}Tc sestamibi and 24-hr delayed ^{201}Tl SPECT images. Evident is a dilated left ventricle with apical anterior septal and inferior defects at stress, which improve at rest and improve further at delayed imaging. The gross and widespread wall motion abnormalities shown on the reconstructed poststress gated perfusion study shown in Figure 150D in anterior and LAO projections are related to ischemic cardiomyopathy and are, at least in part, based in "hibernation." The scintigraphic study, not disadvantaged by wall motion abnormalities, demonstrates that the patient has advanced and extensive CAD and needs aggressive management. Angiography confirmed the advanced CAD (*531,532*).

ITEM 32

Answer: b, c, d, e. Little known is the fact that a single dose of current approved echo contrast agents target the left ventricular cavity, do not always work and generally exceed the per-dose price of current radiopharmaceutical perfusion agents (*865–868*). To this point, echocardiographic contrast agents have had some success visualizing the cavity and enhancing the endocardial

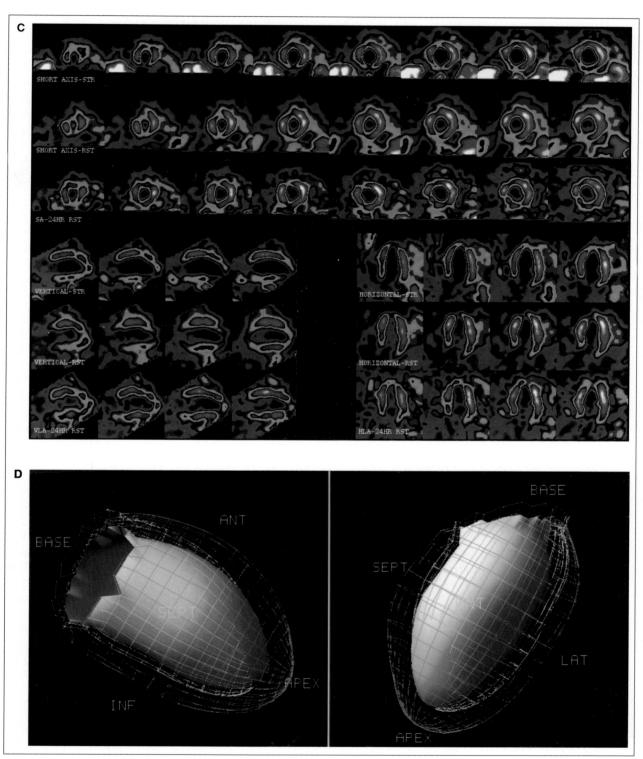

Figure 150

border but have not demonstrated a consistent ability to label myocardial perfusion. The image findings reveal a normal echocardiographic response with a grossly abnormal stress-induced scintigraphic response. LV wall motion was normal, both at rest echocardiography and at rest and poststress gated scintigraphy. Angiographic findings paralleled the scintigraphic findings, and revascularization is planned. The stress echocardiographic method requires recognition of induced wall motion abnormalities, a finding dependent on a multitude of factors, of which insufficient endocardial visualization is only 1, here not sufficiently resolved. The study illustrated shows little evidence of contrast. Did it employ the study agent or the placebo? Regardless, the endocardium was well seen, and the study did not reflect the pathophysiology.